→ In Gratitude for
Gettin[illegible] [illegible]ad-
uate School.
— Adam
January 26, 1983

Radiological Imaging

The Theory of Image Formation,
Detection, and Processing

Volume 2

Radiological Imaging

The Theory of Image Formation, Detection, and Processing

Volume 2

Harrison H. Barrett
William Swindell

Department of Radiology
and
Optical Sciences Center
University of Arizona
Tucson, Arizona

1981

ACADEMIC PRESS

A Subsidiary of Harcourt Brace Jovanovich, Publishers

New York London
Paris San Diego San Francisco
São Paulo Sydney Tokyo Toronto

ACADEMIC PRESS, INC.
111 Fifth Avenue, New York, New York 10003

United Kingdom Edition published by
ACADEMIC PRESS, INC. (LONDON) LTD.
24/28 Oval Road, London NW1 7DX

Library of Congress Cataloging in Publication Data

Barrett, Harrison H.
Radiological imaging.

Includes bibliographies and index.
Contents: v. 1. The theory of image formation, detection, and processing -- v. 2. Tomography, noise, and scattered radiation.
1. Radiography, Medical--Mathematics. 2. Radiography Medical--Image quality. I. Swindell, William. II. Title. [DNLM: 1. Radiography. WN 445 B273r]
RC78.B337 616.07'57 80-69416
ISBN 0-12-079602-3 (vol. 2) AACR2

PRINTED IN THE UNITED STATES OF AMERICA

81 82 83 84 9 8 7 6 5 4 3 2 1

To Cathy, Dave, and Mindy

To Dorothy, Pamela, David, and John

Contents

Preface

This book is an outgrowth of a course that the authors have taught since 1974 at the Optical Sciences Center at the University of Arizona. The students in this course have been advanced graduate students, most of them majoring in optical sciences, but some in physics, mathematics, or electrical engineering. The course is intended to serve two purposes. The first and most obvious is to prepare the student to do research in radiological imaging. The second (and perhaps more important) function is to teach general image science within a radiographic context, to help the student gain fluency with the essential analytical tools of linear systems theory and the theory of stochastic processes that are applicable to any imaging system, radiographic or otherwise.

We have tried to maintain that dual purpose in this book as well. While the specific systems being analyzed are medical diagnostic systems, the principles involved are far broader. To be able to calculate a modulation transfer function or to determine the signal-to-noise ratio in a processed image is a necessary skill for anyone involved in image formation, detection, or processing, whatever the nature of the radiation.

In order to make this work accessible to a wider audience, we have included a certain amount of introductory material that is not normally included in our course. The mathematical material in Appendixes A and B, on the Dirac delta function and the Fourier transform, respectively, is certainly familiar to most graduate students in the sciences, and is included here largely for reference purposes. Similarly, much of the material on radiation physics in Appendix C is often covered in an undergraduate course on modern physics. Chapters 2 and 3 present the essential mathematical techniques needed for the rest of the book. A reader who has taken a graduate course in linear systems will be able to pass lightly over Chapter 2, while a course in random processes will achieve the same result for most of Chapter 3. Perhaps in that case the material on Poisson processes in Chapter 3 should be read more carefully because it is fundamental to radiographic imaging and because it is not often given sufficient attention in the usual graduate course on random processes.

The main task of the book—the analysis of radiographic systems—begins in Chapter 4. The effort in this chapter is aimed at developing a simple yet reasonably realistic model to describe a variety of imaging systems.

The subject of radiographic image detectors, dealt with in Chapter 5, could easily occupy a volume as large as this two-volume work. To reduce the subject to manageable proportions, we have chosen to consider in detail just two detectors—x-ray film (including film–screen systems) and the Anger scintillation camera. In addition to being the most important detectors in diagnostic radiology and nuclear medicine, they also serve as convenient ways to illustrate the important properties of image detectors in general.

In Chapters 6–9 we deal with various aspects of three-dimensional or tomographic imaging. Of these, Chapter 7, on computed tomography, is undeniably the most important in clinical practice. Chapter 6, which contains a brief discussion of what we call classical tomography, is largely of historical interest. In Chapter 8 we cover multiplex or coded-aperture imaging, a topic near and dear to the heart of one of the authors. While the clinical benefits of this imaging method may be debatable, its value as a pedagogical tool seems clear. It is useful to know how to analyze a coded-aperture system even if it is not a part of the clinical routine. Similarly, in Chapter 9 we describe a variety of systems that are now in the research stage or undergoing preliminary clinical trials. This chapter represents one of the forefronts of radiographic imaging research, the effort to find new and better ways of extracting three-dimensional information. To avoid quick obsolescence, we have emphasized basic mathematical principles in this chapter, and have only lightly touched on specific systems that embody these principles.

In Chapter 10 we show how one can analyze the statistical properties of radiographic images that are limited, as they almost always are, by Poisson noise. Included is an all-too-brief discussion of the psychophysics of detection and how it relates to physical measures of image noise. Although we recognize that the observer is as much a part of the imaging system as, say, the detector, limitations of space and our own expertise have forced us to restrict the discussion of psychophysics. Our primary motivation was to include just enough discussion of psychophysics to indicate that the effort expended earlier in the chapter on calculating signal-to-noise ratios was not wasted, that a large SNR was a useful predictor of good observer performance.

In Chapter 11 we discuss scattered radiation and its effect on image quality. There are two distinct questions here: How does one analyze scatter problems, and how does one get rid of scatter?

One of the most difficult parts of writing this book was to achieve a consistent and clear notation. We suspect that we did not really succeed in this endeavor, since subscripts, superscripts, ornaments, and special type fonts abound. However, it may help the reader if we explicitly state some of the conventions we used.

In general, we use boldface roman type for two-dimensional vectors and lightface italics for scalars. It is sometimes necessary to distinguish three-dimensional vectors from two-dimensional ones, and for that purpose we use boldface fraktur type. Lightface fraktur then means the scalar magnitude of a three-dimensional vector. Random variables or processes are printed in boldface sans serif type for both vectors and scalars, and the corresponding lightface italic character indicates a sample function of the random process.

Two conventions are used for Fourier transforms. A function like $f(\mathbf{r})$ denoted by a lowercase letter has its transform denoted by the corresponding uppercase letter, $F(\boldsymbol{\rho})$. Alternatively, a Fourier operator $\mathscr{F}_2$ is also used, so that $F(\boldsymbol{\rho}) = \mathscr{F}_2\{f(\mathbf{r})\}$ and $f(\mathbf{r}) = \mathscr{F}_2^{-1}F(\boldsymbol{\rho})$. The subscript 2 denotes a two-dimensional transform. Frequency-domain variables are denoted by Greek letters, ρ, σ, ξ, η, ζ, ν, etc., while the space or time domain is denoted by Latin variables.

One somewhat peculiar mathematical notation is an integral sign with a subscript ∞. By this we mean an integral over the entire infinite domain of the variable of integration. For example,

$$\int_\infty d^2r = \int_0^\infty r\,dr \int_0^{2\pi} d\theta = \int_{-\infty}^{\infty} dx \int_{-\infty}^{\infty} dy.$$

We also make liberal use of ornaments. A tilde, as in $\tilde{f}(\mathbf{r})$, indicates a scaled version of the function $f(\mathbf{r})$. An overbar indicates some kind of average; $\bar{x}$ may be the statistical expectation value of a random variable x. Angular brackets $\langle\ \rangle$ are also used for averages where necessary, and can refer to spatial or temporal averages as well as statistical averages. A circumflex over a letter, especially over one denoting a random variable, sometimes denotes an estimate of the quantity. For example, $\hat{\boldsymbol{\mu}}$ is an estimate of μ. The circumflex can also denote a unit vector. A dagger indicates a filtered version of some function; $f^\dagger(t)$ is $f(t)$ convolved with some filter function. An asterisk as a superscript denotes complex conjugate, while an asterisk between two functions, as in $f(x) * q(x)$, denotes convolution. A double asterisk, $f(\mathbf{r}) ** g(\mathbf{r})$, denotes two-dimensional convolution. Primes are used for many purposes, one of the most important of which is to denote different planes in the general model set up in Chapter 4, and also used in Chapters 8–10. The conventions used in this model are detailed in Chapter 4.

The list of references by no means constitutes a complete bibliography on radiological imaging. Basically, we have included the works that we found useful in preparing this manuscript, especially review articles, books, and dissertations where the reader can go for a more detailed discussion. Where possible, we have also given a few very recent references to serve as entry points to the current literature, and a few references of historical interest have been given. No systematic attempt has been made to establish historical priorities, and no value judgments are implied by the inclusion or exclusion of a particular work. Our goal was to help the reader, not to either promote or denigrate any individual researcher or group of researchers; we hope we have accomplished the former without inadvertently stumbling into the latter.

The authors could not have written this book without a great deal of help from a great many people. The manuscript was typed by Carolyn Thomas, Susan Kuyper, and Debbie Spargur, but to refer to them as just typists would be an injustice. Their help in editing, organizing, and proofreading was equally invaluable. George Rubalcava very capably prepared most of the line drawings, while Dr. Dennis Patton, Dr. Bruce Hillman, and Dr. Kai Haber helped us assemble some clinical illustrations. Jim Arendt and Ching-Tai Chen contributed some of the computer graphics work. Many of our students read and corrected parts of the manuscript. We are especially indebted to Ming-Yee Chiu, Bob Simpson, John Greivenkamp, and Tony Ervin in this regard. Finally, we are deeply indebted to our families, especially our wives, Cathy and Pam, for the patience and forbearance they have shown during this long project.

Contents of Volume 1

List of Important Symbols

Symbol	Chapter or Appendix	Meaning	Typical Units
$a, a(t)$	3	mean arrival rate	sec^{-1}
a	4, 6, 8, 9, 10	$s_1/(s_1 + s_2)$	—
$a(\ )$	7, 8	space-domain apodizing function	cm^{-2}
A	3, 5, 10, 11	area	cm^{-2}
A	D	radionuclide activity	Curies, disintegrations per sec
A	C	atomic mass number	—
$A(\ )$	7, 8, 9	frequency-domain apodizing function	—
$\mathscr{A}$	9, 10, 11	area	cm^2
$\mathscr{A}$	7	Abel transform operator	—
b	4, 6, 8, 9, 10	$s_2/(s_1 + s_2)$	—
$b(\ )$	7, 9	Summation image	various
c	11	speed of light	$cm\ sec^{-1}$
C	5	count rate	sec^{-1}
C	4, 6, 8, 9, 10	$T[4\pi(s_1 + s_2)^2]^{-1}$	$sec\ cm^{-2}$
C	4, 5	capacitance	μFarad
$\dot{C}$	4	$C/T = [4\pi(s_1 + s_2)^2]^{-1}$	cm^{-2}
d	5, 10	thickness	cm
d	4, 10, 11	diameter	cm
$d(\ )$	4, 10	PSF of detector	cm^{-2}
D	4, 8, 10	diameter	cm
D	5, 7, 10	optical density	—
D	7, 10, D	dose	rad, $J\ kg^{-1}$, $erg\ gm^{-1}$

Symbol	Chapter or Appendix	Meaning	Typical Units
$D(\ )$	4	Fourier transform of $d(\ )$, transfer function of detector	—
$\dot{D}$	D	dose rate	rad sec^{-1}
$e(\ )$	2	edge spread function	various
E	D	energy per unit mass	rad, J kg^{-1}
E	4, 5, 10	film exposure	erg cm^{-2}, J m^{-2}
$\mathscr{E}$	5, 7, 10, 11, C, D	energy	erg, J, eV, keV
$f(\mathbf{r})$	4, 6, 8, 9, 10	2D source function	cm^{-2} sec^{-1}
$f(\ )$	A, B	general function	—
$f(\mathbf{r})$ or $f(\mathbf{r}, z)$ or $f(x, y, z)$	4, 7, 9	3D source function	cm^{-3} sec^{-1}
$f(\mathbf{p}, \mathbf{r}, t)$	11	phase-space distribution function	cm^{-6} gm^{-3} sec^{3}
$F(\ )$	4, 8, 9, 10	Fourier transform of $f(\ )$	various
$\mathscr{F}$	throughout	Fourier operator	—
$g(\ )$	A, B	general function	various
$g(\ )$	7, 9	back-projected image from a single projection	various
$g(\ )$	4, 6, 8, 10	aperture transmission function	—
$g^{\delta}(\ )$	4	impulse aperture transmittance	cm^{-2}
$G(\ )$	4, 8	Fourier transform of $g(\ )$	cm^{-2}
G	5	gain	—
$h(\ )$	3, 4, 6, 8, 10, 11	photon density (fluence)	cm^{-2}
h	3, 5, 11, C	Planck's constant	erg sec
$\dot{h}$	4	flux density h/T (fluence rate)	sec^{-1} cm^{-2}
$h^{\delta}(\ )$	4, 6, 8	photon density for impulse source or impulse aperture	cm^{-2} for impulse source cm^{-4} for impulse aperture
$H(\ )$	4, 8	Fourier transform of $h(\ )$	cm^{-4}
$\mathscr{H}$	7, 8, B	Hankel transform operator	—
i	throughout	$\sqrt{-1}$	—
$i(t)$	4	current	Amperes
I	5	irradiance (energy flux density or energy fluence rate)	Watt m^{-2}, erg sec^{-1} cm^{-2}
$J(\ )$	8, B	Bessel function	—
$\mathbf{J}(\ )$	11	momentum density	gm cm^{-2} sec^{-1}
k	8	magnitude of wave vector $(2\pi/\lambda)$	cm^{-1}
$\mathbf{k}$	8	wave vector	cm^{-1}
$\mathbf{k}$	3	random number	—
$k(\ )$	10	noise kernel	—

Symbol	Chapter or Appendix	Meaning	Typical Units
K	3	number (especially number of counts)	—
$l(\ )$	2	line spread function	various
l	7, 9, 11	path length	cm
L	4, 10	length	cm
$\mathbf{L}$	3, 5, 10	shift variable in 2D autocorrelation function	cm
$L(\ )$	5	Fourier transform of $l(\ )$	various
$\mathscr{L}$	11	general linear operator	—
m	4, 8	magnification	—
m	C, D	mass	gm
M	2, 5	modulation	—
M	2, B	dimensionality of a transform ($M = 1, 2,$ or 3)	—
$M(\ )$	3	characteristic function	—
n	5	index of refraction	—
n	4, 10	number per unit length	cm^{-1}
n	5, 11, C	number per unit volume (especially number of scatterers)	cm^{-3}
$\mathbf{n}$	3	random number	—
$\hat{\mathbf{n}}, \hat{\mathfrak{n}}$	4, 11	unit vectoı	—
N	5, 10	pure number (especially number of photons)	—
N	5	noise	—
N_0	7, C	Avogadro's number	mol^{-1}
$\mathbf{N}$	3, 5, 10	random number	—
$\mathfrak{p}$	11	magnitude of momentum vector	gm cm sec^{-1}
$\boldsymbol{\mathfrak{p}}$	11	momentum	gm cm sec^{-1}
$p(\ )$	throughout	impulse response (especially PSF)	various
$P(\ )$	throughout	Fourier transform of $p(\ )$, transfer function	various
pr( )	3	probability density function	various
Pr( )	3, 5, 11	probability	—
$q(\ )$	4, 7, 8, 9, 10	impulse response of filter	various
Q	D	charge	Coulombs
$Q(\ )$	7, 8, 9, 10	Fourier transform of $q(\ )$, transfer function of filter	various
r	throughout	radius, magnitude of $\mathbf{r}$	cm
$\mathbf{r}$	throughout	2D position vector	cm
$\mathfrak{r}$	4, 11, A	magnitude of $\boldsymbol{\mathfrak{r}}$	cm
$\boldsymbol{\mathfrak{r}}$	4, 9, 11, A	3D position vector	cm

Symbol	Chapter or Appendix	Meaning	Typical Units
R	4, 6, 8, 10	radius	cm
R	4	resistance	Ω
$R(\ )$	3,5,10	statistical autocorrelation function	various
$\mathscr{R}(\ )$	3	temporal autocorrelation function	various
s_1	4, 6, 8, 9, 10, 11	distance from source to aperture	cm
s_2	4, 6, 8, 9, 10, 11	distance from aperture to detector	cm
S	5	film speed	
S	5	signal	various
S	4	planar sensitivity	$\mu Ci^{-1}\,cm^2\,sec^{-1}$
$S(\mathscr{E})$	7, D	Spectral Energy fluence	cm^{-2}
$S(\ )$	3, 5, 10	Power spectral density	various
$\mathscr{S}$	5	Selwyn's granularity constant	cm
t	throughout	Time	sec
t	8	transmittance (especially amplitude transmittance)	—
T	3, 4, 6, 8, 9, 10, 11	time interval (especially exposure time)	sec
T	5, 7	transmittance (especially film transmittance)	—
u	2, B	general independent variable (time or position)	various
$u(\ )$	B	general function	various
$u(\ )$	11	volume density of photons	cm^{-3}
$\mathbf{u}(\ )$	3, 10	2D Poisson random process (sequence of impulses)	cm^{-2}
$U(\ )$	B	Fourier transform of $u(\ )$	various
$v, v(\ )$	2, 4	voltage	V
v	4, 10	speed	$cm\,sec^{-1}$
$v(\ )$	B	general function	various
V	4, 5	voltage	V
V	C	volume	cm^3
$V(\ )$	B	Fourier transform of $v(\ )$	various
w	5, 7	weighting factor	—
w	C	energy density	$J\,m^{-3}$, $erg\,cm^{-3}$
$w(\ )$	2, B	general function (especially input or output of linear system)	various
$\mathbf{w}(\ )$	3	general random process (especially input or output of linear system)	various

Symbol	Chapter or Appendix	Meaning	Typical Units
W	7	width	cm
$W(\ )$	B	Fourier transform of $w(\ )$	various
x	throughout	Cartesian coordinate	cm
x	A, B	general variable (not necessarily a coordinate)	various
x_m	C	mass per unit area	$gm\ cm^{-2}$
$\mathbf{x}$	3	general random variable (not necessarily a coordinate)	various
X	5, D	x-ray exposure	R
$\dot{X}$	D	exposure rate	$R\ sec^{-1}$
y	throughout	Cartesian coordinate	cm
$\mathbf{y}$	3	general random variable (not necessarily a coordinate)	various
z	throughout	Cartesian coordinate	cm
$\mathbf{z}(t)$	3	1D Poisson random process process (sequence of impulses)	sec^{-1}
Z	11, C	atomic number	—
α	C	$h\nu/m_0c^2$	—
α_{pf}	4, 10	packing fraction	—
γ	5, 10	slope of H–D curve	—
Γ	5, 7	maximum slope of H–D curve	—
δ	4, 5, 8, 10	resolution distance (FWHM of PSF)	cm
$\delta(\ )$	throughout	Dirac delta function	various
Δ	throughout	change in something	—
ε	4, 10	small distance	cm
ζ	9	spatial frequency component conjugate to z	cm^{-1}
η	throughout	spatial frequency component conjugate to y	cm^{-1}
η	5,10	quantum efficiency	—
θ	throughout	angle (especially polar coordinate)	—
κ	2, B	general frequency variable (1D, 2D, or 3D)	various
κ	11	diffusion constant	cm^{-1}
λ	3	frequency variable in characterstic function	various
λ	8, 11	wavelength	cm, Å
$\lambda(\ )$	7, 9, 10	projection	various

Symbol	Chapter or Appendix	Meaning	Typical Units
$\Lambda(\ )$	7, 9	Fourier transform of projection	various
$\mu, \mu(\ )$	4, 5, 7, 10, 11, C, D	linear attenuation coefficient	cm^{-1}
μ_m	7	mass attenuation coefficient, μ/ρ	$cm^2\ gm^{-1}$
$M(\ )$	7	Fourier transform of $\mu(\ )$	cm
ν	3, 4, 5, 11, C	temporal frequency	sec^{-1}
ξ	throughout	spatial frequency component conjugate to x	cm^{-1}
π	throughout	3.14159	—
ρ	5, 10, C, D	density	$gm\ cm^{-3}$
ρ	throughout	magnitude of $\boldsymbol{\rho}$	cm^{-2}
$\boldsymbol{\rho}$	throughout	2D spatial frequency vector	cm^{-2}
σ	5, 11, C	cross section	cm^2
σ	3, 5, 10	standard deviation (square root of variance)	various
σ^2	3, 5, 10	variance	various
σ	9	magnitude of $\boldsymbol{\sigma}$	cm^{-3}
$\boldsymbol{\sigma}$	9	3D spatial frequency vector	cm^{-3}
τ	10	time constant	sec
τ	3	shift variable in temporal autocorrelation function	sec
ϕ	throughout	angle (phase angle or azimuthal coordinate)	—
Φ	5, 7, 10, 11, C, D	particle fluence	cm^{-2}
$\dot{\Phi}$	D	particle fluence rate	$cm^{-2}\ sec^{-1}$
$\Phi_{\mathscr{E}}(\mathscr{E})$	5	spectral density of particle fluence	$cm^{-2}\ keV^{-1}$
$\psi(\ )$	8	wave amplitude	unspecified
Ψ	C, D	energy fluence	$keV\ cm^{-2}$, $J\ m^{-2}$
$\dot{\Psi}$	D	energy fluence rate	$keV\ cm^{-2}\ sec^{-1}$, $J\ m^{-2}\ sec^{-1}$ (W/m^2)
ω	6, 8	radian frequency	sec^{-1}
Ω	4, 5, 8, 9, 11, C	solid angle	—

Named Functions

Name	Meaning
circ(r)	$\begin{cases} 1 & \text{if } r < 1 \\ 0 & \text{if } r > 1 \\ \text{undefined} & \text{if } r < 0 \end{cases}$
comb(x)	$\sum_{n=-\infty}^{\infty} \delta(x - n)$
rect(x)	$\begin{cases} 1 & \text{if } \lvert x\rvert < \frac{1}{2} \\ 0 & \text{if } \lvert x\rvert > \frac{1}{2} \end{cases}$
sgn(x)	$\begin{cases} 1 & \text{if } x > 0 \\ -1 & \text{if } x < 0 \end{cases}$
sinc(x)	$\sin(\pi x)/\pi x$
step(x)	$\begin{cases} 1 & \text{if } x > 0 \\ 0 & \text{if } x < 0 \end{cases}$
tri(x)	$\begin{cases} 1 - \lvert x\rvert & \text{if } \lvert x\rvert < 1 \\ 0 & \text{if } \lvert x\rvert > 1 \end{cases}$
GR	grid ratio
LSF	line spread function
MTF	modulation transfer function
PSF	point spread function
SNR	signal-to-noise ratio
SPR	scatter-to-primary ratio
TF	transfer function

6

Classical Tomography

6.1 PRINCIPLES OF CLASSICAL TOMOGRAPHY

In our three-dimensional world the human visual system is occupied with the task of viewing the outer surfaces of three-dimensional objects. In order to visualize the internal structure of an opaque object, we must resort either to cutting it open or to probing the intact object by passing radiation through it. The internal structure can then be deduced from the manner in which the object absorbs and scatters the radiation.

The usual x-ray image is a two-dimensional representation of the three-dimensional body, and necessarily a great deal of information has been irretrievably lost. It is easy to see why. Consider the body to be composed of a large number of contiguous thin slices. When a thin pencil beam of x rays passes through the object, it is attenuated in part by each slice through which it passes, and yet only one piece of information, namely the final intensity, is measured. The individual sets of information regarding each plane have been superimposed on a single plane. Depth information has been destroyed. The picture is quite unlike our normal visual perception of the solid universe. We are looking "through" and "into" a solid object; internal, spatially separated features are confounded, and although the more strongly absorbing body tissues such as bone and nonabsorbing gas-filled spaces are easily recognized from their outline, it takes years of training and experience to properly analyze the content of such a radiographic image.

Tomography is a technique in which a selected layer of an object is clearly imaged and the overlying and underlying structure are seen either only in blurred form or not at all. The intention is to remove the confusion of superimposed images that occurs in a normal projection radiograph so that individual attention can be given to the particular anatomical section of interest.

We distinguish between classical tomography and computed tomography. Classical tomography has been in clinical use for over 40 years. The plane of interest is singled out by arranging for the images of all other planes to be blurred to such an extent that they contribute no useful information. The blur is introduced by moving the x-ray source and detector during the exposure. It should be realized that spatial information from the out-of-focus planes has not been removed from the image, but simply coded by motion blur to be less obtrusive.

This is in distinction to computed tomography, the subject of Chapter 7, in which the plane of interest is imaged without any interference from neighboring structures because the incident x rays are confined to lie within that plane. The resulting images, which must be reconstructed using computer techniques are, ipso facto, free from such interference.

Classical tomography excels in the delineation of very small (i.e., submillimeter), high-contrast structures such as the bones of the inner ear. Note that it is precisely this kind of object that creates problems in computed tomography, where dose considerations limit the achievable resolution to approximately 1 mm, and beam hardening and edge ringing phenomena can limit the fidelity of reconstruction of high-contrast subject matter.

The underlying principle of classical motion tomography is demonstrated in Fig. 6.1. The patient is radiographed by a moving x-ray source, and the image is recorded on a moving film-screen detector system. In the most commonly used arrangement, the source motion is confined to a horizontal plane, the source plane, and the detector motion is likewise confined to a horizontal plane, the detector plane. The relative motion of the source and detector is constrained by mechanical linkages such that a straight line drawn from the source to a fiducial point on the detector always passes through a fixed point in space. This fulcrum point also defines the location of the horizontal fulcrum plane. Another common arrangement allows the source and detector to move in opposition over spherical segments that are concentric with the fulcrum point. There is no essential difference between these systems, and we shall consider only the former. The patient is positioned so that the anatomical section of interest is located in the fulcrum plane, and a time exposure is made during which the source and detector move through a predetermined trajectory. It follows from the geometry of similar triangles that the x-ray image of all structures in the fulcrum plane, such as point A, will remain stationary with respect to the moving detector. Provided that a point x-ray source is used, these structures will be sharply

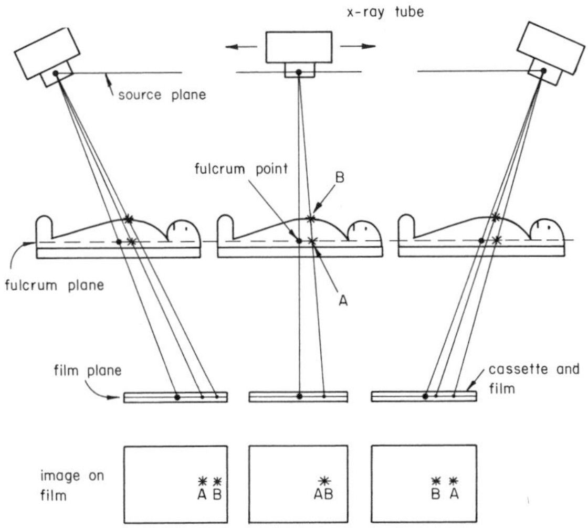

Fig. 6.1 Three positions of the source, patient, and detector during the continuous exposure of a conventional tomogram. Points such as A lying in the fulcrum plane will be sharply imaged. The image of point B (which is in an out-of-focus plane) will move relative to the detector and thus it will appear blurred.

imaged. Now consider point B, which lies above the fulcrum plane. Its image moves over the detector during the exposure. The actual track of the image point or, in other words, the out-of-focus PSF, will be a scaled-down version of the trajectory of the source during exposure. The dimensional scale factor will be directly proportional to the distance from the point to the fulcrum plane. Thus, the manner in which the unwanted object planes are displayed in superposition with the desired sectional image can be controlled by varying the source trajectory.

The choice of spread function depends upon many parameters, some of which relate to the subjective biases of the radiologist. However, a few general comments can be made.

There is an inverse relationship between the size of a small object and the minimum density difference it must have with respect to the background before it can be detected. If a characteristic dimension of the object is Δl, the contrast in the image is about $\Delta\mu\,\Delta l$. When low-contrast features are imaged tomographically, small angular motions of the source should be used. This permits a relatively thick section of the patient to be "essentially" in focus, thus allowing sufficient image contrast to be obtained. Unfortunately, this is just the condition that results in reduced blur for other planes, and it is a general observation that classical motion tomography is of limited use in isolating tomographic sections for low-contrast subject detail.

Large angular motions can be employed when the object contrast is large. Correspondingly, high degrees of spatial isolation can be achieved. Thus the widest application for classical motion tomography is in studies of the skeletal systems, the air-filled spaces of the head, and the lungs.

Linear motion blur is the easiest to implement from the mechanical standpoint, but it is generally the least satisfactory from the clinical imaging point of view since structure with edges parallel to the motion direction will be sharply imaged, independent of the depth at which it is located. It could even lie tilted across several planes and still appear sharp. Thus the out-of-focus point spread function is severely anisotropic and gives images that are hard to interpret. The ideal blurring function appears to be a uniform circular disk or similar pattern. Such a pattern is hard to achieve by mechanical scanning, but a close approximation, the Archimedean spiral, is available on some commercial machines. Another pattern used commercially is the hypocycloid. This pattern again attempts to approximate a solid disk, but with rather less success. Very "dilute" approximations to a filled disk, such as a simple ring created by circular motion, are generally to be avoided. These dilute blur functions can give serious image artifacts under certain conditions. For example, a circular-ring out-of-focus PSF can combine with a circular anatomic or pathologic feature in an out-of-focus plane to create a sharp pointlike feature in the final image.

The "optimum" shape of the blur function, if such a thing exists, has not yet been defined. Harding *et al.* (1978) have indicated some of the factors that must be taken into consideration. Any definite statement concerning the "best" or "optimum" profile would have to be substantiated with a psychophysical evaluation. For a thorough review of the clinical applications of classical tomography, see Littleton *et al.* (1976).

6.2 THE PSF IN CLASSICAL MOTION TOMOGRAPHY

In this section we use the methods developed in Chapter 4 to derive an expression for the PSF for the completely general case of arbitrary source distribution and arbitrary motion.

The geometry is shown in Fig. 6.2. In the absence of motion, the photon distribution in the film plane is given by (4.13):

$$h(\mathbf{r}'') = C \int_\infty f(\mathbf{r}) g(a\mathbf{r}'' + b\mathbf{r})\, d^2\mathbf{r}, \tag{6.1}$$

where

$$a = \frac{s_1}{s_1 + s_2}, \qquad b = \frac{s_2}{s_1 + s_2}, \qquad C = \frac{T}{4\pi(s_1 + s_2)^2} \tag{6.2}$$

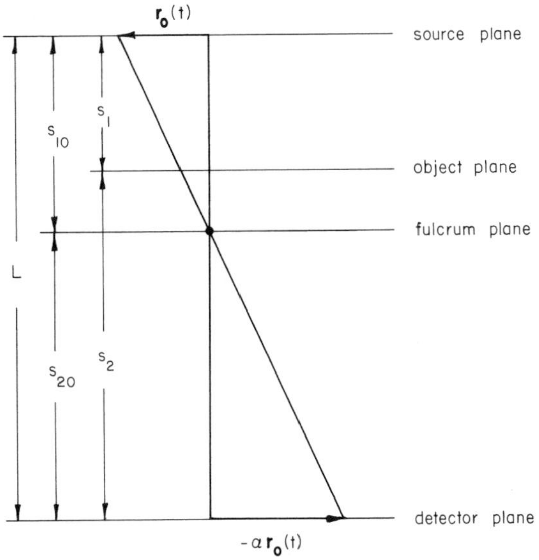

Fig. 6.2 Geometry used for calculating the PSF for motion tomography.

and T is the time over which the exposure is made. The source function $f(\mathbf{r})$ describes the number of photons per square centimeter emitted into 4π steradians per second. Note that s_1 and s_2 define the plane of the object $g(\ )$. This, in general, is different from the fulcrum plane, which is defined by s_{10} and s_{20}. Equation (6.1) applies only to planar objects. This is legitimate since we are calculating the PSF of the imaging system for a given layer in the object. We can explore how the PSF changes for different layers simply by changing a and b.

When in motion, the source position is described by a time-varying displacement vector $\mathbf{r}_0(t)$, so the source function becomes

$$f_t(\mathbf{r}) = f[\mathbf{r} - \mathbf{r}_0(t)]. \tag{6.3}$$

For a given offset $\mathbf{r}_0(t)$, the detector is moved in its own plane by an amount

$$\mathbf{r}_0''(t) = -\alpha\mathbf{r}_0(t), \tag{6.4}$$

where $\alpha = s_{20}/s_{10}$.

Since we are looking for image motion relative to the detector, it is convenient to define a coordinate system $\mathbf{r}_{\mathrm{d}}''(t)$ attached to the detector,

$$\mathbf{r}_{\mathrm{d}}''(t) = \mathbf{r}'' + \alpha\mathbf{r}_0(t), \tag{6.5}$$

and determine the system imaging properties relative to this coordinate system.

It follows from (6.1) that the instantaneous arrival rate of photons (in photons per square centimeter per second) is

$$\frac{d}{dt}(h(\mathbf{r}'')) = \frac{C}{T}\int_{\infty} f_t(\mathbf{r})g(a\mathbf{r}'' + b\mathbf{r})\,d^2\mathbf{r}. \tag{6.6}$$

To convert to the detector coordinate system, we note that the photon density in that system $h_{\mathrm{d}}(\mathbf{r}_{\mathrm{d}}'')$ is given by

$$h_{\mathrm{d}}(\mathbf{r}_{\mathrm{d}}'') \equiv h(\mathbf{r}'') = h(\mathbf{r}_{\mathrm{d}}'' - \alpha\mathbf{r}_0). \tag{6.7}$$

Substituting (6.7), (6.5), and (6.3) into (6.6) and integrating over the exposure time, we obtain the complete expression for the photon density in the detector-fixed coordinate system for arbitrary source function $f(\ )$, transmittance $g(\ )$, and motion vector $\mathbf{r}_0(t)$:

$$h_{\mathrm{d}}(\mathbf{r}_{\mathrm{d}}'') = \frac{C}{T}\int_0^T dt \int_{\infty} f[\mathbf{r} - \mathbf{r}_0(t)]g\{a[\mathbf{r}_{\mathrm{d}}'' - \alpha\mathbf{r}_0(t)] + b\mathbf{r}\}\,d^2\mathbf{r}. \tag{6.8}$$

We now determine the point spread function of the system by requiring that the transmission function $g(\ )$ be a δ function:

$$g(\mathbf{r}') \to g^{\delta}(\mathbf{r}') = \delta(\mathbf{r}') \tag{6.9}$$

Note that the dimensions of $g^{\delta}(\mathbf{r}')$ are L^{-2}. The image-plane photon density is given by substituting (6.9) into (6.6) and using the sifting property of the δ function to perform the integration:

$$h_{\mathrm{d}}^{\delta}(\mathbf{r}_{\mathrm{d}}'') = \frac{C}{b^2 T}\int_0^T f\left(-\frac{a}{b}(\mathbf{r}_{\mathrm{d}}'' - \beta\mathbf{r}_0(t))\right)dt, \tag{6.10}$$

where $\beta = \alpha - (b/a) = (s_{20}/s_{10}) - (s_2/s_1)$. For $\beta \ll 1$, it is easy to show that $\beta \approx L(s_{20} - s_2)/s_{10}^2$, i.e., β is proportional to the "out-of-focus" distance of the plane in question. To get the PSF referred to the object dimensions, $h_{\mathrm{d}}^{\delta}(\mathbf{r}_{\mathrm{d}}'')$ must be scaled to the object (not fulcrum) plane. This gives

$$p(\mathbf{r}') = \frac{1}{a^2}h_{\mathrm{d}}^{\delta}(\mathbf{r}'/a) = \frac{C}{a^2 b^2 T}\int_0^T f\left(-\frac{1}{b}[\mathbf{r}' - a\beta\mathbf{r}_0(t)]\right)dt \tag{6.11}$$

as the general expression for the PSF of any motion tomography system in which the source and detector motions are in two parallel planes.

If the source is a δ function, $f(\mathbf{r}) = f_0\delta(\mathbf{r})$, then

$$p(\mathbf{r}') = \frac{Cf_0}{a^2T}\int_0^T \delta[\mathbf{r}' - a\beta\mathbf{r}_0(t)]\,dt. \tag{6.12}$$

When the fulcrum and object planes coincide, $\beta = 0$ and $p(\mathbf{r}')$ is simply a stationary δ function. For out-of-focus planes, $p(\mathbf{r}')$ is seen to be an appropriately scaled version of the source trajectory. Quantities $p(\mathbf{r}')$ and $h^\delta(\mathbf{r}_a'')$ both have dimensions L^{-4}. This is in agreement with the general behavior of a PSF defined by "image equals object convolved with PSF," since in this case the object is dimensionless (a transmission function), and the image has dimensions L^{-2} (photons per square centimeter). (The extra L^{-2} comes from the convolution integral.)

We can illustrate the use of (6.12) by considering a circular scan

$$\mathbf{r}_0(t) = r_0[\hat{\mathbf{x}}\cos\omega t + \hat{\mathbf{y}}\sin\omega t], \tag{6.13}$$

where $\hat{\mathbf{x}}$ and $\hat{\mathbf{y}}$ are Cartesian unit vectors. In Cartesian coordinates, the two-dimensional δ function factors into one-dimensional δ functions, and (6.12) becomes

$$p(\mathbf{r}') = \frac{Cf_0}{a^2T}\int_0^T dt\,\delta(x' - a\beta r_0\cos\omega t)\,\delta(y' - a\beta r_0\sin\omega t). \tag{6.14}$$

By repeated use of (A.24), the integral can be evaluated, giving

$$p(\mathbf{r}') = \frac{Cf_0}{a^2T}\frac{\delta(r' - R')}{R'}, \tag{6.15}$$

where $\delta(r' - R')$ is a one-dimensional ring δ function (discussed also in Section 8.2.1), whose radius R' is

$$R' = a\beta r_0. \tag{6.16}$$

In evaluating (6.14), it is necessary to assume that either $T \gg \omega^{-1}$ or $T = (2\pi/\omega) \times$ integer.

6.3 VARIATIONS ON THE THEME

6.3.1 Multiple-Film Method

There is a method that permits the recording of several images simultaneously, each with a different fulcrum plane (see Fig. 6.3). Several films spaced apart are positioned under the patient. There is no relative motion between the films, but the whole cassette assembly is translated parallel to the source by a mechanical linkage that keeps the source A, a fulcrum B,

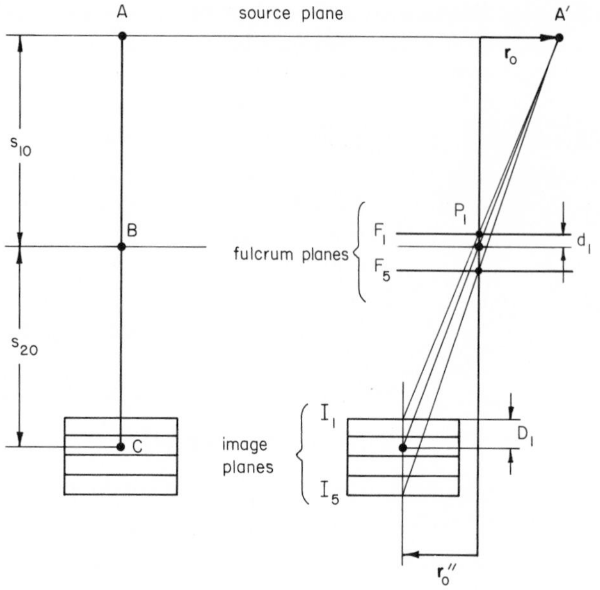

Fig. 6.3 A multiple-film method that allows several discrete tomographic planes to be imaged simultaneously.

and a point C on the cassette collinear. Although B is the fulcrum of the lever ABC, it is not generally the fulcrum of the tomographic images recorded on the various films. Consider the top photographic film in the stack located at image plane I_1. When the source is at A' the stack as a whole will have translated $\mathbf{r}_0'' = -(s_{20}/s_{10})\mathbf{r}_0$. The point P_1 on AB in the object, whose image lies on I_1 at a displacement $\mathbf{r}_0''$, defines the fulcrum plane F_1 for that image plane. The shadow of P_1 will always fall at the same point on the moving film located in image plane I_1. Similarly, for each image plane I_n, there is a corresponding fulcrum plane F_n. From Fig. 6.3 it can be seen that the displacement d_n of the tomographic fulcrum planes from the mechanical fulcrum B is given by

$$d_n = \left(\frac{s_{10}}{s_{10} + s_{20}}\right) D_n, \tag{6.17}$$

where D_n is the corresponding displacement between the nth image plane and the cassette pivot point C.

The principal disadvantage of this method is that each detector must be relatively transparent to the x-ray photons (i.e., inefficient) in order that all detectors receive useful exposure. Low-efficiency detectors, such as photographic film without a fluorescent intensifying screen, result in an increased dose to the patient. We shall see shortly that this penalty of increased dose for multiple tomographic planes need not be accepted.

6.3.2 Transverse Tomographic System

The systems described so far are most suitable for obtaining images of longitudinal sections of the body (i.e., those sections containing the long axis of the body). It is difficult, if not impossible, to obtain transverse sections using the sort of equipment described earlier.

One way to overcome this problem is shown in Fig. 6.4. Suppose the source to be stationary and let both the patient and the film holder rotate synchronously at the same angular velocity about vertical axes. The ray from the point source that intersects the film at its center of rotation also intersects the axis of rotation of the patient at a point that defines the tomographic plane. As the patient and film rotate, the image of the tomographic plane remains stationary with respect to the rotating film. Other horizontal sections are blurred with a ring-δ-function PSF. In clinical practice it is preferable to keep the patient stationary and horizontal. In that case both source and detector rotate about the patient while maintaining the relative geometries described above.

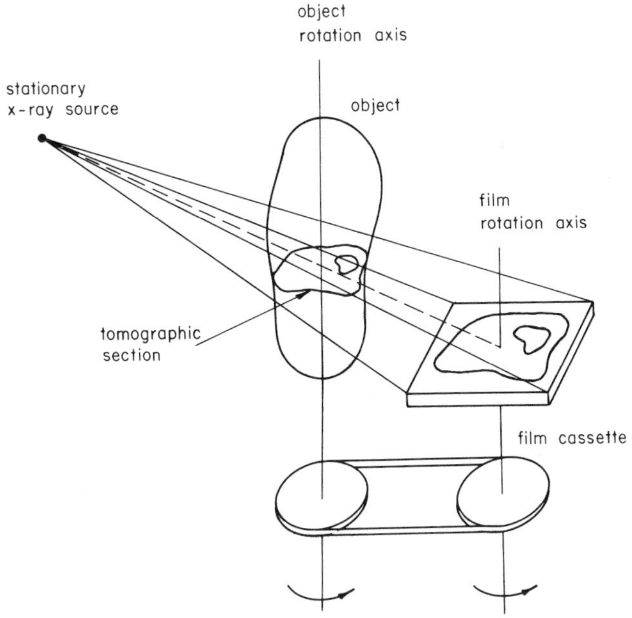

Fig. 6.4 A system that permits transverse tomographic images to be recorded.

6.3.3 Multiple-Exposure Method

In the methods described previously, it is necessary to repeat the study or otherwise incur a higher patient dose if multiple images with differing tomographic fulcrum planes are desired. We shall now show that by taking a series of separate film exposures, each with a different source–patient–film geometry, essentially any tomographic fulcrum plane can be selected for imaging. We shall also show that there is little or no penalty in dose for this flexibility.

Consider multiple source positions as shown in Fig. 6.5. At each position the source is flashed and a radiograph taken; a fresh film is used for each exposure. Suppose initially that the object consists of a single point absorber. On each film that point will show as a dot. If all the films are superimposed it will be possible by carefully positioning each one to align all of the dot

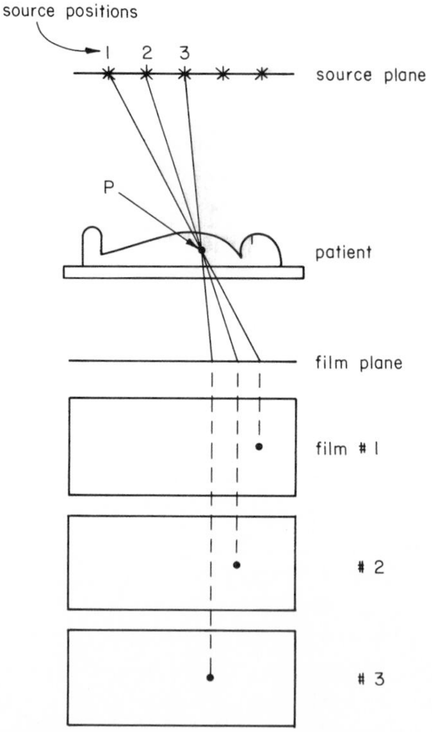

Fig. 6.5 The principle of tomosynthesis is shown. A separate film is taken at each of several source positions. For viewing, the films are superimposed with a shift so that detail from a given plane such as the one containing the point *P* is brought into registration. Any desired plane can be tomographically imaged by applying the appropriate shifts.

images. For more complicated planar objects, it follows that multiple images of any other structure in the same plane as the absorbing point will also be registered together. Viewing the N superimposed films in transmission will demonstrate a sharp image of the planar object. The plane of interest can be located anywhere between the source plane and the film plane in a continuous fashion; there is no relationship between N and the possible number of fulcrum planes. However, when considering three-dimensional objects, the number and separation of the source points does determine the out-of-focus point spread function. Consider two point absorbers A and B at different depths. When the images of point A are superimposed, the images of point B will form an array of dots which is a scaled replica of the spatial arrangement of the source points. For any arbitrary pattern of source positions $\mathbf{r}_1, \mathbf{r}_2, \ldots, \mathbf{r}_n$ with exposure times $t_1, t_2, \ldots, t_n$, it follows from (6.12) that the PSF from the out-of-focus plane containing point B, referred to the scale of the in-focus plane containing point A, is given by

$$p(\mathbf{r}') = \frac{Cf_0}{a^2} \sum_{n=1}^{N} t_n \delta(\mathbf{r}' - a\beta\mathbf{r}_n) \Big/ \sum_{n=1}^{N} t_n, \tag{6.18}$$

where, using the notation of Fig. 6.2,

$$a = s_1/(s_1 + s_2) \tag{6.19}$$

and

$$\beta = (s_{20}/s_{10}) - (s_2/s_1). \tag{6.20}$$

Thus, in principle, the out-of-focus PSF can be made to approximate any desired function by appropriate choice of the t_n and $\mathbf{r}_n$ while retaining the capability of selecting, after exposure, any desired fulcrum plane. It is apparent that the out-of-focus PSF more closely approximates a smooth continuous function as N increases, and it would seem desirable to make N as large as possible.

We now show that the increased flexibility is achieved without a significant increase in dose to the patient. This can be seen most easily by considering a photon-counting detector rather than a photographic film. Suppose an average value of M photons per pixel or resolution element is required to give the desired signal-to-noise ratio in the final image. It makes no difference whether the M photons arrive at the detector in one continuous exposure, or in N independent exposures with M/N photons per exposure. With Poisson statistics governing the fluctuations in the number of photons the variance for the independent-multiple-exposure case will simply be the sum of the individual variances, i.e., $\sum^N (\sqrt{M/N})^2 = M$, which is the variance in the single-exposure case also. Therefore the signal-to-noise ratio is the same in both cases.

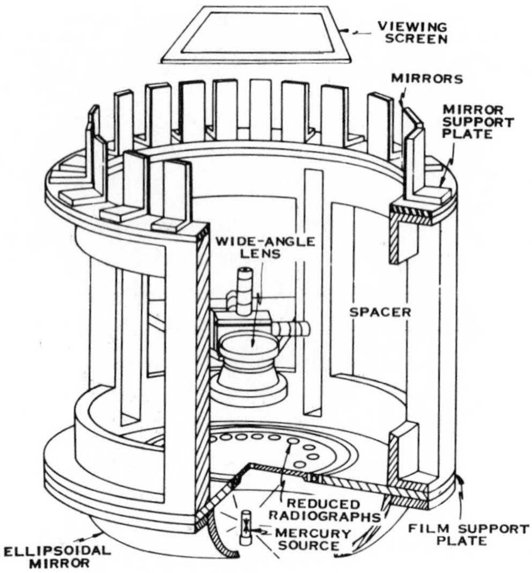

Fig. 6.6 Three-dimensional projector for viewing twenty radiographs taken with a circular scan geometry. (From Grant, 1972.)

There have been reported several ways of implementing the principle of multiple-exposure tomography. The Dynatome (CFC Products Inc.) exposes ten films sequentially. A viewing device allows the films to be superimposed and translated with respect to each other in order to select the required fulcrum plane. A problem with film methods is the rapid buildup of "base-plus-fog" density when a large number of films are superimposed and viewed in transmission; also, low-gamma film must be used.

Grant (1972) has described a system called Tomosynthesis in which 20 radiographs are taken using a single-ring geometry for the sources. Images of photographic reductions of the radiographs are projected into a viewing space (see Fig. 6.6). Folding mirrors ensure that the images overlap and are in a common region where they can be optically summed on a ground-glass screen. Moving the ground-glass screen along the optical axis of the special projector changes the degree of overlap between the images, which is equivalent to selecting different fulcrum planes. A wide-angle lens with a high f number (to give a wide depth of field) is required. One interesting feature is that complete tomographic images from tilted fulcrum planes may be observed simply by tilting the viewing screen. This follows since each point in the volume where the reconstructions are being made is conjugate to a point in the original object. Thus any plane in the reconstruction space can be thought of as a tomographic image plane.

A variant on this system has been described by Bailey *et al.* (1974). In his system a set of projection images are recorded using an x-ray image intensifier tube and TV camera. Each image is stored on a disk recorder. For playback, each image is recalled in turn and summed with the appropriate spatial shift on an analog silicon storage target. The shifts are determined by the position of the corresponding projection and the desired reconstruction fulcrum layer. After summation, the composite image is recorded for subsequent viewing on a TV monitor. By storing many reconstructions and playing them in rapid succession, it is possible to move "through" a three-dimensional reconstruction of the object. This enables an enhanced appreciation of depth to be obtained.

Next we mention a holographic method described by Kock and Tiemens (1973) in which individual radiographs (up to 48 in number) are obtained from a circular line source geometry. A hologram is formed from each radiograph and, in the reconstruction phase, the individual holograms are coherently illuminated to produce emerging wave fronts equivalent to the wave fronts that would emanate from the original radiographs. The wave fronts from each hologram form real images in the reconstruction volume, so they can be captured on a diffusing screen for observation. The system is equivalent to Grant's system except that the data are stored as a hologram rather than as direct projection images.

6.4 METHODS IN NUCLEAR MEDICINE

Because of the classification system used in this book, many of the tomographic γ-ray imaging systems are described elsewhere. For example, the rectilinear scanner with a focused collimator (Section 4.4.5) is inherently tomographic in nature, as are the coded apertures described in Chapter 8; however, there are still several other devices designed to give (clinical) tomographic images that deserve mention, and we give brief details of two of them here.

6.4.1 Multiplane Tomographic Scanner

This system uses a focused collimator attached to a scanning γ-ray scintillation camera. The commercial version allows six tomographic images to be simultaneously obtained. To describe the principle of operation, we shall consider initially just a single point source P located beneath the scanning collimator (see Fig. 6.7). As the collimator scans from right to left, the image of the point source will move uniformly from A' to B' on the camera face as

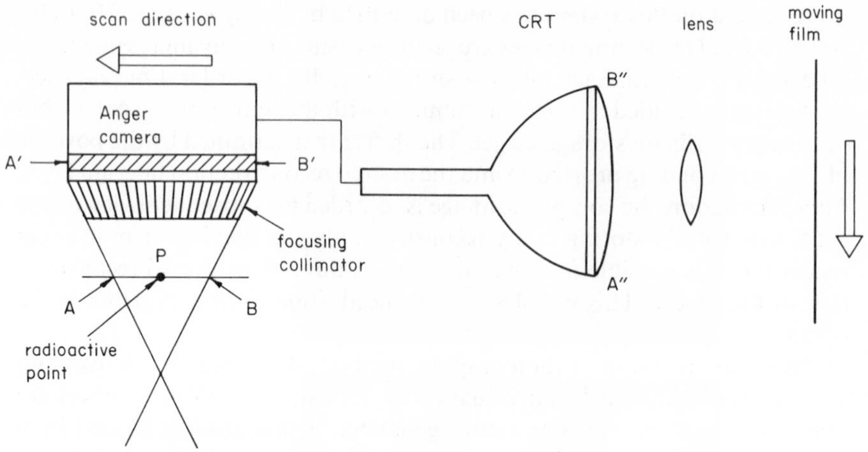

Fig. 6.7 A scanning focused collimator on an Anger camera can be used as a tomographic imaging system. See text for details.

the source traverses the collimator field from A to B. The camera output is displayed on a CRT as described in Section 5.4, and the display spot moves synchronously from A'' to B''. This display is imaged onto a moving film by a stationary lens L, and by choosing the appropriate lens position and focal length, the image of the moving display spot can be made stationary with respect to the film. The patient is scanned in a boustrophedonic fashion and the film motion is synchronized to scanner motion. Thus, whenever the point source appears in the field of the collimator its image will fall at the same point on the film throughout the whole exposure. It follows that if instead of a single spot there is a distributed planar object located in the plane of P, it also will be sharply imaged onto the film. For a point source not located in that plane, its moving image on the CRT will not synchronize with the film motion and the integrated image will be a circular disklike pattern whose diameter is proportional to the distance between the object point and the fulcrum plane defined by P. Different fulcrum planes can be selected simply by changing the lens system. In Anger's version of the device, six lens systems are used to simultaneously create six different images, side by side, on a single piece of film (Anger, 1974). Note that for any given point source, neglecting attenuation losses, the same mean number of scintillations will be detected during a complete scan irrespective of the depth of the source. Thus a given plane is emphasized only by sharpening the detail rather than by selectively weighting the counts from different depths. This is analogous to the methods of classical x-ray tomography. The depth discrimination capability is shown in Fig. 6.8.

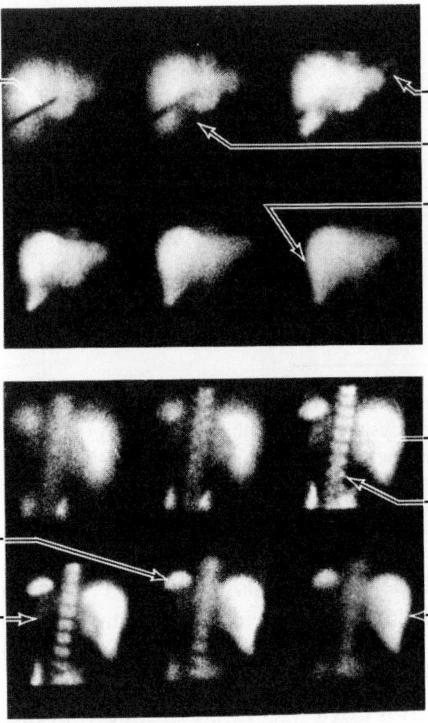

Fig. 6.8 Six-plane tomograms of a patient with liver cirrhosis. Tomograms are focused 1, 2, 3, 4, 5, and 6 in. from the collimator. (From Anger, 1974.)

6.4.2 The Tomo Camera

In this system (Muehllehner, 1971), a standard γ camera is fitted with a rotating parallel-slant-hole collimator. As the collimator rotates, a given point on the scintillation crystal will be illuminated by sources that lie on the surface of a cone as shown in Fig. 6.9. Consider a planar object that lies parallel to and beneath the collimator. If the object is translated (but not rotated) with a circular motion that is synchronized to the collimator rotation and of the appropriate radius, then the image of the object will be stationary on the camera crystal. It can then be displayed using the usual camera display methods. When the system is mechanically focused in this manner for a given plane, the out-of-focus PSF for other planes will be a ring-shaped pattern that is traced out in synchronization with the collimator rotation. However, it is straightforward to add compensating deflection circuitry to the CRT display that will circularly translate the final image in synchronism with the collimator rotation and in effect cancel the circular motion

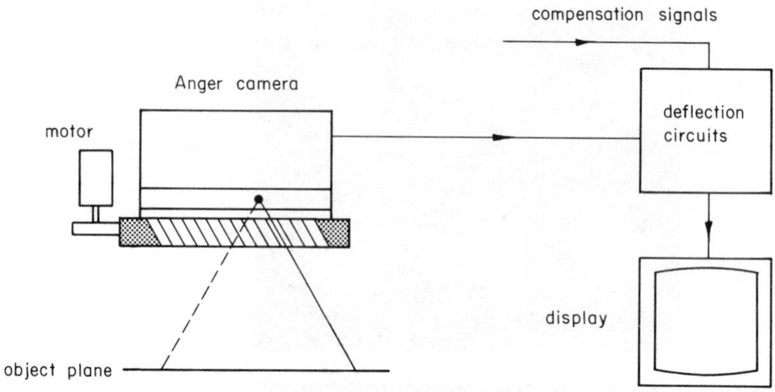

Fig. 6.9 Tomocamera for nuclear medicine based on a rotating slant-hole collimator. The examination table moves synchronously with the collimator rotation to mechanically stabilize the image from a chosen depth on the camera face. Electronically derived shift signals stabilize the image from slices at other depths of the patient on the CRT display. The data from out-of-focus sections is blurred by a ringlike PSF.

associated with the out-of-focus PSF. This enables the images from planes other than the mechanically focused plane to be made stationary on the CRT. Thus tomographic depth selection can be continuously varied simply by changing the amplitude of the compensating scan voltages. The out-of-focus PSF is still a circular ring. It is obvious that the output from the camera can be multiplexed into several simultaneous displays, each showing a different (electronically derived) fulcrum plane. The clinical version of this device produces four separate images. It is simply a matter of mechanical expedience that requires the bed rather than the camera head to undergo the translatory motion, and if large enough camera heads were available, no mechanical translations at all would be necessary.

7

Computed Tomography

7.1 INTRODUCTION

A conventional projection x-ray image can be thought of as a superposition of many discrete images, each one of a different slice of the object. As we saw in Chapter 6, the methods of classical tomography allow some of the confusion caused by overlapping images to be removed. Interference from unwanted slices is reduced by means of motion blurring.

Computed tomography (CT) is a technique by which each slice of the object can be viewed in total isolation, that is, with complete freedom of clutter from adjacent slices. The difficulty is that in measuring a property at a given internal point of a solid body, the radiation must also pass through a series of other points. Without cutting the object open, it is impossible to make independent measurements at each point. However, this does not mean that it is impossible to collect data that will allow clutter-free reconstructions to be made. The required data are obtained from transmission measurements whose paths are restricted to lie within the plane of interest. Therefore, any estimate (reconstruction) of the object distribution in that plane must be free of artifacts generated by other parts of the object since only points within the slice of interest are involved in generating the data set.

The tissue property that is actually computed is the linear attenuation coefficient μ. Even though most soft tissues in the body are composed mainly of water, there is sufficient variation to result in significant differences among the attenuation coefficients. Computed tomography is able to detect and display these differences, and the radiologist is thus presented with a picture which, in addition to showing a cross section of the anatomy, contains quantitative information, which may be used for a variety of purposes.

The ability to discriminate small differences has resulted in the creation of the hounsfield (H) as the unit of attenuation coefficient. One hounsfield represents 0.1% of the attenuation coefficient of water, and the zero on the scale is H(water) = 0.

$$\mathrm{H} = \frac{\mu(\text{tissue}) - \mu(\text{water})}{\mu(\text{water})} \times 1000. \tag{7.1}$$

Thus air has $\mathrm{H} = -1000$ and bone has $\mathrm{H} \approx +1000$. (An earlier definition using 0.2% as opposed to 0.1% has fallen into disuse.)

Nearly all manufacturers claim essentially equivalent performance figures for their equipment. These are: 0.5% density discrimination (i.e., 5 H) and 1- to 2-mm spatial resolution, but it should be realized that these limits are not achieved simultaneously. The spatial resolution figure is achieved with high-contrast objects, while the density discrimination of 5 H can only be observed with reasonable certainty over an area several times larger ($\sim$4) than a single resolution element (see Section 10.7.1). We shall see later that these figures are determined by the statistical nature of the photon flux (rather than the hardware systems) and that the only way to improve upon them significantly is to increase the x-ray patient dose to unacceptable levels. It seems likely that even if powerful nonlinear algorithms are introduced into the CT software arsenal, there will not be dramatic improvement over the currently demonstrated limits.

To illustrate the detection sensitivity of CT, we compare film-recorded projection radiographs and CT when used to detect small low-contrast lesions. Consider a 1 cm ($= \Delta x$) lesion with $\Delta\mu = 0.01\mu(\text{water})$, i.e., $\Delta \mathrm{H} = 10$. This lesion would be readily discernible on a CT image. If the same lesion were imaged using projection radiography, then the fractional change in transmittance, $\Delta T/T$, due to the lesion would be

$$\Delta T/T = \Gamma \Delta\mu \, \Delta x = 2 \times 0.01 \times 0.2 \times 1 = 0.004, \tag{7.2}$$

where we have assumed a film gamma Γ of 2. Since a 4% contrast change is about the threshold of visual discrimination, this lesion of contrast one-tenth that amount would certainly be missed. The film gamma can be increased to improve the discrimination, but not by much since doing so severely compromises the dynamic range of exposures that the film can record. For example, it is not unusual to have an exposure dynamic range of 100:1. Even for $\Gamma = 2$, which is a reasonable value, this exposure range would require a maximum density $D_{\max}$ of 4 simply to record the incident information. A $D_{\max}$ of 4 is virtually useless for direct viewing. Thus there is a basic incompatibility between dynamic range and density discrimination requirements. This is unfortunate because, as has been shown by Motz and Danos (1978), the needed information is actually contained in the transmitted photon flux (see also Section 10.4). It is simply the limitations of film as a detector and the eye as a discriminator, along with the problems of overlapping image detail, that prevent film from yielding all of the information that has been recorded.

On the other hand, the CT image easily displays the lesion. Such systems allow the reconstructed image to be displayed with a selectable portion of the image dynamic range being used to fully modulate the brightness of the display tube. The width of this data window and the central value are under operator control. If we select the width equal to 20 H, the lesion will occupy 50% of the total gray scale of the display, equivalent to a $\Delta T/T$ value of 0.5 for purposes of comparing to film. Looked at in a slightly different way, the equivalent film would need a Γ of 250.

For a discourse on the mathematical aspects of CT, the reader should consult Herman (1980). A comprehensive collection of relevant FORTRAN program listings has been provided by Huesman *et al.* (1977).

7.2 ANALYTICAL THEORY OF RECONSTRUCTING FROM PROJECTIONS

7.2.1 Projections

Figure 7.1 shows the simplest configuration for recording CT projection data. It consists of a source and a single detector. By a series of translations and rotations, a large number of transmission measurements are made. These measurements are the raw data. Although modern systems may have multiple sources and large detector arrays for parallel data gathering, it is just the same data set that is ultimately gathered.

We define two coplanar reference frames: the x–y frame, which is fixed with respect to the object, and the x_r–y_r frame, in which the y_r direction is the direction of the incident x-ray beam. The origin of both systems is located at the center of rotation of the scanning gantry. The x_r–y_r frame is rotated by angle ϕ counterclockwise with respect to the x–y frame (see Fig. 7.2).

The following notation will be used throughout this chapter: $\mu(\mathbf{r})$ is a generalized expression for the linear attenuation coefficient at position vector $\mathbf{r}$. To show the different functional forms of μ in the various coordinate systems, we shall use square brackets [ ] to denote Cartesian coordinates, round brackets ( ) to denote polar coordinates, and subscript r to denote a

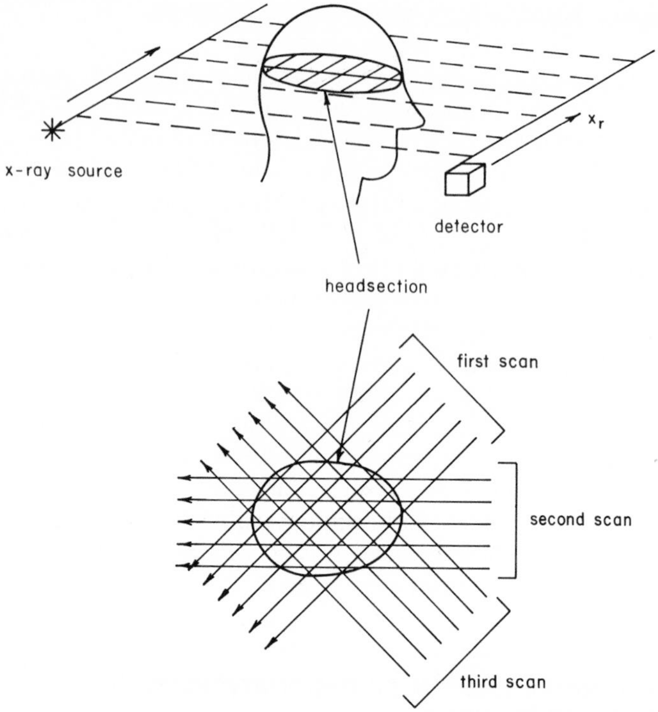

Fig. 7.1 Simple scanning system for transaxial tomography. A pencil beam of x rays passes through the object and is detected on the far side. The source-detector assembly is scanned sideways to generate one projection $\lambda_\phi(x_r)$. This is repeated at many viewing angles and the required set of projection data is obtained.

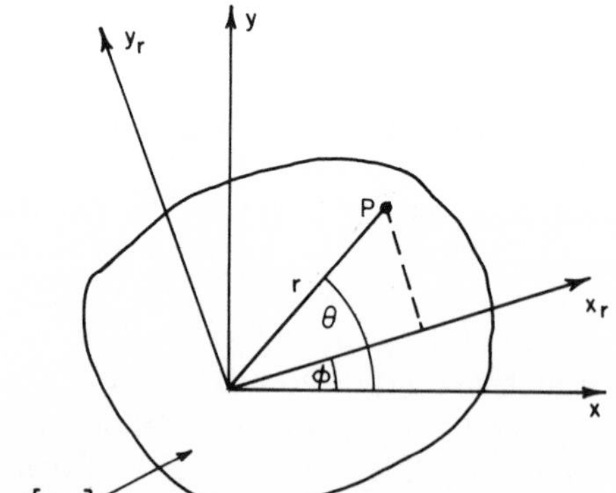

Fig. 7.2 Object is represented as a two-dimensional distribution of linear attenuation coefficient $\mu[x, y]$. The x-ray source and detector rotate with the x_r–y_r frame, with the x-rays traveling parallel to y_r. P is the general point in the object.

rotated frame of reference. Thus we have the following equivalences:

$$\mu(\mathbf{r}) \equiv \mu[x, y] \equiv \mu_r[x_r, y_r] \equiv \mu(r, \theta) \equiv \mu_r(r_r, \theta_r) \tag{7.3}$$

with

$$x = r\cos\theta, \qquad y = r\sin\theta, \tag{7.4}$$

$$x_r = r_r\cos\theta_r = x\cos\phi + y\sin\phi, \qquad y_r = r_r\sin\theta_r = -x\sin\phi + y\cos\phi, \tag{7.5}$$

$$r_r = r, \qquad \theta_r = \theta - \phi, \tag{7.6}$$

and

$$\mathbf{r} = x\hat{\mathbf{x}} + y\hat{\mathbf{y}} = x_r\hat{\mathbf{x}}_r + y_r\hat{\mathbf{y}}_r, \tag{7.7}$$

where $\hat{\mathbf{x}}$, $\hat{\mathbf{y}}$, $\hat{\mathbf{x}}_r$, and $\hat{\mathbf{y}}_r$ are the appropriate unit vectors.

For a pencil beam of monochromatic x rays traversing a medium of constant linear attenuation coefficient μ for a distance x, the beam is attenuated in accordance with Beer's law,

$$\Phi = \Phi_0 \exp(-\mu x), \tag{7.8}$$

where Φ and Φ_0 are the transmitted and the incident photon fluences, respectively. When the medium is nonhomogeneous, we must integrate along the absorption path,

$$\Phi = \Phi_0 \exp\left(-\int_l \mu(\mathbf{r})\, dl\right), \tag{7.9}$$

where l is the straight line joining the source and detector. In the complete data set, each transmission measurement is identified by the projection angle ϕ and the lateral position of the individual measurement x_r (see Fig. 7.3), and is written

$$\Phi_\phi(x_r) = \Phi_0 \exp\left(-\int_l \mu(\mathbf{r})\, dy_r\right). \tag{7.10}$$

The equations are linearized by taking the natural logarithms of both sides, giving rise to a new function $\lambda_\phi(x_r)$ which is a line integral of $\mu(\mathbf{r})$:

$$\lambda_\phi(x_r) = -\ln\left(\frac{\Phi_\phi(x_r)}{\Phi_0}\right) = \int_l \mu(\mathbf{r})\, dy_r. \tag{7.11}$$

The quantity $\lambda_\phi(x_r)$ is called the *Radon transform* or the *projection* of $\mu(\mathbf{r})$, and the whole task of reconstructing slices of objects from their projections is simply that of inverting (7.11). This is the subject of this chapter.

In practice, the transmission data are sampled both in x_r and ϕ, but for the time being we shall regard $\lambda_\phi(x_r)$ as being either a continuous one-dimensional function of x_r for a given projection angle ϕ, or a continuous

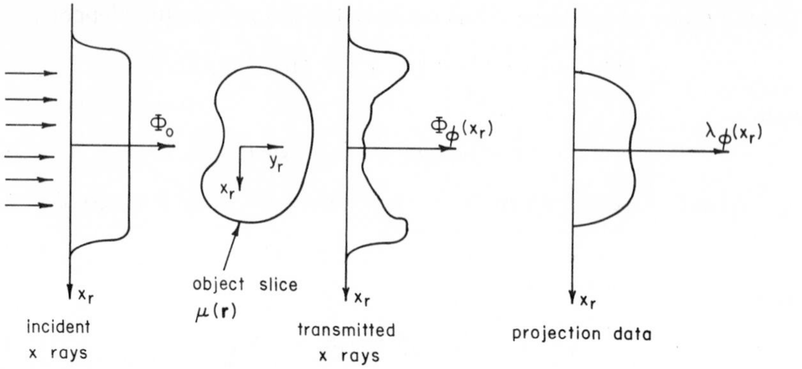

Fig. 7.3 Incident x rays of fluence Φ_0 are attenuated to a level $\Phi_\phi(x_r)$ in passing through the object slice. The projection data set $\lambda_\phi(x_r) = -\ln[\Phi_\phi(x_r)/\Phi_0]$ is the line integral of the x-ray linear attenuation coefficient taken through the slice in the direction of y_r.

two-dimensional function of ϕ and x_r. The effects of sampling will be discussed later.

It is instructive to see how data are mapped from the x–y space of real objects to the x_r–ϕ space of the projection data. Projection space may be represented either in polar or Cartesian form using coordinates x_r and ϕ. In the polar representation, which is often called the *Radon-space* representation, each point represents a line integral taken through the object. The vector from the origin to that point in Radon space is equal to the pedal vector of the projection in real space, and the value of the function in Radon space at point (x_r, ϕ) is given by $\lambda_\phi(x_r)/|x_r|$. [The denominator term $|x_r|$ comes from the nonlinear compression of data into the polar map (see Fig. 7.4a)]. Since each point in Radon space represents a path of line integration in object space, the equivalence between the two spaces is further illustrated by considering how a point in object space is mapped into Radon space. We must determine the locus of all line-integral paths that pass through the point in question. From Fig. 7.4b it is seen that for the general point P, or (r, θ), in object space, the x_r value is given by

$$x_r = r\cos(\theta - \phi). \tag{7.12}$$

This is the equation of a circle in Radon space. It is completely specified by its diameter, the end points of which are the origin and the point $x_r = r, \phi = \theta$.

If the projection data are mapped using x_r and ϕ as Cartesian coordinates, we again have a one-to-one correspondence between points in the projection space and line-integral paths in object space. We need consider only values of ϕ given by $0 < \phi < \pi$; all projection data are included in this range. The

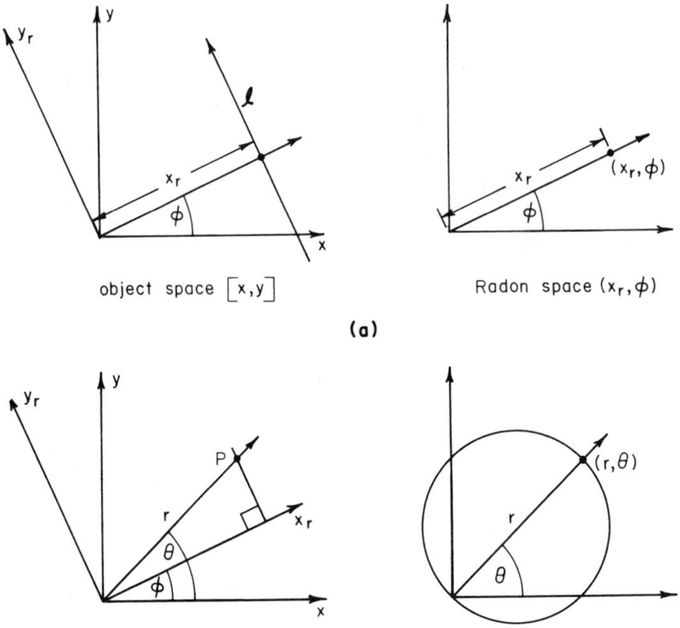

Fig. 7.4 Mapping between object and Radon space. (a) The line integral path l transforms to a point (x_r, ϕ) in Radon space. (b) The locus of all projections passing through $P(r, \theta)$ is a circle of diameter r centered on $(r/2, \theta)$.

locus of all projections passing through a given point in the object is again given by (7.12), which this time is a cosine curve. The radius r and azimuth θ of the object point are encoded directly as the amplitude and spatial phase of the cosine curve. This particular display of the projection data is called *sinogram* format (see Fig. 7.5).

There are several interesting properties concerning the data set $\lambda_\phi(x_r)$:

(1) It is bounded. Unlike some other integral transform pairs, $\mu(\mathbf{r})$ and $\lambda_\phi(x_r)$ share the same minimum circle of support. This is just the opposite of the Fourier transform, for example, where a narrowing in one domain implies a broadening in the other.

(2) There are certain symmetry considerations that result from the fact that the source and detector can be interchanged without affecting the value of a transmission measurement. In other words, all possible projection data are contained in projections gathered over a continuous semicircle of projection angles. Thus

$$\lambda_\phi(x_r) = \lambda_{\phi+\pi}(-x_r). \tag{7.13}$$

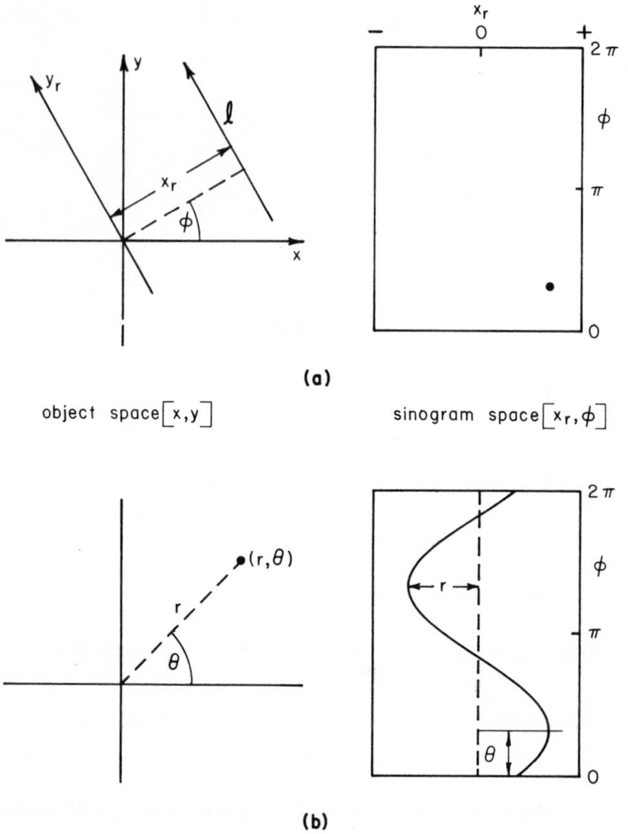

Fig. 7.5 Mapping between object and sinogram space. (a) A single projection data point defined by line l maps to a point $[x_r, \phi]$ in sinogram space, where (x_r, ϕ) denotes the pedal vector of l in object space. (b) The locus of all line integrals passing through point (r, θ) is a cosine wave of amplitude r and phase θ.

(3) There is an additional constraint on the projection data:

$$\int_{-\infty}^{\infty} \lambda_\phi(x_r)\, dx_r = W = \text{const.} \tag{7.14}$$

This follows immediately from the definition of $\lambda_\phi(x_r)$:

$$\int_{-\infty}^{\infty} \lambda_\phi(x_r)\, dx_r = \int_{-\infty}^{+\infty} \int_{-\infty}^{\infty} \mu(\mathbf{r})\, dy_r\, dx_r \tag{7.15}$$

and the right-hand side is seen to be the two-dimensional integral of the object over all space. This integral is clearly independent of the orientation of the frame in which the integration is carried out. There are several con-

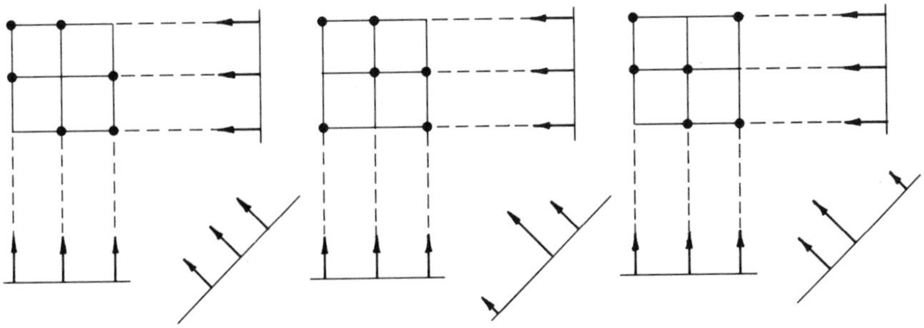

Fig. 7.6 Three different objects composed of points that have the same horizontal and vertical projections. A third projection such as the diagonal shown here is needed to distinguish between them.

sequences of this fact. One is that points in data space are not mutually independent as they are, for example, in Fourier space. Also, (7.15) may be used as a data consistency check. (There are many practical reasons why the data may not be self-consistent. These include photon noise statistics, x-ray tube instability, patient motion, sampling artifacts, and the effects of beam divergence.)

We now pose the question, How many projections are needed in order to reconstruct the object? For the special case of an object that consists only of a single absorbing point, two projections at different angles are enough. The location of the point may be found by a technique equivalent to the triangulation method used by surveyors.

When the object consists of an assembly of points, two projections are not, in general, sufficient to allow an unambiguous reconstruction. Figure 7.6 shows three different distributions of points that all have the same vertical and horizontal projections. If a third projection is taken along a diagonal, the ambiguity is resolved immediately. There is clearly a relationship between object complexity and the required number of projections. In Section 7.2.2 we shall show that

(1) any object is completely described by the continuous set of its projections, i.e., even the most complicated object can be reconstructed from its projections;

(2) there is a straightforward interpretation of the information that is contained in each projection; and

(3) the insight provided by (2) gives rise to many equivalent analytical methods for solving (7.11).

The question of how many samples are actually needed in practice is discussed in Section 7.3.2.

7.2.2 The Central Slice Theorem

We start by proving a theorem. Consider the expression for a single projection through the object at angle ϕ,

$$\lambda_\phi(x_r) = \int_{-\infty}^{+\infty} \mu_r[x_r, y_r]\, dy_r. \tag{7.16}$$

The one-dimensional Fourier transform of $\lambda_\phi(x_r)$, namely $\Lambda_\phi(\xi_r)$, is given by

$$\begin{aligned}\Lambda_\phi(\xi_r) &= \int_{-\infty}^{+\infty} \lambda_\phi(x_r)\exp(-2\pi i\xi_r x_r)\, dx_r \\ &= \int_{-\infty}^{+\infty}\int_{-\infty}^{+\infty} \mu_r[x_r, y_r]\exp(-2\pi i\xi_r x_r)\, dx_r\, dy_r,\end{aligned} \tag{7.17}$$

where we have taken $[\xi_r, \eta_r]$ to be the Fourier-space variables conjugate to $[x_r, y_r]$.

The previous equation can be rewritten

$$\begin{aligned}\Lambda_\phi(\xi_r) &= \int_{-\infty}^{\infty}\int_{-\infty}^{\infty} \mu_r[x_r, y_r]\exp[-2\pi i(\xi_r x_r + \eta_r y_r]\, dx_r\, dy_r\big|_{\eta_r=0} \\ &= \mathscr{F}_2\{\mu(\mathbf{r})\}\big|_{\eta_r=0} = \mathrm{M}_r[\xi_r, 0].\end{aligned} \tag{7.18}$$

The right-hand side of this expression is recognizable as the *two-dimensional* Fourier transform of the object, $\mathrm{M}_r[\xi_r, \eta_r]$, evaluated along the line $\eta_r = 0$. (Note that M is a capital Greek mu.) Thus, the one-dimensional Fourier transform of a projection is equal to a particular section of the two-dimensional Fourier transform of the object itself. That particular section is the ξ_r axis (which is the conjugate to the x_r axis along which the projection is specified). This is the *central slice theorem*.

To illustrate the theorem, consider a general, bounded object. This object can always be synthesized from a linear superposition of all of its two-dimensional spatial frequency components. Now, consider just one of those cosinusoidal frequency components (see Fig. 7.7a). Only when the projection direction is parallel to the wave crests does the projection differ from zero. However, for that particular direction, the full cosine distribution is projected onto the x_r axis. The Fourier transform of this one component is shown in Fig. 7.7b. The original object is a superposition of many component waves of various phases, periods and directions, and it follows that only those waves that are parallel to the first one will have their transforms located on the ξ_r axis, and that these are the only waves that will change the form of $\lambda_\phi(x_r)$. Thus, the transform of the slice *is* identical to the corresponding section (or slice) of the full two-dimensional transform.

There are two important consequences of this theorem. The first is that the projections do contain sufficient information to allow the general object to be reconstructed. The second is that in order to be able to do this, an

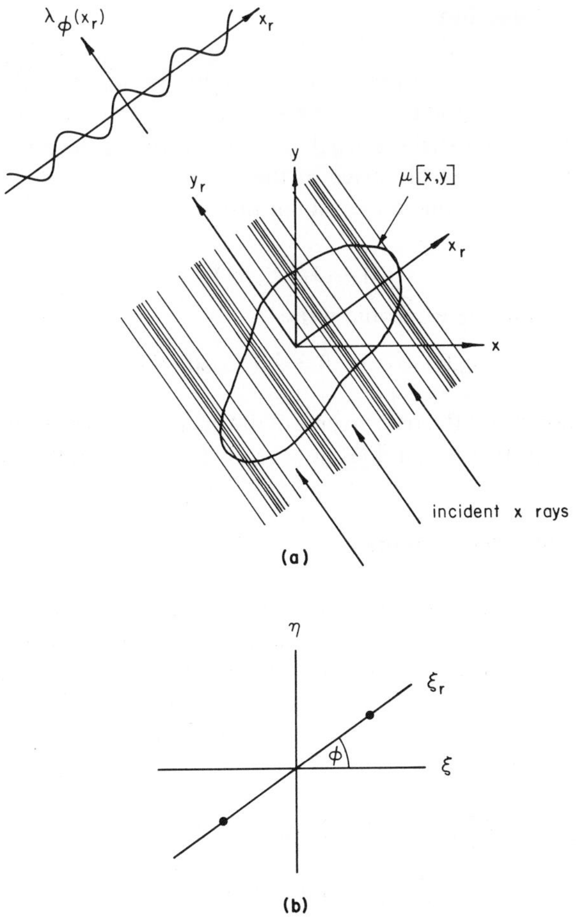

Fig. 7.7 (a) General object distribution $\mu(\mathbf{r})$ can be decomposed into Fourier components of the form $\sin 2\pi\boldsymbol{\rho} \cdot \mathbf{r}$ or $\cos 2\pi\boldsymbol{\rho} \cdot \mathbf{r}$. One of the latter is depicted here. There is only one direction ϕ for which the projection of this component is nonzero, and at this particular ϕ the component is fully mapped onto the projection. (b) The Fourier transform of this component is a pair of δ functions (shown here by dots) located on the ξ_r axis.

infinite number or continuum of projection data is required (at least in theory) since this is the only way to completely determine the Fourier space, and hence, through Fourier transformation, the real-space distribution of the object. In practice, however, the finite size of the x-ray beam, and other considerations, effectively bandlimit the data, and satisfactory reconstructions can be obtained using a finite number of projection angles (typically a few hundred) and finite number of samples of each projection.

7.2.3 Back-Projection

Back-projection is the opposite of projection in the sense that we take a one-dimensional function of x_r, namely the projection data, and create from it a two-dimensional distribution $g_\phi[x_r, y_r]$ by smearing the one-dimensional function uniformly over all space in the y_r direction. Stated formally, the back-projection of the one-dimensional projection $\lambda_\phi(x_r)$ is given by

$$g_\phi[x_r, y_r] = \lambda_\phi(x_r). \tag{7.19}$$

In the unrotated frame we would write

$$g_\phi(\mathbf{r}) = g_\phi(r, \theta) = \lambda_\phi(r\cos(\theta - \phi)). \tag{7.20}$$

Back-projection is not the true inverse of the projection operation. Projection followed by back-projection does not reconstruct the original object.

7.2.4 The Summation Image

The process of combining many back-projections creates a new two-dimensional image, the summation image. If we take a discrete number of back-projections corresponding to a set of object projections at angles ϕ_i, the summation image is simply the arithmetic sum of the individual back-projections. Denoting this discretely formed summation image by $b_d(\mathbf{r})$, $b_d(r, \theta)$, etc., as appropriate, we have

$$\begin{aligned} b_d(\mathbf{r}) = b_d(r, \theta) &= \sum_i g_{\phi_i}[x_r, y_r] = \sum_i \lambda_{\phi_i}(x_r) \\ &= \sum_i \lambda_{\phi_i}(r\cos(\theta - \phi_i)). \end{aligned} \tag{7.21}$$

This procedure is illustrated in Fig. 7.8.

In the case of continuous data sets, the appropriate operation is integration, and we define the continuous summation image $b(\mathbf{r})$, $b(r, \theta)$, etc., as follows:

$$\begin{aligned} b(\mathbf{r}) = b(r, \theta) &= \frac{1}{\pi}\int_0^\pi g_\phi[x_r, y_r]\, d\phi = \frac{1}{\pi}\int_0^\pi \lambda_\phi(x_r)\, d\phi \\ &= \frac{1}{\pi}\int_0^\pi \lambda_\phi(r\cos(\theta - \phi))\, d\phi. \end{aligned} \tag{7.22}$$

The ϕ integration extends over a range of π rather than 2π because all available information is contained in this range of projection angles. As a

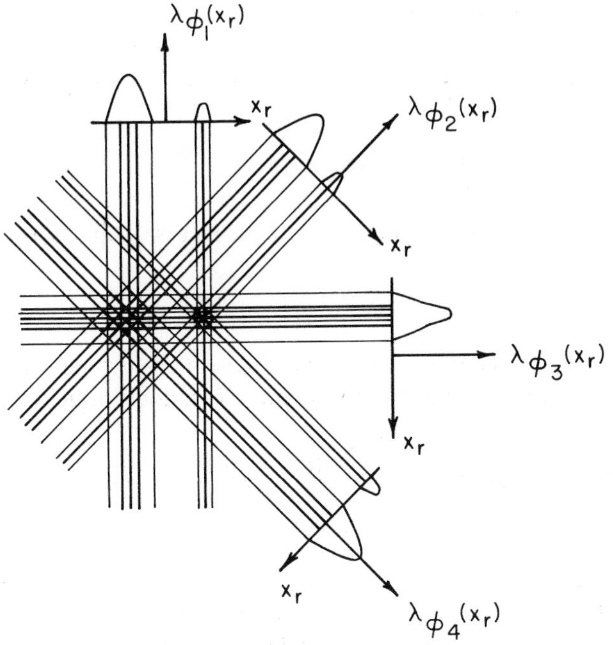

Fig. 7.8 Back-projection is the operation in which a one-dimensional projection data set is smeared uniformly back into two-dimensional space. Shown here are four projections $\lambda_{\phi_i}(x_r)$ ($i = 1$ to 4) and the summation image which is formed by summing the four corresponding back-projections. The original object was two absorbing disks of different sizes.

note of caution, we point out that many authors do not distinguish between the separate operations of back-projection, (7.19) and (7.20), and summation, (7.21) and (7.22), preferring to call the combined operation "back-projecting" and $b(\mathbf{r})$ the "back-projected image." Occasionally, the name "layergram" is also used to describe $b(\mathbf{r})$.

We now examine the relationship between the summation image and the original object $\mu(\mathbf{r})$. Since we are dealing with a linear shift-invariant system, this is most easily done by considering the special case of a point object located at the origin. The object is thus represented by $\mu^\delta[x_r, y_r] = \delta(x_r)\delta(y_r)$, where $\delta(\ )$ is the Dirac delta function. The resulting expression for $b(\mathbf{r})$ will be the point spread function $p_u(\mathbf{r})$ (subscript u denotes unfiltered) of the summation image.

From (7.11) and (7.22), we can write

$$b(\mathbf{r}) = \frac{1}{\pi} \int_0^\pi d\phi \int_{-\infty}^{\infty} dy_r\, \mu(\mathbf{r}). \tag{7.23}$$

For the special case of the point object we have

$$p_u(r) = \frac{1}{\pi}\int_0^{\pi} d\phi \int_{-\infty}^{\infty} dy_r\, \delta(y_r)\,\delta(x_r) = \frac{1}{\pi}\int_0^{\pi} \delta(x_r)\,d\phi$$

$$= \frac{1}{\pi}\int_0^{\pi} \delta(r\cos(\theta - \phi))\,d\phi. \tag{7.24}$$

To evaluate this integral, we make use of the fact (see Appendix A) that

$$\delta[f(x)] = \sum_i \left|\frac{df}{dx}\right|_{x=x_i}^{-1} \delta(x - x_i), \tag{7.25}$$

where $f(x_i) = 0$. In the present problem, $f(\phi) = r\cos(\theta - \phi)$, which has only one root $\phi = \phi_i$ in the range of integration. It follows immediately that

$$p_u(r) = \frac{1}{\pi|r\sin(\theta - \phi_i)|}\int_0^{\pi} \delta(\phi - \phi_i)\,d\phi = \frac{1}{\pi}\frac{1}{|r\sin(\theta - \phi_i)|}$$

$$= \frac{1}{\pi r}, \tag{7.26}$$

since $|\sin(\theta - \phi_i)| = 1$ if $\cos(\theta - \phi_i) = 0$. This result can be understood by considering the summation image to be formed from a large number of line delta functions all passing through the origin (see Fig. 7.9). The increasing density of lines toward the center represents the point spread

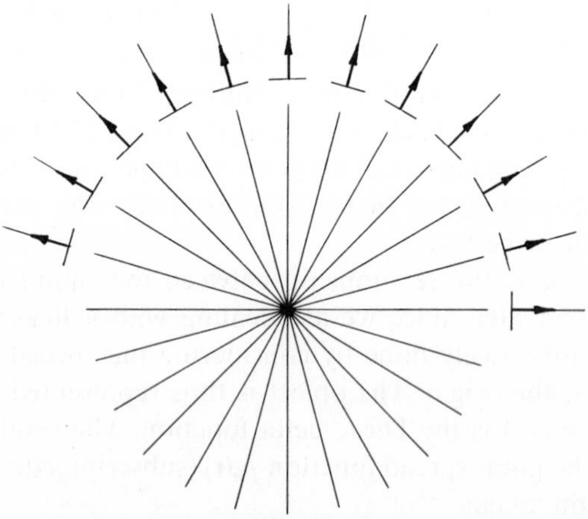

Fig. 7.9 Large number of back-projected δ functions results in a point spread function that approaches a $1/r$ functional form as indicated by the increasing line density toward the center of the pattern.

function and accounts for the $1/r$ distribution. Equation (7.26) is an important result for it shows a clear relationship between the object and the summation image. For a general distribution of attenuation coefficient $\mu(\mathbf{r})$, we can write

$$b(\mathbf{r}) = \mu(\mathbf{r}) ** p_u(\mathbf{r}) = \mu(\mathbf{r}) ** (1/\pi r). \tag{7.27}$$

As before, we have used the symbol $**$ to denote two-dimensional convolution. Because of the extended skirts on the PSF, $b(\mathbf{r})$ as given by (7.27), will not be a good representation of the original object. In fact, it will normally be a very badly blurred rendition that is quite unsuitable for applications in medical diagnosis.

Equation (7.27) is dimensionally inconsistent if we want b and μ to have the same dimensions, which would be reasonable from a physical point of view. In real life, of course, b and μ do not have the same dimensions; μ, an attenuation coefficient, has dimensions L^{-1}, and b, which represents a reconstructed image, will have whatever dimensions are consistent with the actual physical manifestation of the display, e.g., watts per square centimeter per steradian if the display is a CRT phosphor. Certainly we never reconstruct, in a literal sense, the original object. However, we should inquire as to why (7.27) is dimensionally incorrect. It stems from a rather loose definition for the back-projection operation, (7.19). Recall that $\lambda_\phi(x_r)$ has the dimensions of $[O]L$, where $[O]$ is the dimension set characteristic of the object and the L is an additional length dimension brought about from the projection (line integral) operation. Equation (7.19), as it stands, endows $g_\phi(\mathbf{r})$ with exactly the same dimensions as $\lambda_\phi(x_r)$, and since $b(\mathbf{r})$ is simply a superposition of various $g_\phi(\mathbf{r})$ functions, it follows that $b(\mathbf{r})$ and the original object are dimensionally inconsistent. There is another problem stemming from the definition given by (7.19). Whereas $\lambda_\phi(x_r)$ was obtained by averaging over a finite object, the value of that line integral is now back projected over an infinitely long line in the y_r direction. Thus, any image formed by summation of the various $g_\phi(\mathbf{r})$ values will have an infinite weight compared to the original object. This observation is confirmed by examining the expression for the point spread function, (7.26), where it is seen that the integral of $p_u(\mathbf{r})$ over all space is infinite. The solution to both of these problems is to redefine back projection in a more appropriate manner. The following definition would suffice:

$$g_\phi[x_r, y_r] = \lim_{L\to\infty} \left[\frac{1}{L} \lambda_\phi(x_r) \right], \tag{7.28}$$

where L is the length in real space over which the function $\lambda_\phi(x_r)$ is smeared out.

Mathematically this patches up the problems of scale and dimensionality, but it is so cumbersome that we shall not use it, preferring, for simplicity, the original statement (7.19). Thus, inconsistencies of this nature will pervade the rest of this chapter (as indeed they do the majority of published work on the subject). They are of little consequence, relating only to discrepancies in an overall brightness factor and the image dimensionality. The fact that real systems display images rather than reconstruct actual bodies justifies our neglect of these details.

7.2.5 Filtered Summation Image

We have just seen that the (unfiltered) summation image is equivalent to the object convolved with a $1/r$ point spread function. By appropriately filtering the summation image we can improve the quality of the reconstruction.

First, we look at frequency-domain filtering. Fourier transforming (7.27) gives

$$B(\boldsymbol{\rho}) = \mathscr{F}_2\{b(\mathbf{r})\} = \mathrm{M}(\boldsymbol{\rho})/\pi\rho \tag{7.29}$$

since $\mathscr{F}_2\{r^{-1}\} = \rho^{-1}$ [see (B.109)]. Here $b(\mathbf{r})$ is the unfiltered summation image defined in (7.23), and $M(\boldsymbol{\rho})$ is the (two-dimensional) transform of $\mu(\mathbf{r})$, given by

$$\mathrm{M}(\boldsymbol{\rho}) = \mathrm{M}[\xi, \eta] = \int_{-\infty}^{\infty}\int_{-\infty}^{\infty} \mu[x, y] \exp[-2\pi i(\xi x + \eta y)]\, dx\, dy. \tag{7.30}$$

We wish to find a filter $Q_2(\boldsymbol{\rho})$ which, when applied to $B(\boldsymbol{\rho})$, will yield a better representation of the transform of $\mu(\mathbf{r})$. It is tempting simply to write $Q_2(\boldsymbol{\rho}) = \pi\rho$, which (mathematically) generates $\mathrm{M}(\boldsymbol{\rho})$ and hence $\mu(\mathbf{r})$ in a totally uncontaminated condition. However, practical considerations require that we do not boost higher and higher frequencies with ever increasing weight, that is, use a "ρ filter," but rather use, in addition, an *apodizing function* $A_2(\boldsymbol{\rho})$ to control the high-frequency behavior. The filter thus has the form

$$Q_2(\boldsymbol{\rho}) = \pi\rho A_2(\boldsymbol{\rho}). \tag{7.31}$$

Subscripts on $Q_2(\boldsymbol{\rho})$ and $A_2(\boldsymbol{\rho})$ serve to emphasize that the functions are two-dimensional, a distinction that will become important later.

The filtered-image Fourier spectrum $\hat{\mathrm{M}}(\boldsymbol{\rho})$ is given by

$$\hat{\mathrm{M}}(\boldsymbol{\rho}) = Q_2(\boldsymbol{\rho})B(\boldsymbol{\rho}) = \mathrm{M}(\boldsymbol{\rho})A_2(\boldsymbol{\rho}) = \mathscr{F}_2\{\hat{\mu}(\mathbf{r})\}, \tag{7.32}$$

where $\hat{\mu}(\mathbf{r})$ is the estimated value of the original object, i.e., it is the image. It follows at once that

$$\hat{\mu}(\mathbf{r}) = \mu(\mathbf{r}) ** a_2(\mathbf{r}). \tag{7.33}$$

The quantity $a_2(\mathbf{r})$, the inverse transform of the apodizing filter, is thus the point spread function of the system, $p(\mathbf{r})$. To be more explicit, we can write

$$p(\mathbf{r}) = a_2(\mathbf{r}) = \mathscr{F}_2^{-1}\{Q_2(\boldsymbol{\rho})/\pi\rho\} = \mathscr{F}_2^{-1}\{A_2(\boldsymbol{\rho})\}. \tag{7.34}$$

In principle, arbitrarily perfect reconstructions could be made (in the absence of noise). This would happen, for example, if we chose $A_2(\boldsymbol{\rho})$ to have a Gaussian form where the width approached infinity, in which case $a_2(\mathbf{r})$ would approach a delta function and allow a perfect reconstruction.

There is an equivalent real-space filtering operation in which $b(\mathbf{r})$ is convolved with a processing function $q_2(\mathbf{r})$:

$$\hat{\mu}(\mathbf{r}) = b(\mathbf{r}) ** q_2(\mathbf{r}). \tag{7.35}$$

Rewriting this with the help of (7.27) as

$$\hat{\mu}(\mathbf{r}) = \mu(\mathbf{r}) ** (\pi r)^{-1} ** q_2(\mathbf{r}), \tag{7.36}$$

we see that the point spread function of the reconstruction is given by

$$p(\mathbf{r}) = q_2(\mathbf{r}) ** (\pi r)^{-1}. \tag{7.37}$$

This equation is simply a restatement of (7.34).

7.2.6 Summation of Filtered Back-Projections

In Section 7.2.5 we saw that by appropriately filtering the summation image, arbitrarily good reconstructions are possible. (We are still considering noisefree continuous data sets.) Summation and filtering are both linear operations; thus we should be able to reverse the order and filter the projections before summing. Note that the filtering will now necessarily be a one-dimensional operation since it will be applied to the one-dimensional functions $\lambda_\phi(x_r)$. It is this method of *filtered back-projection* that is favored by the majority of manufacturers of CT equipment.

The method requires that each projection be convolved with a filter function $q_1(x_r)$, yielding $\lambda_\phi^\dagger(x_r)$:

$$\lambda_\phi^\dagger(x_r) = \int_{-\infty}^{\infty} \lambda_\phi(x_r')q_1(x_r - x_r')\,dx_r' \equiv \lambda_\phi(x_r) * q_1(x_r). \tag{7.38}$$

Note the subscript on $q_1(x_r)$, denoting a one-dimensional function. The dagger superscript denotes a filtered function. These filtered projections are now back-projected and summed to yield the image $\hat{\mu}(\mathbf{r})$, given by

$$\hat{\mu}(\mathbf{r}) = \frac{1}{\pi}\int_0^\pi d\phi[\lambda_\phi(x_r) * q_1(x_r)]. \tag{7.39}$$

In polar coordinates, this equation becomes

$$\hat{\mu}(r,\theta) = \frac{1}{\pi}\int_0^\pi d\phi \int_{-\infty}^{\infty} \lambda_\phi(x_r')q_1(x_r - x_r')\,dx_r'\big|_{x_r = r\cos(\theta-\phi)}. \tag{7.40}$$

In terms of the original object distribution,

$$\hat{\mu}(r,\theta) = \frac{1}{\pi}\int_0^\pi d\phi \int_{-\infty}^{\infty} dy_r \int_{-\infty}^{\infty} dx_r'\,\mu_r[x_r', y_r]q_1(r\cos(\theta-\phi) - x_r'). \tag{7.41}$$

It is now straightforward to deduce the point spread function of the system by substituting the pointlike object $\mu^\delta = \delta(x_r)\delta(y_r)$ for $\mu_r[x_r, y_r]$ and evaluating (7.41). We immediately obtain

$$p(\mathbf{r}) = \frac{1}{\pi}\int_0^\pi q_1(r\cos(\theta-\phi))\,d\phi. \tag{7.42}$$

This important result states that the point spread function is given, quite simply, by the summation image of the one-dimensional filter function. It is apparent that unipolar functions $q_1(x_r)$ are unsuitable for filtering the data. For any function that is everywhere greater than zero, the point spread function thus generated would be spatially extended and give rise to a blurred reconstruction. The filter function *must* have negative sidelobes. Only in this way can the resulting point spread function be made compact.

7.2.7 Equivalence Between One- and Two-Dimensional Filtering

We next derive a relationship between the one-dimensional filter $q_1(\ )$ of Section 7.2.6, which is assumed to be a real, even function of x_r, and the two-dimensional filter $q_2(\ )$ of Section 7.2.5. From (7.42) we have

$$p(\mathbf{r}) = \frac{1}{\pi}\int_0^\pi q_1(r\cos\phi)\,d\phi. \tag{7.43}$$

There is no loss in generality in evaluating (7.42) for $\theta = 0$ since $p(\mathbf{r})$ is rotationally symmetric. Next we write $q_1(x_r)$ in terms of its one-dimensional Fourier transform $Q_1(\xi_r)$, yielding

$$p(\mathbf{r}) = \frac{1}{\pi}\int_0^\pi d\phi \int_{-\infty}^{\infty} d\xi_r\,Q_1(\xi_r)\exp(2\pi i\xi_r r\cos\phi). \tag{7.44}$$

The integration over ϕ gives [cf. (B.99)]

$$p(\mathbf{r}) = \int_{-\infty}^{\infty} Q_1(\xi_r) J_0(2\pi\xi_r r)\, d\xi_r. \tag{7.45}$$

Since $q_1(x_r)$ is real and symmetric, $Q_1(\xi_r) = Q_1(-\xi_r)$, and (7.45) can be written

$$p(\mathbf{r}) = 2\int_0^{\infty} J_0(2\pi\xi_r r)\left[\frac{Q_1(\xi_r)}{|\xi_r|}\right]|\xi_r|\, d\xi_r, \tag{7.46}$$

which is recognized as the Hankel transform of $Q_1(\xi_r)/|\xi_r|$ (see Section B.8). This latter quantity is rotationally symmetrical, so we can replace the Hankel transform with a two-dimensional inverse Fourier transform, giving

$$p(\mathbf{r}) = (1/\pi)\, \mathscr{F}_2^{-1}\{[Q_1(\xi_r)/|\xi_r|]_{|\xi_r|=\rho}\}. \tag{7.47}$$

We now compare (7.47) with (7.34), rewritten here as

$$p(\mathbf{r}) = (1/\pi)\, \mathscr{F}_2^{-1}\{[Q_2(\boldsymbol{\rho})/\rho]\}. \tag{7.48}$$

Notice that in (7.47) the operand of $\mathscr{F}_2^{-1}$ must be two dimensional, hence the formal substitution $|\xi_r| = \rho$.

The relationship between $Q_1(\ )$ and $Q_2(\ )$ has now been shown. If $Q_1(\ )$ and $Q_2(\ )$ have the same functional form, then they will result in identical point spread functions and hence identical image reconstructions. By analogy with (7.31), a one-dimensional apodizing function $A_1(\xi_r)$ can be defined by the relation

$$Q_1(\xi_r) = \pi|\xi_r| A_1(\xi_r). \tag{7.49}$$

Substituting (7.49) into (7.47), we obtain

$$p(\mathbf{r}) = \mathscr{F}_2^{-1}\{A_1(\xi_r)|_{|\xi_r|=\rho}\}. \tag{7.50}$$

By comparing (7.50) and (7.34) we see that exactly the same relationship applies between the one- and two-dimensional apodizing functions as applied between the total filter functions $Q_1(\ )$ and $Q_2(\ )$.

For later use we note a particular result. For the abrupt-cutoff ρ filter defined by

$$A_2(\rho) = \operatorname{circ}(\rho/\rho_m) = \begin{cases} 1 & \text{if} \quad \rho \leqslant \rho_m \\ 0 & \text{if} \quad \rho > \rho_m, \end{cases} \tag{7.51}$$

the PSF is immediately obtained from (7.34) and (B.114):

$$p(\mathbf{r}) = \pi\rho_m^2 \frac{2J_1(2\pi\rho_m r)}{2\pi\rho_m r}. \tag{7.52}$$

7.2.8 Fourier Methods

In Section 7.2.2 it was shown that the projection data are related to the Fourier transform of the object in a particularly simple manner. The result expressed in (7.18) is restated here as

$$\Lambda_\phi(\xi_r) = \int_{-\infty}^{+\infty} \int_{-\infty}^{+\infty} \mu[x_r, y_r] \exp[-2\pi i(x_r\xi_r + y_r\eta_r)]\, dx_r\, dy_r\big|_{\eta_r=0}$$

$$= \mathrm{M}_r(\xi_r, 0). \tag{7.53}$$

In this section we shall show how the full two-dimensional function $\mathrm{M}(\xi, \eta)$ can be assembled from these slices through the origin in frequency space.

The two-dimensional function in frequency space that corresponds to the one-dimensional function $\Lambda_\phi(\xi_r)$ is $\Lambda_\phi(\xi_r)\,\delta(\eta_r)$. If we assemble all of these two-dimensional functions by integrating over ϕ, we obtain the two-dimensional function $B(\boldsymbol{\rho})$, given by

$$B(\boldsymbol{\rho}) = \frac{1}{\pi} \int_0^\pi \Lambda_\phi(\xi_r)\,\delta(\eta_r)\, d\phi. \tag{7.54}$$

This quantity is not the Fourier transform of the object distribution however. The image $\hat{\mu}(\mathbf{r})$ is obtained by multiplying $B(\boldsymbol{\rho})$ by a factor ρ and any desired apodizing function $A(\rho)$ before performing the inverse two-dimensional transform:

$$\hat{\mu}(\mathbf{r}) = \frac{1}{\pi} \mathscr{F}_2^{-1} \left\{ \rho A(\rho) \int_0^\pi \Lambda_\phi(\xi_r)\,\delta(\eta_r)\, d\phi \right\}. \tag{7.55}$$

The factor ρ is needed to compensate for the variation of sample density with radius. Note that we can now leave the subscript off $A(\rho)$ in light of the results of Section 7.2.7. Equation (7.55) is the principal result of this section.

We can formally justify the inclusion of the factor ρ by showing that (7.55) is exactly equivalent to the reconstruction algorithm using convolution methods, (7.39). Equation (7.55) can be rewritten

$$\hat{\mu}(\mathbf{r}) = \frac{1}{\pi} \int_0^\pi \int_{-\infty}^{\infty} \int_{-\infty}^{\infty} \exp[2\pi i(x\xi + y\eta)] \rho A(\rho) \Lambda_\phi(\xi_r)\,\delta(\eta_r)\, d\eta\, d\xi\, d\phi. \tag{7.56}$$

Now we transform the integrals over ξ and η to integrals over ξ_r and η_r and obtain

$$\hat{\mu}(\mathbf{r}) = \frac{1}{\pi} \int_0^\pi \int_{-\infty}^{\infty} \int_{-\infty}^{\infty} \exp[2\pi i(x_r\xi_r + y_r\eta_r)][\xi_r^2 + \eta_r^2]^{1/2}$$

$$\times A[(\xi_r^2 + \eta_r^2)^{1/2}] \Lambda_\phi(\xi_r)\,\delta(\eta_r)\, d\eta_r\, d\xi_r\, d\phi. \tag{7.57}$$

Integrating over η_{r} is easy:

$$\hat{\mu}(\mathbf{r}) = \frac{1}{\pi} \int_0^{\pi} \int_{-\infty}^{\infty} \exp[2\pi i x_{\mathrm{r}} \xi_{\mathrm{r}}] \, |\xi_{\mathrm{r}}| \, A(|\xi_{\mathrm{r}}|) \Lambda_{\phi}(\xi_{\mathrm{r}}) \, d\xi_{\mathrm{r}} \, d\phi. \tag{7.58}$$

The ξ_{r} integral is in the form of a one-dimensional Fourier transform of the product $|\xi_{\mathrm{r}}| \, A(|\xi_{\mathrm{r}}|)\Lambda_{\phi}(\xi_{\mathrm{r}})$, so we can write

$$\hat{\mu}(\mathbf{r}) = \frac{1}{\pi} \int_0^{\pi} [q_1(x_{\mathrm{r}}) * \lambda_{\phi}(x_{\mathrm{r}})] \, d\phi, \tag{7.59}$$

where $q_1(x_{\mathrm{r}}) = \mathscr{F}_1^{-1}\{|\xi_{\mathrm{r}}| \, A(\xi_{\mathrm{r}})\}$, and the modulus bars on the argument have been dropped since A is invariably chosen to be even. Equation (7.59) is identical to the expression of the summation of filtered back-projections given by (7.39).

7.2.9 The Inverse Radon Transform

The direct inversion of (7.11) can be obtained by making use of the central slice theorem (7.18) which states that the one-dimensional Fourier transform of a projection is equal to a corresponding section of the object itself. Formally, this is written

$$\Lambda_{\phi}(\xi_{\mathrm{r}}) = \mathrm{M}_{\mathrm{r}}[\xi_{\mathrm{r}}, \eta_{\mathrm{r}}]_{\eta_{\mathrm{r}}=0}, \tag{7.60}$$

or in polar coordinates,

$$\Lambda_{\phi}(\xi_{\mathrm{r}}) = \mathrm{M}(\rho, \theta_{\rho})\big|_{\rho=\xi_{\mathrm{r}}, \, \theta_{\rho}=\phi}, \qquad \xi_{\mathrm{r}} \geqslant 0, \quad 0 < \phi \leqslant \pi, \tag{7.61}$$

and

$$\Lambda_{\phi}(\xi_{\mathrm{r}}) = \mathrm{M}(\rho, \theta_{\rho})\big|_{\rho=-\xi_{\mathrm{r}}, \, \theta_{\rho}=\phi+\pi}, \qquad \xi_{\mathrm{r}} \leqslant 0, \quad \pi < \phi \leqslant 2\pi. \tag{7.62}$$

The two equations are necessary because the polar coordinates of Fourier space are defined over the limits $\rho \geqslant 0$, $0 < \theta_{\rho} \leqslant 2\pi$, whereas the coordinates ϕ and ξ_{r} relating to the data-collecting frame need to be defined over the limits $-\infty < \xi_{\mathrm{r}} < \infty$ and $0 \quad \phi \leqslant \pi$ (see Fig. 7.10).

Now we write down the expression for the two-dimensional inverse Fourier transform in polar coordinates,

$$\mu(r, \theta) = \int_0^{2\pi} d\theta_{\rho} \int_0^{\infty} \rho \, d\rho \, \mathrm{M}(\rho, \theta_{\rho}) \exp[2\pi i \rho r \cos(\theta_{\rho} - \theta)]. \tag{7.63}$$

The next step is to substitute (7.61) and (7.62) into (7.63). From here it is easy to express the object function explicitly in terms of its projections $\lambda_{\phi}(x_{\mathrm{r}})$, which is the task of this section.

The first detail of this procedure is to separate (7.63) into two parts:

$$\mu(r, \theta) = I_1 + I_2, \tag{7.64}$$

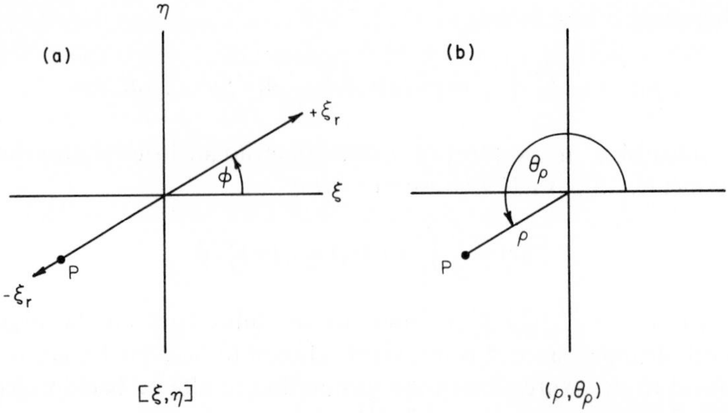

Fig. 7.10 General point P in Fourier space can be described either by polar coordinates (ρ, θ_ρ) or coordinates (ξ_r, ϕ) which relate to the data-taking frame of reference.

where

$$I_1 = \int_0^\pi d\theta_\rho \int_0^\infty \rho\, d\rho\, \mathrm{M}(\rho, \theta_\rho) \exp[2\pi i \rho r \cos(\theta_\rho - \theta)], \tag{7.65a}$$

and

$$I_2 = \int_\pi^{2\pi} d\theta_\rho \int_0^\infty \rho\, d\rho\, \mathrm{M}(\rho, \theta_\rho) \exp[2\pi i \rho r \cos(\theta_\rho - \theta)]. \tag{7.65b}$$

The integral I_1 is over the upper half plane of Fourier space, and according to (7.61), we can substitute ξ_r for ρ and ϕ for θ_ρ:

$$I_1 = \int_0^\pi d\phi \int_0^\infty \xi_r\, d\xi_r \mathrm{M}(\xi_r, \phi) \exp[2\pi i \xi_r r \cos(\phi - \theta)]. \tag{7.66}$$

By use of the central-slice theorem (7.61), I_1 can be written

$$I_1 = \int_0^\pi d\phi \int_0^\infty \xi_r\, d\xi_r\, \Lambda_\phi(\xi_r) \exp[2\pi i \xi_r x_r], \tag{7.67a}$$

where we have made use of the general expression, $x_r = r\cos(\theta - \phi)$ (see Fig. 7.2).

I_2 is evaluated by making substitutions appropriate to the lower half-space, i.e, $-\xi_r = \rho$ and $\phi = \theta_\rho - \pi$, and we obtain

$$I_2 = -\int_0^\pi d\phi \int_{-\infty}^0 \xi_r\, d\xi_r\, \Lambda_\phi(\xi_r) \exp(2\pi i \xi_r x_r). \tag{7.67b}$$

Combining (7.67) and (7.64), we obtain

$$\mu(r, \theta) = \int_0^\pi d\phi \int_{-\infty}^\infty d\xi_r\, |\xi_r|\, \Lambda_\phi(\xi_r) \exp(2\pi i \xi_r x_r), \tag{7.68}$$

where it is implicitly assumed that the integral is evaluated at $x_r =$

$r\cos(\theta - \phi)$. The final step is to recognize this expression as the one-dimensional inverse Fourier transform of a product of $|\xi_r|$ and $\Lambda_\phi(\xi_r)$, which is conveniently evaluated by rewriting (7.68)

$$\mu(r,\theta) = \frac{1}{2\pi i}\int_0^\pi d\phi\left(\frac{\partial}{\partial x_r}\int_{-\infty}^{\infty} d\xi_r \operatorname{sgn}(\xi_r)\Lambda_\phi(\xi_r)\exp(2\pi i\xi_r x_r)\right), \quad (7.69)$$

where

$$\operatorname{sgn}(\xi_r) = \begin{cases} +1 & \text{for} \quad \xi_r > 0 \\ 0 & \text{for} \quad \xi_r = 0 \\ -1 & \text{for} \quad \xi_r < 0. \end{cases} \quad (7.70)$$

Note that $|\xi_r| = \xi_r \operatorname{sgn}(\xi_r)$. The convolution theorem can now be applied to (7.69), and we obtain

$$\mu(r,\theta) = \frac{1}{2\pi^2}\int_0^\pi d\phi\left\{\frac{\partial}{\partial x_r}\left[\lambda_\phi(x_r) * \mathscr{P}\left(\frac{1}{x_r}\right)\right]\right\}_{x_r = r\cos(\theta-\phi)}. \quad (7.71)$$

In deriving this result, we make use of the fact that

$$\mathscr{F}_1^{-1}\{\operatorname{sgn}(\xi_r)\} = \mathscr{P}(-1/i\pi x_r),$$

where $\mathscr{P}$ denotes the Cauchy principal value [see (B.32)].

From the definition of the convolution, it is easy to show that

$$(\partial/\partial x)[f(x) * g(x)] = f'(x) * g(x),$$

where $f'(x) = \partial f(x)/\partial x$. Thus (7.71) can also be written

$$\mu(r,\theta) = \frac{1}{2\pi^2}\int_0^\pi d\phi\, \mathscr{P}\int_{-\infty}^{\infty} \frac{\partial\lambda_\phi(x_r')/\partial x_r'}{r\cos(\theta-\phi) - x_r'}\, dx_r', \quad (7.72)$$

which is one representation of the inverse two-dimensional *Radon transform*. The relationships between object, Fourier, and Radon space are shown in Fig. 7.11.

Now we state a theorem regarding the convolution of high-order derivatives of functions, namely that

$$f^{(m)}(x) * g(x) = f^{(m-1)}(x) * g^{(1)}(x) = \cdots = f^{(1)}(x) * g^{(m-1)}(x) = f(x) * g^{(m)}(x),$$

where $f^{(m)}(x)$ is the mth derivative of $f(x)$ with respect to x. Applying this theorem, which follows from (B.23) and (B.52), to (7.71), we obtain the following expression for the inverse Radon transform:

$$\begin{aligned} \mu(r,\theta) &= \frac{-1}{2\pi^2}\int_0^\pi d\phi\left(\lambda_\phi(x_r) * \frac{1}{x_r^2}\right)_{x_r = r\cos(\theta-\phi)} \\ &= \frac{-1}{2\pi}\int_0^\pi d\phi\int_{-\infty}^{\infty} \frac{\lambda_\phi(x_r')}{[r\cos(\theta-\phi) - x_r']^2}\, dx_r', \end{aligned} \quad (7.73)$$

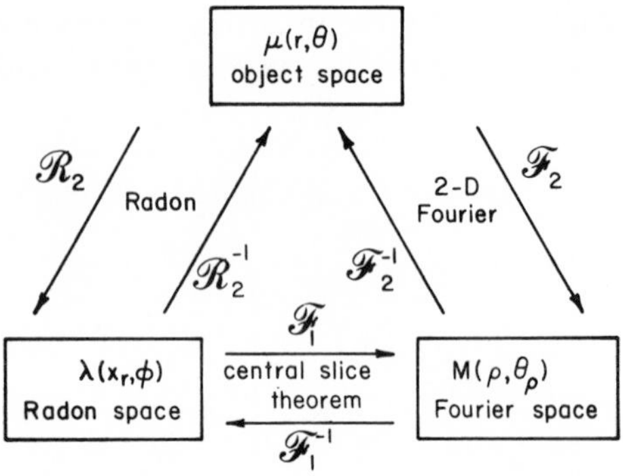

Fig. 7.11 Showing the transform relationships between object space, Radon space and Fourier space. $\mathscr{R}_2$ and $\mathscr{R}_2^{-1}$ are the Radon and inverse Radon transform operators defined by (7.11) and (7.72), respectively.

where $1/x_r^2$ must be interpreted as a generalized function. The problem in interpretation stems from the singularity that occurs in (7.72) or (7.73) when $x_r' = r\cos(\theta - \phi)$. The meaning becomes clearer if we replace the $(1/x_r)$ of (7.71) by a function $h(x_r)$ that approaches $\mathscr{P}(1/x_r)$ in some limit, and then proceed by evaluating an estimate $\hat{\mu}(r, \theta)$ using (7.71). In the limit $h(x_r) \rightarrow \mathscr{P}(1/x_r)$ we have $\hat{\mu}(r, \theta) \rightarrow \mu(r, \theta)$.

A suitable choice for $h(x_r)$ is

$$h(x_r) = \begin{cases} x_r/\varepsilon^2 & \text{if } |x_r| \leqslant \varepsilon \\ 1/x_r & \text{if } |x_r| > \varepsilon. \end{cases} \tag{7.74}$$

We also define a function $q_R(x_r)$ (where R stands for Radon) by

$$q_R(x_r) = \frac{1}{2\pi}\frac{d}{dx_r}h(x_r) = \begin{cases} 1/(2\pi\varepsilon^2) & \text{if } |x_r| \leqslant \varepsilon \\ -1/(2\pi x_r^2) & \text{if } |x_r| > \varepsilon. \end{cases} \tag{7.75}$$

Functions h and q_R are shown in Fig. 7.12.

A reconstruction based on using $h(x_r)$ in place of $\mathscr{P}(1/x_r)$ will give an estimate $\hat{\mu}(r, \theta)$ of the object, according to (7.71), of

$$\hat{\mu}(r, \theta) = \frac{1}{2\pi^2}\int_0^{\pi} d\phi \, \frac{\partial}{\partial x_r}\left[\lambda_\phi(x_r) * h(x_r)\right]_{x_r = r\cos(\theta - \phi)}, \tag{7.76}$$

which is equivalent to

$$\hat{\mu}(r, \theta) = \frac{1}{\pi}\int_0^{\pi} d\phi \left[\lambda_\phi(x_r) * q_R(x_r)\right]_{x_r = r\cos(\theta - \phi)}. \tag{7.77}$$

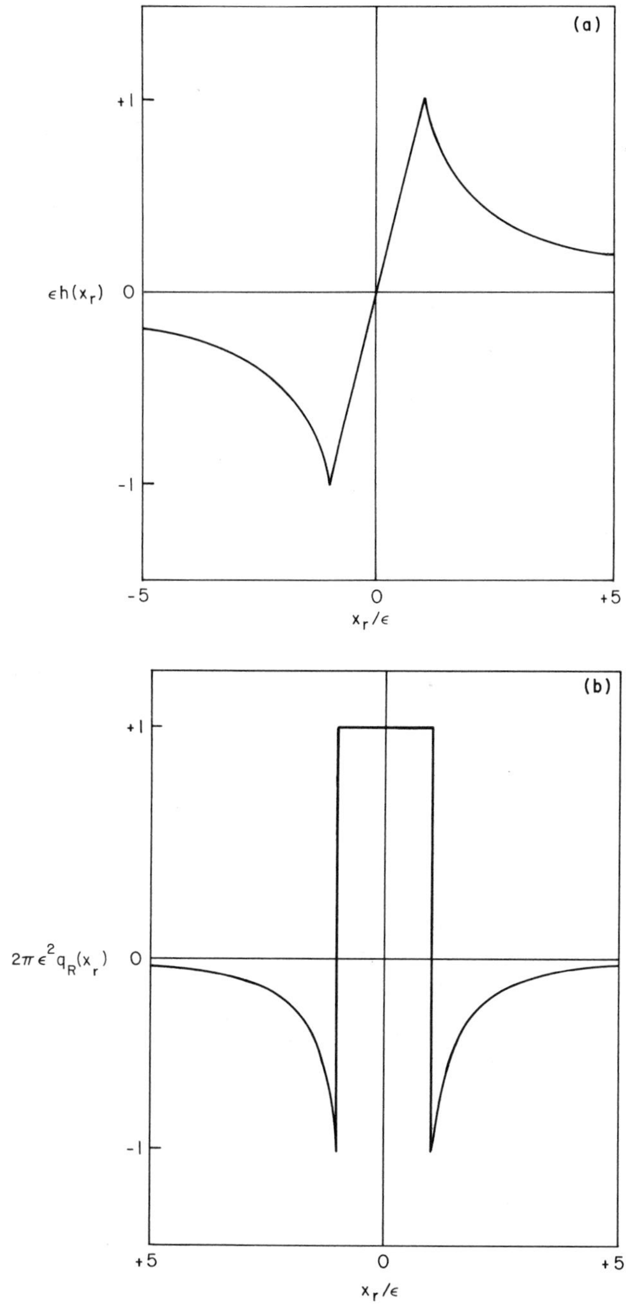

Fig. 7.12 (a) $h(x_r)$ as defined by (7.74) is a function that closely resembles $\mathscr{P}(1/x_r)$. (b) $q_R(x_r) = (1/2\pi)\, dh(x_r)/dx_r$ is the filter function derived from $h(x_r)$.

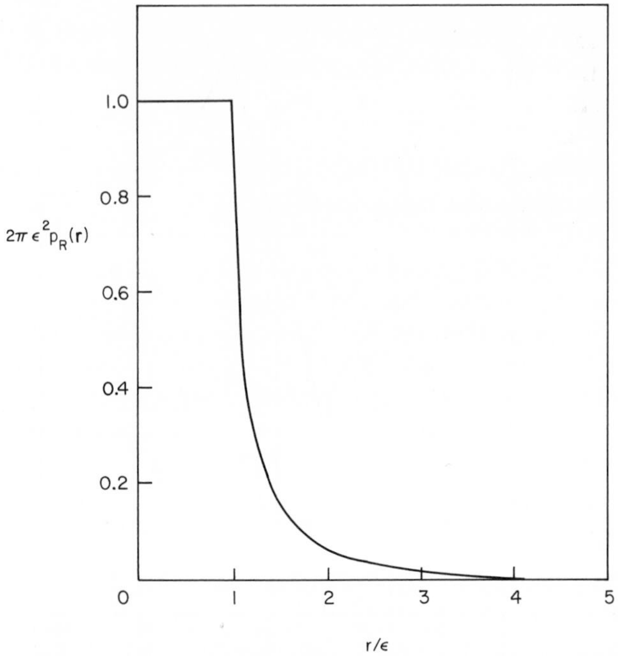

Fig. 7.13 $p_R(\mathbf{r})$ is the point spread function obtained by continuously summing $q(x_r)$ over ϕ, $0 \leqslant \phi < \pi$. In the limit $\varepsilon \to 0$, $p_R(\mathbf{r})$ becomes a δ function.

This is precisely in the form of the filtered-back-projection expression (7.39). Thus $q_R(x_r)$ is an appropriate filter function to apply in this technique, and in the limit $\varepsilon \to 0$ the reconstruction will be perfect. This can be shown by computing the point spread function using (7.43):

$$p_R(\mathbf{r}) = \begin{cases} 1/(2\pi\varepsilon^2) & \text{if} \quad r \leqslant \varepsilon \\ \dfrac{1}{\pi^2\varepsilon^2}\left[\sin^{-1}\left(\dfrac{\varepsilon}{r}\right) - \dfrac{\varepsilon(r^2-\varepsilon^2)^{1/2}}{r^2}\right], & \text{if} \quad r > \varepsilon. \end{cases} \tag{7.78}$$

This quantity, shown in Fig. 7.13, approaches a delta-function-like distribution as $\varepsilon \to 0$.

In the limit $\varepsilon \to 0$, (7.77) becomes

$$\mu(r, \theta) = \frac{1}{\pi}\int_{\phi=0}^{\pi} d\phi \left[\lambda_\phi(x_r) * \lim_{\varepsilon \to 0} q_R(x_r)\right]_{x_r = r\cos(\theta-\phi)}. \tag{7.79}$$

The interpretation of (7.73) now becomes clear by comparing (7.73) and (7.79). The function $(-1/x_r)^2$ must be interpreted at its face value for $x_r \neq 0$ and as a positive, infinite-weight delta function for $x_r = 0$. The weight of the delta function is such that $\int_{-\infty}^{\infty} (-1/x_r^2)\,dx_r = 0$ as required by the central ordinate theorem, see (B.15).

7.2.10 Circular Harmonic Decomposition

In Section 7.2.6 we discussed a reconstruction algorithm based on the decomposition of sinogram data space into horizontal strips, each strip representing one projection (see Fig. 7.14a). In this section we look at a method, introduced by Cormack (1963), in which the initial decomposition of the data set is into vertical strips of sinogram space, which correspond to annular rings in Radon space (see Fig. 7.14b). Each annular ring of data $\lambda(x_r, \phi)$ is periodic in ϕ with period 2π. Thus it can be written in terms of a

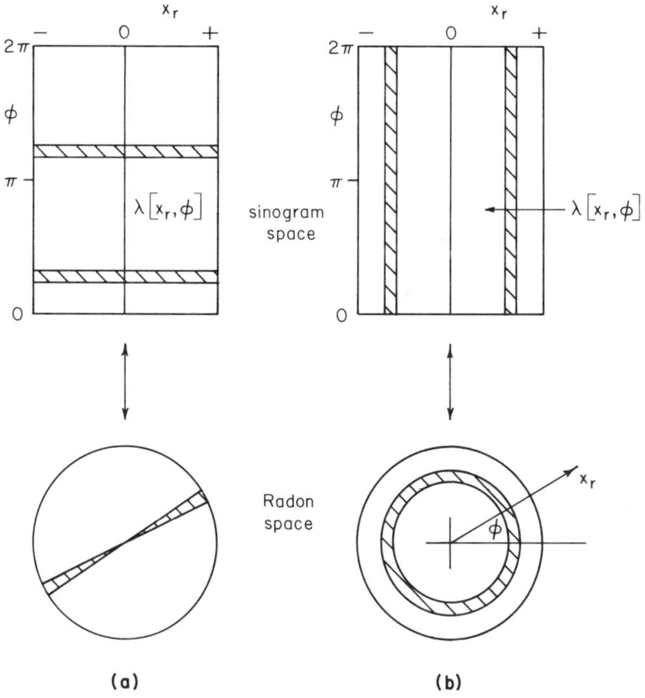

Fig. 7.14 (a) One projection set in sinogram space maps to a segment in Radon space. (b) A vertical strip of data in sinogram space maps to an annulus. All nonredundant projection data are contained in the range $0 < \phi \leqslant \pi$. Thus there are two regions in sinogram space shown here that map redundantly to the same region of Radon space.

Fourier series:

$$\lambda(x_r, \phi) = \sum_{n=-\infty}^{\infty} \lambda_n(x_r) \exp(in\phi), \tag{7.80}$$

with

$$\lambda_n(x_r) = \frac{1}{2\pi} \int_0^{2\pi} \lambda(x_r, \phi) \exp(-in\phi)\, d\phi. \tag{7.81}$$

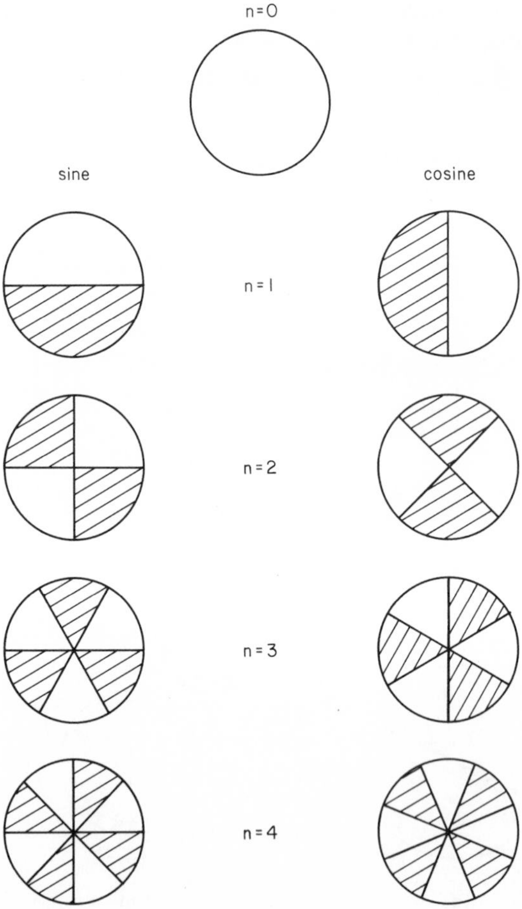

Fig. 7.15 Showing the DC, sine, and cosine components of the complex exponential terms in the circular harmonic expansion for $N = 0$–4. Shaded areas indicate where the functions are negative.

For obvious reasons, the $\lambda_n(x_r)$ are called circular harmonic coefficients. Note also the slight notational change from $\lambda_\phi(x_r)$ to $\lambda(x_r, \phi)$. These quantities are the same. The first few cosine and sine components of the series (7.80) are depicted in Fig. 7.15.

The object $\mu(r, \theta)$ can also be decomposed into circular harmonic components,

$$\mu(r, \theta) = \sum_{n=-\infty}^{\infty} \mu_n(r) \exp(in\theta), \tag{7.82}$$

with

$$\mu_n(r) = \frac{1}{2\pi} \int_0^{2\pi} \mu(r, \theta) \exp(-in\theta)\, d\theta. \tag{7.83}$$

We shall now derive a relationship between the circular harmonic coefficients $\lambda_n(x_r)$ and $\mu_n(r)$. We repeat the fundamental projection equation,

$$\lambda(x_r, \phi) = \int_{-\infty}^{\infty} \mu(r, \theta)\, dy_r, \tag{7.84}$$

and it is understood that the line integral is along the line $x_r = r\cos(\theta - \phi)$. The integral in (7.84) can be broken into two parts (refer to Fig. 7.16):

$$\lambda(x_r, \phi) = \int_0^{\infty} \mu(r, \theta)\, dy_r + \int_{-\infty}^{0} \mu(r, \theta)\, dy_r. \tag{7.85}$$

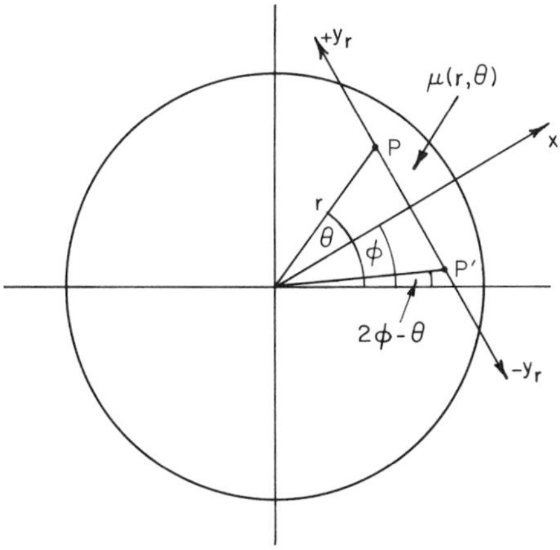

Fig. 7.16 For each point $P(r, \theta)$ on the line integral path $y_r > 0$ there is a point P' with the same radius whose polar angle is $(2\phi - \theta)$.

The first integral covers the region $\phi + \pi/2 > \theta \geqslant \phi$ and the second $\phi > \theta \geqslant \phi - \pi/2$. The change of variables $y_r \to -y_r$ which changes θ to $2\phi - \theta$ in the second integral yields

$$\lambda(x_r, \phi) = \int_0^\infty [\mu(r, \theta) + \mu(r, 2\phi - \theta)]\, dy_r. \tag{7.86}$$

Next we make use of the circular harmonic expansions (7.80) and (7.82) and obtain

$$\sum_{n=-\infty}^{\infty} \lambda_n(x_r) \exp(in\phi) = \int_0^\infty \sum_{n=-\infty}^{\infty} \mu_n(r) \{\exp(in\theta) + \exp[in(2\phi - \theta)]\}\, dy_r$$

$$= 2 \int_0^\infty \sum_{n=-\infty}^{\infty} \mu_n(r) \exp(in\phi) \cos[n(\theta - \phi)]\, dy_r. \tag{7.87}$$

The next step is to use the change of variable $r^2 = x_r^2 + y_r^2$. Noting that $\theta - \phi = \cos^{-1}(x_r/r)$, we can write

$$\sum_{n=-\infty}^{\infty} \lambda_n(x_r) e^{in\phi} = 2 \sum_{n=-\infty}^{\infty} e^{in\phi} \int_{|x_r|}^{\infty} \frac{\mu_n(r) \cos[n \cos^{-1}(x_r/r)]}{\sqrt{r^2 - x_r^2}}\, r\, dr. \tag{7.88}$$

Because of the orthogonality of circular harmonic transforms, this equation must hold term by term, i.e.,

$$\lambda_n(x_r) = 2 \int_{|x_r|}^{\infty} \frac{\mu_n(r) T_n(x_r/r)}{\sqrt{r^2 - x_r^2}}\, r\, dr, \tag{7.89}$$

where $T_n(u) = \cos(n \cos^{-1} u)$ denotes a Tschebycheff polynomial of the first kind. This is an important intermediate result. It remains to solve this equation for $\mu_n(r)$ so that the expansion coefficients of the object are expressed explicitly. The solution, which involves the orthogonality relationships of the Tschebycheff polynomials, is straightforward but tedious, and we give only the result here. Interested readers should consult Cormack (1963) for details.

$$\mu_n(r) = -\frac{1}{\pi} \frac{d}{dr} \int_r^\infty \frac{r \lambda_n(x_r) T_n(x_r/r)\, dx_r}{(x_r^2 - r^2)^{1/2}\, x_r}. \tag{7.90}$$

We call (7.89) and (7.90) the Cormack and inverse-Cormack transforms, respectively.

It is also possible to expand the object Fourier transform in a circular harmonic series:

$$M(\rho, \theta_\rho) = \sum_{n=-\infty}^{\infty} M_n(\rho) \exp(in\theta_\rho), \tag{7.91}$$

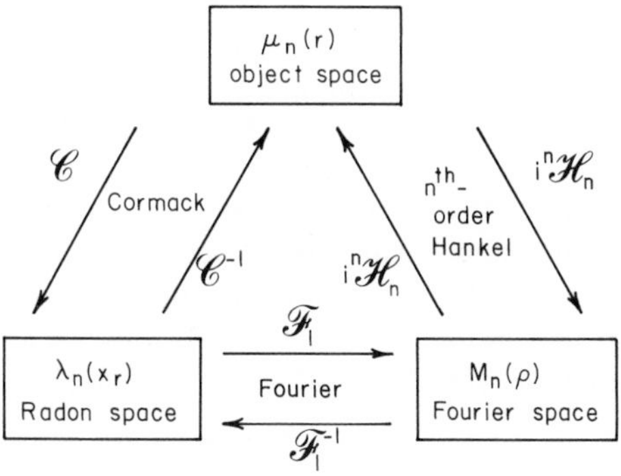

Fig. 7.17 The transform relationships between the coefficients of the circular harmonic decompositions of object, Radon and Fourier spaces. $\mathscr{C}$ and $\mathscr{C}^{-1}$ are operators for the Cormack and inverse Cormack transforms.

with

$$M_n(\rho) = \frac{1}{2\pi}\int_0^{2\pi} M(\rho, \theta_\rho)\exp(-in\theta_\rho)\,d\theta_\rho. \tag{7.92}$$

The relation between the coefficients $M_n(\rho)$ and the previously used $\mu_n(r)$ is

$$M_n(\rho) = i^n 2\pi \int_0^\infty \mu_n(r) J_n(2\pi r\rho) r\,dr, \tag{7.93}$$

$$\mu_n(r) = i^{-n} 2\pi \int_0^\infty M_n(\rho) J_n(2\pi\rho r)\rho\,d\rho. \tag{7.94}$$

These two equations are called nth-order Hankel transforms. The complete set of interrelationships is shown in Fig. 7.17.

7.2.11 Objects with Circular Symmetry

From a radiological standpoint, circularly symmetrical objects are not very important. Indeed, they form a subset of the general class of objects and are thus amenable to analysis by any of the methods described in this chapter. Mathematically, however, there are some interesting observations to be made.

Let the object be represented by the distribution $\mu(r)$ and let it be identically zero for all values of r greater than r_0. Note that $\mu(r)$ is now an even function of a single variable r even though it represents a two-dimensional object distribution.

The projection of the object onto the x axis is given by

$$\lambda(x) = \int_{-\infty}^{\infty} \mu(r)\,dy. \tag{7.95}$$

Using the substitution $y = (r^2 - x^2)^{1/2}$, we obtain

$$\lambda(x) = 2 \int_{|x|}^{\infty} \frac{\mu(r) r\, dr}{(r^2 - x^2)^{1/2}} \equiv \mathscr{A}\{\mu(r)\}. \tag{7.96}$$

This is the expression for the *Abel transform* of the object function $\mu(r)$.

To reconstruct the object from its projection, we must determine the inverse Abel transform. The expression for the inverse transform can be derived directly from Radon's formula, (7.72), but we shall derive it here starting with a statement of the central slice theorem (7.18):

$$\Lambda(\xi) = \mathscr{F}_1\{\lambda(x)\} = \mathscr{H}\{\mu(r)\}. \tag{7.97}$$

The two-dimensional Fourier transform in (7.18) has been replaced with the zero-order Hankel transform expressed by the operator $\mathscr{H}$ (see Section B.8). The Hankel conjugate of r is ξ, and because the Hankel transform is its own inverse, it follows that

$$\mu(r) = 2\pi \int_0^{\infty} \xi J_0(2\pi\xi r)\left(\int_{-\infty}^{\infty} \lambda(x) \exp(-2\pi i \xi x)\, dx\right) d\xi. \tag{7.98}$$

The projection $\lambda(x)$ is even, i.e., $\lambda(x) = \lambda(-x)$, so that

$$\begin{aligned} \mu(r) &= \int_0^{\infty} J_0(2\pi\xi r)\left(\int_{-\infty}^{\infty} \lambda(x) 2\pi\xi \cos(2\pi\xi x)\, dx\right) d\xi \\ &= \int_0^{\infty} J_0(2\pi\xi r)\left(\int_{-\infty}^{\infty} \lambda(x) \frac{d}{dx} \sin(2\pi\xi x)\, dx\right) d\xi. \end{aligned} \tag{7.99}$$

Integrating by parts, we obtain

$$\mu(r) = -\int_0^{\infty} J_0(2\pi\xi r)\left(\int_{-\infty}^{\infty} \frac{d\lambda}{dx} \sin(2\pi\xi x)\, dx\right) d\xi. \tag{7.100}$$

To evaluate the integral over ξ, we make use of the following standard result:

$$\int_0^{\infty} J_0(at) \sin bt\, dt = \begin{cases} 0, & b < a \\ \dfrac{1}{(b^2 - a^2)^{1/2}}, & b > a, \end{cases} \tag{7.101}$$

which gives the final answer,

$$\mu(r) = -\frac{1}{\pi} \int_r^{\infty} \frac{d\lambda/dx}{(x^2 - r^2)^{1/2}}\, dx \equiv \mathscr{A}^{-1}\{\lambda(x)\}, \tag{7.102}$$

where $\mathscr{A}^{-1}$ is the inverse Abel operator.

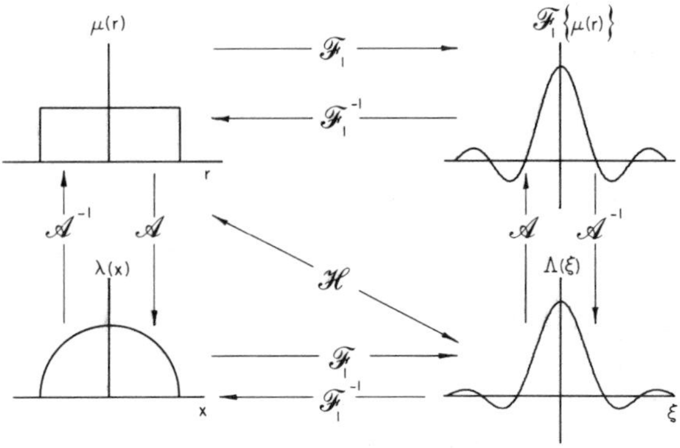

Fig. 7.18 For circularly symmetrical objects $\mu(r)$, the projection $\lambda(x)$ and section $\Lambda(\xi)$ of the object's 2D Fourier (i.e., Hankel) transform are related through the Abel ($\mathcal{A}$), 1D Fourier ($\mathcal{F}_1$), and Hankel ($\mathcal{H}$) transforms. Note that for these even functions $\mathcal{F}_1 = \mathcal{F}_1^{-1}$. There is an equivalent set of relationships between $\mu(r)$, its *one-dimensional* Fourier transform, and $\Lambda(\xi)$. The relations are illustrated for a uniform disk object.

In operator notation, (7.98) is written

$$\mu = \mathcal{H}\mathcal{F}_1\mathcal{A}\{\mu\}. \tag{7.103}$$

In words, this operator equation says that the Fourier transform of the Abel transform is the same as the inverse Hankel transform. Since the Hankel transform is its own inverse, the following relationships hold:

$$\mathcal{H}\mathcal{F}_1\mathcal{A} = \mathcal{A}\mathcal{H}\mathcal{F}_1 = \mathcal{F}_1\mathcal{A}\mathcal{H} = \mathcal{I}, \tag{7.104}$$

$$\begin{aligned} \mathcal{F}_1 &= \mathcal{A}\mathcal{H}, & \mathcal{F}^{-1} &= \mathcal{H}\mathcal{A}^{-1}, \\ \mathcal{A} &= \mathcal{F}_1\mathcal{H}, & \mathcal{A}^{-1} &= \mathcal{H}\mathcal{F}_1^{-1}, \\ \mathcal{H} &= \mathcal{F}_1\mathcal{A}, & \mathcal{H}^{-1} &= \mathcal{A}^{-1}\mathcal{F}_1^{-1}, \end{aligned} \tag{7.105}$$

where $\mathcal{I}$ is the identity operator. Note also that $\mathcal{F} = \mathcal{F}^{-1}$ when it operates on real even functions. This cyclic behavior is illustrated in Fig. 7.18.

7.2.12 Summary

We have studied many ways of reconstructing a two-dimensional object from the set of line integrals passing through it (see Fig. 7.19). In principle, all of these methods lead to perfect reconstructions. In practice, the effects of noise, equipment limitations, data sampling schemes, patient motion, etc., result in less than perfect reconstructions being possible. These limitations are studied in Section 7.3.

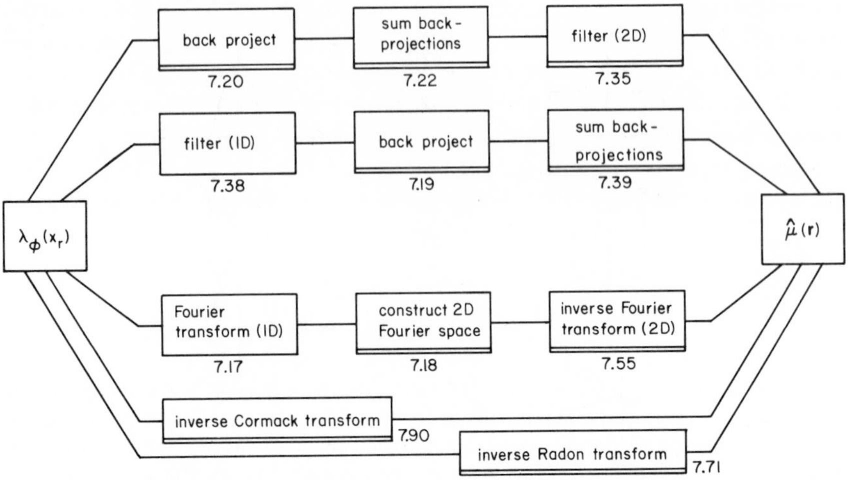

Fig. 7.19 Summary of the analytic methods in Section 7.2 for obtaining an estimate (reconstruction) $\hat{\mu}(\mathbf{r})$ of object distribution $\mu(\mathbf{r})$ from its projections $\lambda_\phi(x_r)$. The double line in some boxes indicates the two-dimensional nature of the operation. Numbers refer to equations in the text.

7.3 PRACTICAL CONSIDERATIONS

7.3.1 Data-Gathering Hardware

Source-Detector Geometries

There are many different arrangements for the source-detector assembly (see Fig. 7.20). In Fig. 7.20a we see the single-source single-detector arrangement that appeared on the original EMI Mark I CT1000 head scanner. Although slow ($\sim 4\frac{1}{2}$ minutes per complete scan), it has the advantage of being easily calibrated and it offers the best possibility for rejecting scattered radiation. The source and detector can both be pipe-collimated on a common axis, and there is only one beam passing through the patient at any one time. Thus there can be no scattering from primary radiation that was aimed initially in a different direction. This is the only system that achieves this degree of scatter rejection since all others have multiple detectors operating simultaneously. The system shown in Fig. 7.20b was the first attempt to speed up the operation by having several detectors operating with a single source. The fan-shaped beam of x rays covers a relatively small angular subtense, and patient coverage is provided by laterally scanning the source-detector gantry. After one lateral scan, the gantry is rotated by a coarse increment equal to the fan angle, which is about 10°. By stepping the source-detector array off to one side of the patient, it is possible to recalibrate each detector several times during the scanning process, should this be considered desirable. As with the system in Fig. 7.20a, efficient pipe collimation is possible since each detector views only in a fixed direction.

The systems shown in Figs. 7.20c–e have only one motion. In Fig. 7.20c the system is similar to that in Fig. 7.20b except that the detector array is

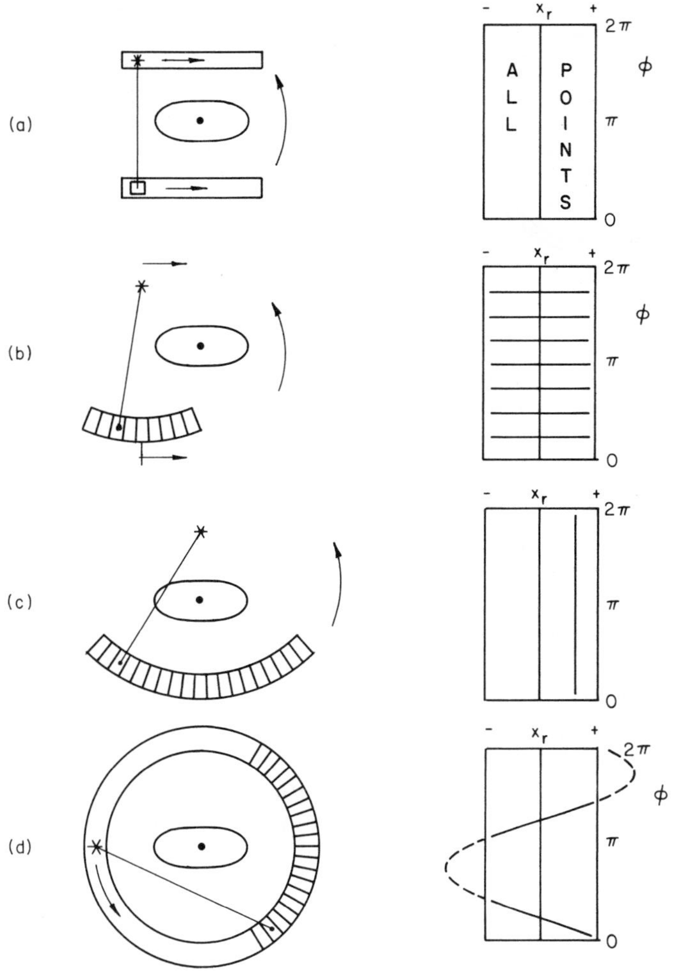

Fig. 7.20 Some of the source-detector geometries that have been utilized in commercial CT scanners and the corresponding regions of sinogram space associated with the output of a single detector.

(e)

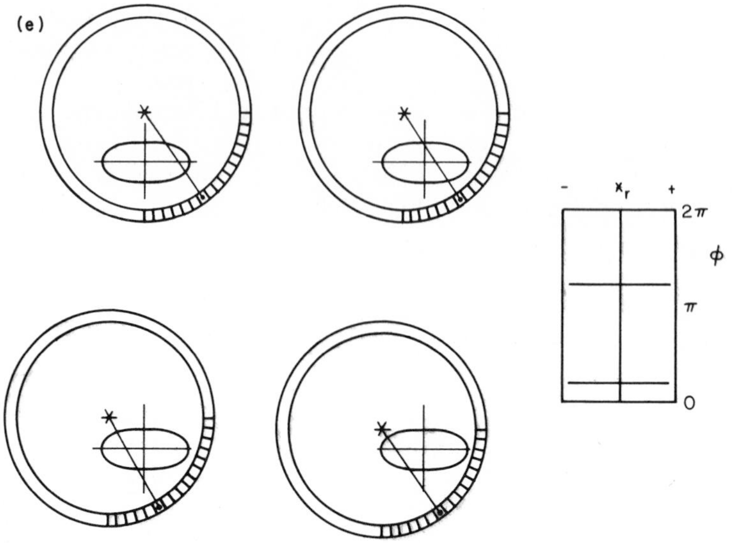

Fig. 7.20 *(continued)*

enlarged so that the patient is covered by the resulting wide-angle fan and the lateral scan is no longer necessary. Both the x-ray source and the detectors rotate about the patient simultaneously. The system is mechanically simpler than that in Fig. 7.20b, but it is no longer possible to calibrate the detector array during a run since normally the patient is always obstructing the primary beam.

In Fig. 7.20d, a stationary detector ring with several hundred detectors simplifies the mechanical aspects even more. Calibration is possible, but collimation against scattered radiation is harder to achieve since each detector receives primary photons from a wide angular range. The system in Fig. 7.20e seems to combine most of the advantages of the previous ones. The complete ring of detectors does not rotate but it does translate such that its center makes a complete circular path around the patient. The x-ray tube is located at the center of the detector array and directs a wide fan beam directly toward the patient. It can be seen that each detector can be pipe-collimated toward the source and that calibration during a run is possible.

Beam Shape

At the source end the beam shape is defined by the focal spot or line of the x-ray tube. At the other end it is determined by the entrance face of the detector or collimator. The detectors are usually rectangular and closely spaced so as not to waste photons. We designate the height and width of each detector by h_d and w_d, respectively, and next consider the factors that affect the choice of a value for h_d. Initially we assume that $\mu(r, \theta)$ is not a function of z, where z is the direction perpendicular to the slice. (In the human body, this is to some extent a reasonable assumption since most of the large bones and major tubular structures are axially oriented.) In Section 10.5.3 it is shown that in order to achieve a spatial resolution δ with a signal-to-noise ratio (SNR), which is the reciprocal of the fractional density discrimination, a certain linear photon density $\bar{n}$ (photons per unit length of projection) is required. Neglecting the constant terms, the equation is [cf. (10.193)]

$$\bar{n} \propto (\mathrm{SNR})^2/\delta^3. \tag{7.106}$$

Since patient dose is determined by spatial fluence (photons per unit area), the patient dose is minimized by making the slice thickness large, thus spreading the photons into a thicker slice. A large slice thickness will also be useful in view of the fact that fewer slices will be needed to cover any predetermined portion of the body. The problem, of course, is that the body is not homogeneous in the axial direction. Any feature running obliquely through the slice will be blurred in the final image. This can be seen by considering a thick slice to be composed of many superimposed thin slices, in each of which the oblique feature will have a different location. Another problem with thick slices is that small objects may not completely run through the full thickness. Consider a small feature that fills a fraction α of the slice thickness. Because of averaging over the slice, its apparent density difference with respect to its surroundings will be reduced to α times the true density difference. This would especially be a problem if the quantitative output from the CT machine were being used for tissue identification purposes.

We have also assumed that all of the radiation is parallel to the faces of the slice. But the source emits diverging radiation, and this too can cause problems. Consider the line source of length h_s and detector of height h_d shown in Fig. 7.21. The sensitivity of this system to a small absorbing object depends upon the location of the object. Imagine an opaque screen with a small slit in it placed between the source and detector. The slit, parallel to the plane of the fan, will serve to probe the spatial sensitivity of the system. If the slit is translated past the source, the detector response will be a rect function. The same result applies if the slit moves over the detector face. However, the peak response will be different since the slit will obscure a different fraction of the source than of the detector if the source and detector have different dimensions. If the slit is moved anywhere in the region between source and detector, the sensitivity is directly proportional to the angle that

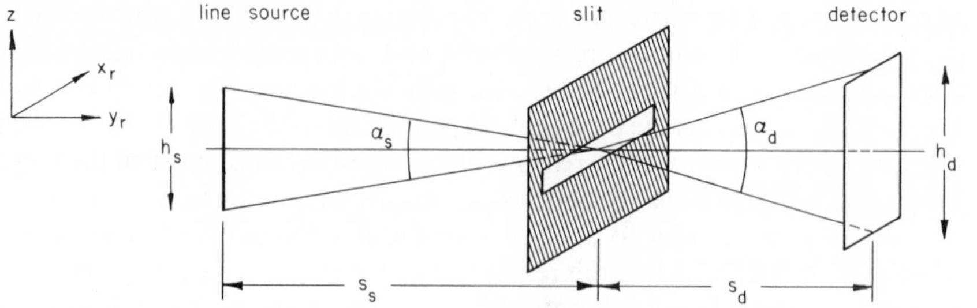

Fig. 7.21 Geometry used in evaluating the spatial sensitivity of a line source and rectangular detector.

is subtended in common by source and detector at the slit. For the line joining the midpoints of the source and detector, this angle is the smaller of $\alpha_s = h_s/s_s$ and $\alpha_d = h_d/s_d$. For other points, penumbra effects may reduce the system sensitivity. The result of this varying sensitivity is that small objects located exactly at the center of a slice will be imaged more strongly than objects located at the top or bottom of a slice (see Fig. 7.22). The worst case would be with $h_s = h_d$, where the image of *contiguously scanned* slices would not reveal a small, high-contrast object if it just happened to lie on the interface between the slices and close to the center of rotation. The final comment on beam height is concerned with the overall nonparallelism of the beam that occurs when h_s and h_d are markedly different. In this case, image artifacts may occur because some projections see a high-contrast object that just dips into the beam at one angle, yet is not seen by the beam at some

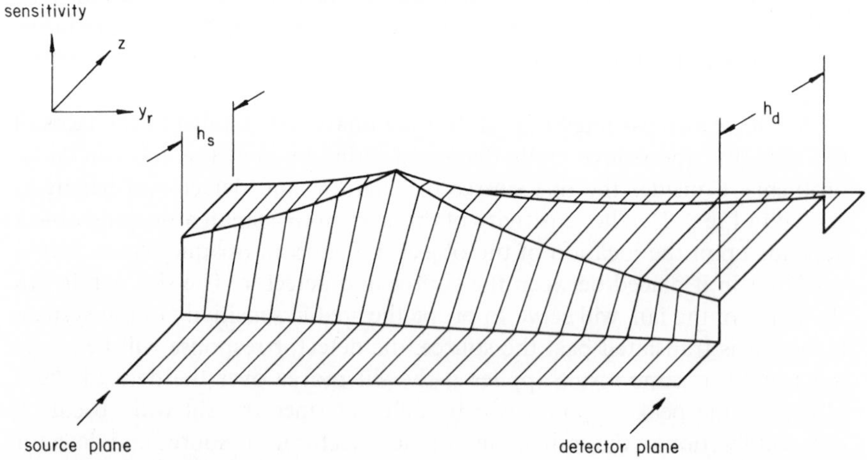

Fig. 7.22 A plot of the sensitivity of the source, slit, and detector configuration of Fig. 7.21.

other angle, thus giving rise to an inconsistent data set. This problem is effectively dealt with by taking 360° of projection data and averaging projections taken in opposing directions. Artifacts arising from this problem are called *partial volume* artifacts.

7.3.2 Data Sampling

Number of Samples

In this section we consider only parallel-beam data-gathering geometry such as shown in Fig. 7.20a. The x-ray projection $\lambda_\phi(x_r)$ has to this point, been regarded as a continuous, two-dimensional quantity. In order to implement digital reconstruction methods, it is necessary to form discrete samples from this distribution. We need to know the increments d (in x_r) and $\Delta\phi$ (in ϕ) at which the samples should be taken. Note that d, the spacing between samples, is not in general equal to the width of the detector w_d. If we consider the object to be contained in a circular region of diameter $2a$, then the number of samples per projection is

$$N_s = 2a/d. \tag{7.107}$$

The number of projections N_ϕ is given by

$$N_\phi = \pi/\Delta\phi. \tag{7.108}$$

The numerator is π and not 2π because of the redundancy of the projection data for $\pi < \phi \leqslant 2\pi$.

Intuitively, one might argue that the angular increments should be such that the corresponding linear increment of any given detector-source line should, at the circle perimeter, also be d, i.e.,

$$\Delta\phi = d/a. \tag{7.109}$$

We shall justify this step later. The total number of data points is simply

$$N = N_s N_\phi = (\pi/2)(2a/d)^2. \tag{7.110}$$

Dose versus Resolution

The smallest resolvable object dimension δ in the reconstruction will be directly proportional to (and approximately equal to) d, and there is no reason in principle why d should not be made arbitrarily small so that high-resolution pictures will result. In practice, cost and patient dose considerations limit d. Suppose it is required to scan a cylindrical object in contiguous transaxial slices of height h. From the discussion in Section 10.5.4, we can approximate the dose D and the integrated dose D_{int} as follows:

$$D \propto \frac{(\mathrm{SNR})^2}{\delta^3 h} \quad \mathrm{rad} \tag{7.111}$$

and

$$D_{int} = k_1 DM \quad \mathrm{rad\ gm} \tag{7.112}$$

The dose D is a measure of the absorbed energy in the irradiated slice during primary irradiation of that slice per gram of tissue, and D_{int} integrates this dose over the mass M of tissue in the cylinder. Factor k_1 ($k_1 \sim 3$) is to account for energy that is scattered out of the irradiated section and absorbed elsewhere in the cylinder.

Quantities δ and h should be proportional to each other. Ideally the slice thickness h should not exceed the resolution distance δ if small structures that are oriented obliquely to the tomographic axis are not to be unduly blurred in the reconstructed image. A practical compromise is reached in commercial machines with h being typically 5 to 10 times δ. The benefits arising from this compromise are (i) lower dose per slice, (ii) lower integrated dose, and (iii) fewer scans for a required total image volume. It is important to realize that a machine that has a claimed (and even demonstrated) minimum resolved distance of 1 mm or less will not provide this performance in normal clinical use. Human body parts simply do not resemble the axially oriented bundles of high-contrast rods, with which the resolution specifications are obtained.

Typical values encountered with commercial machines are $D = 1$ rad for SNR ≈ 200 and $\delta \approx 2$ mm. If slice thickness h is assumed to be directly proportional to δ, then both dose and integrated dose are seen to depend upon the inverse fourth power of δ. This fact precludes the possibility of seeking reconstructed clinical sections with significantly greater detail, say $\delta \approx 0.2$ mm, which would make the image almost as sharp as a conventional projection radiograph, since for the same density discrimination, the dose and integrated dose would be several orders of magnitude greater than that deemed acceptable. This result is a consequence of the statistical properties of the photon beam, and there appears to be no way significantly to improve the fourth-power trade-off.

Aliasing

We now show that the very act of sampling the data introduces errors into the reconstruction. If the projection of the object is sampled at N_s evenly spaced points, then the Fourier-space representation of the projection can also be determined at N_s discrete points by using the discrete Fourier transform:

$$\Lambda_\phi^s(\xi_r = m\Delta\xi) = \frac{1}{N_s} \sum_{n=-N_s/2+1}^{N_s/2} \lambda_\phi^s(x_r = nd)\exp(-2\pi inm/N_s). \quad (7.113)$$

The superscript is to remind us that this is a discrete (sampled) representation of the projection and its Fourier transform. The spacing of samples in Fourier space is given by $\Delta\xi = (2a)^{-1}$, and in real space by $d = (2\xi_{max})^{-1} = (N_s\,\Delta\xi)^{-1}$.

The $\Lambda_\phi^s(\xi_r)$ sample values are not, however, equal to sampled values of the (continuous) Fourier transform of $\lambda_\phi(x_r)$ sampled at the corresponding frequency, i.e.,

$$\Lambda_\phi^s(\xi_r) \neq \Lambda_\phi(\xi_r), \quad (7.114)$$

and there is no way, in general, in which the true values can be extracted from the discrete Fourier transform values. As shown in Section 2.5, the sample values in frequency space Λ_ϕ^s are formed by a summation of samples of shifted versions of the continuous Fourier transform [cf. (2.79)]:

$$\Lambda_\phi^s(\xi_r) = \sum_{j=-\infty}^{\infty} \Lambda_\phi(\xi_r + jN_s\,\Delta\xi). \quad (7.115)$$

This *aliasing* effect is illustrated in Fig. 7.23.

The only way to prevent aliasing is to limit the extent of the Fourier spectrum of the projection so that the overlap in frequency space does not occur, i.e., $\Lambda_\phi(\xi_r) = 0$ for $|\xi_r| \geqslant N_s\,\Delta\xi/2$. Unfortunately, for a finite-sized object, the Fourier spectrum extends to $\pm\infty$ and aliasing is unavoidable.

However, it is possible to prefilter the projection data so that an insignificant amount of information is contained in the region $|\xi_r| \geqslant N_s\,\Delta\xi/2$. Functions of this type, which have finite extent in real space and essentially finite extent in Fourier space, are called *essentially* bandlimited functions.

The required filtering process is done automatically by the detector. For collimated parallel radiation the detector supplies a signal that represents

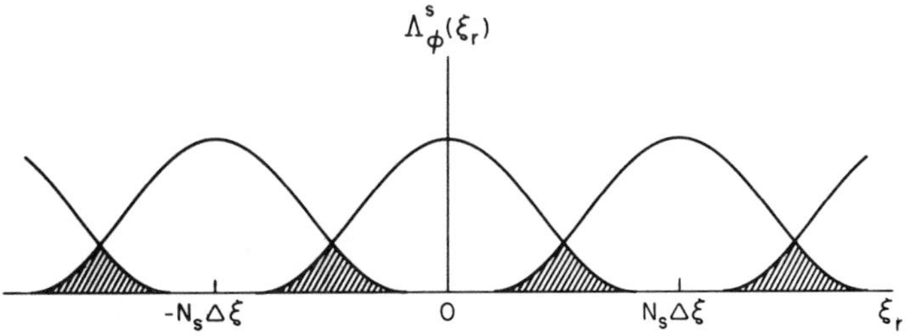

Fig. 7.23 Aliasing in the Fourier transform of the sampled function occurs when there is overlap (shaded regions) between the shifted versions of the Fourier transforms of that function.

the line integral of the attenuation coefficient averaged over the rectangular aperture of the detector. In the x–y plane the projection is convolved (filtered) with a rect function,

$$\lambda_\phi^\dagger(x_r) = \lambda_\phi(x_r) * \text{rect}(x_r/w_d), \tag{7.116}$$

before the sampling process takes place. [Strictly speaking, the transmitted *intensity* is convolved with a rect, and then the logarithm is taken to get $\lambda_\phi^\dagger$. But if the intensity variations across the detector face are small compared to the average intensity, (7.116) is a good approximation.] The width of the rect function is just the width of the detector. Additional low-pass filtering is provided as a result of having a finite source size. Thus it is reasonable to assume that the original projection data become bandlimited to the region $-\xi_D < \xi_r < \xi_D$ by this averaging process, where ξ_D is the first zero of the Fourier transform of the detector aperture function:

$$\xi_D = 1/w_d. \tag{7.117}$$

We can now determine the intervals d at which the $\lambda_\phi^\dagger(x_r)$ should be sampled. The sampling theorem (see Section 2.5) gives us the answer immediately. In order to completely specify a function that is bandlimited to the region $-\xi_D < \xi < \xi_D$, samples must be taken at intervals not exceeding $(2\xi_D)^{-1}$. In our case, with $\xi_D = 1/w_d$, the required increment is

$$d \leqslant w_d/2. \tag{7.118}$$

The detector-source line of sight should be stepped in increments of half the detector width or less.

In practice, it turns out that this requirement is too stringent. Samples are normally taken at twice this interval; adjacent samples are taken from adjacent detectors in a close packed configuration. The aliasing that results from this procedure does not significantly affect the quality of the reconstructed image, probably because of the low-pass prefiltering afforded by the finite source size and the effect of averaging the object transmission measurement over the z direction.

Since the width of the sampled object field is $2a$, the sampling interval in Fourier space is $\Delta\xi = (2a)^{-1}$. If we presume that the system is optimized so that this is the Nyquist limit, it follows that in order to completely sample all of Fourier space, the spacing between samples in the azimuthal direction must also be $\leqslant (2a)^{-1}$. Setting the angle between projections $\Delta\phi$ equal to

$$\Delta\phi = \Delta\xi/\xi_{\max} = (2a)^{-1}/(2d)^{-1} = d/a \tag{7.119}$$

satisfies this requirement (see Fig. 7.24). This equation justifies our intuitive approach in (7.109). The interior portions of Fourier space are unavoidably oversampled in the azimuthal direction.

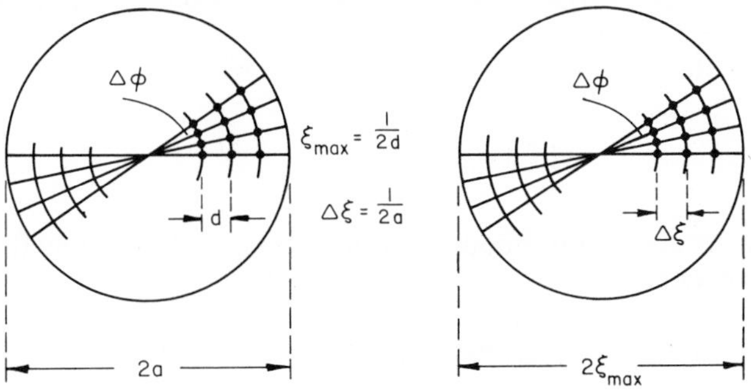

Fig. 7.24 Radon space of radius a is sampled at lateral increments d and angular increments $\Delta\phi$. The corresponding sample points in Fourier space are shown on the right.

In summary, if the data are bandlimited to $\pm\xi_{\max}$, the number of evenly spaced samples per projection N_s need not exceed the space-bandwidth product $4a\xi_{\max}$. The number of azimuthal samples N_ϕ is given by

$$N_\phi = \frac{\pi}{\Delta\phi} = \frac{\pi a}{d} = 2\pi a\xi_{\max} = \frac{\pi N_s}{2}. \tag{7.120}$$

Theoretically, a detector of width w_d will approximately bandlimit the data to $\xi_D = 1/w_d$, which would require samples spaced $w_d/2$ apart. In practice, a sample spacing of w_d appears to be satisfactory.

7.3.3 Digital Filtering

For the filtered-back-projection algorithm, the projection data are filtered by means of a discrete convolution process in which the filter function is simply the sampled version of the continuous filter function $q(x_r)$ of Section 7.2.6. The discrete version of (7.38) is written

$$\lambda_j^{\dagger s}(x_i) = \sum_l \lambda_j^s(x_l) q^s(x_i - x_l), \tag{7.121}$$

where the superscript s denotes a sampled function that is defined only at the sample points and subscript j is the index of the projection angle ϕ_j.

The digital process (7.121) is entirely equivalent to the continuous filtering (7.38) inasmuch as $\lambda_\phi^\dagger(x_r)$ can be reconstructed exactly from $\lambda_\phi^{\dagger s}(x_i)$ by sinc-function interpolation (assuming of course perfect sampling and no noise). A sufficient requirement is that both $\lambda_\phi(x_r)$ and $q_1(x_r)$ be bandlimited and sampled at the Nyquist rate or better so that they are properly represented by their sampled versions $\lambda_j^s(x_i)$ and $q^s(x_i)$.

Consider the abrupt-cutoff $|\xi_r|$ filter defined by

$$Q(\xi_r) = \begin{cases} \pi|\xi_r|, & |\xi_r| \leqslant \xi_{max} \\ 0, & |\xi_r| > \xi. \end{cases} \tag{7.122}$$

The one-dimensional continuous filter function $q(x_r)$ is given by the Fourier transform of $Q(\xi_r)$,

$$q(x_r) = 2\pi\xi_{max}^2 \operatorname{sinc}(2\xi_{max}x_r) - \pi\xi_{max}^2 \operatorname{sinc}^2(\xi_{max}x_r). \tag{7.123}$$

This filter was first given by Bracewell and Riddle (1967).

The discrete form, $q^s(x_i)$ is given by $q(x_r)$ evaluated at sample points $x_i = i/2\xi_{max}$,

$$q^s(x_i) = \begin{cases} \pi\xi_{max}^2, & i = 0 \\ \dfrac{-4}{\pi}\dfrac{\xi_{max}^2}{i^2}, & i = \pm 1, \pm 3, \pm 5, \ldots \\ 0, & i = \pm 2, \pm 4, \pm 6, \ldots . \end{cases} \tag{7.124}$$

This discrete filter was first used by Ramachandran and Lakshminarayanan (1971).

Another frequently used filter is one that was introduced by Shepp and Logan (1974). It is equivalent to the Ramachandran–Lakshminarayanan (RL) filter with an additional $\operatorname{sinc}(\xi_r/2\xi_{max})$ apodizing filter. Thus the maximum frequency ξ_{max} passed by the filter is attenuated by $2/\pi$ relative to the RL filter. The filter is described by

$$\begin{aligned} Q_{SL}(\xi_r) &= Q(\xi_r)\operatorname{sinc}(\xi_r/2\xi_{max}) \\ &= \pi|\xi_r|\operatorname{rect}(\xi_r/2\xi_{max})\operatorname{sinc}(\xi_r/2\xi_{max}). \end{aligned} \tag{7.125}$$

The corresponding space domain filter $q_{SL}(x_r)$ is given by

$$\begin{aligned} q_{SL}(x_r) &= \mathscr{F}^{-1}\{Q_{SL}(\xi_r)\} \\ &= 2\xi_{max} q(x_r) * \operatorname{rect}(2\xi_{max}x_r) \\ &= 2\xi_{max}\int_{x_r-(4\xi_{max})^{-1}}^{x_r+(4\xi_{max})^{-1}} q(x_r')\,dx_r', \end{aligned} \tag{7.126}$$

where the second stage follows from the first with the use of (7.125) and (B.52). This integral is readily evaluated using (7.123). Using the change of variable $p = 2\pi\xi_{\max}x_r'$ and writing $\theta = 2\pi\xi_{\max}x_r$ we have

$$q_{SL}(x_r) = 2\xi_{\max}^2 \int_{\theta-\pi/2}^{\theta+\pi/2} \left[\frac{\sin p}{p} - \frac{1-\cos p}{p^2}\right] dp$$

$$= 2\xi_{\max}^2 \left[\frac{1-\cos p}{p}\right]_{\theta-\pi/2}^{\theta+\pi/2}. \tag{7.127}$$

In terms of the original variables we have after evaluating (7.127)

$$q_{SL}(x_r) = \frac{-8\xi_{\max}^2}{\pi}\left[\frac{1-4\xi_{\max}x_r\sin(2\pi\xi_{\max}x_r)}{16\xi_{\max}^2x_r^2-1}\right]. \tag{7.128}$$

The digital form of this filter function is obtained by evaluating $q_{SL}(x_r)$ at the sample points $x_i = i/2\xi_{\max}$:

$$q_{SL}^s(x_i) = \frac{-8\xi_{\max}^2}{\pi}\left[\frac{1}{4i^2-1}\right], \qquad i = 0, \pm 1, \pm 2, \ldots . \tag{7.129}$$

This is the form in which the filter is usually applied in digital reconstruction methods. Because of the additional apodization, it does not quite have the same sharpness as the RL filter; however, it does handle noisy data in a somewhat better fashion. The continuous and discrete versions of the RL and SL filters are shown in Fig. 7.25.

Because of the discrete nature of the digital data, a problem arises in the back-projection operation. It is usual to describe the reconstructed section as a two-dimensional matrix of square picture elements (pixels), $\hat{\mu}(k)$, $k = 1, \ldots, K$. During the back-projection operation a particular data value must be assigned to each of these elements. There are basically two ways in which this can be done. One way (see Fig. 7.26) is to assign a fraction of the value of the point being back projected, $\lambda_j^{\dagger s}(x_i)$, where the weighting factor w_{ijk} is determined by some geometrical construct:

$$\hat{\mu}_j(k) = \sum_i w_{ijk}\lambda_j^{\dagger s}(x_i), \tag{7.130}$$

where $\hat{\mu}_j(k)$ is the contribution to $\hat{\mu}(k)$ from the projection at angle ϕ_j. For example, w_{ijk} can be made proportional to the length of the back-projected ray path contained in the kth image cell. A simpler scheme sets $w_{ijk} = 0$ or 1 according to whether the back-projection line intersects a circle of a given radius that is centered on the kth image cell. Whatever scheme is chosen, the w_{ijk} can be compiled and stored for all time. The final image is obtained by summation over j:

$$\hat{\mu}(k) = \sum_j \hat{\mu}_j(k). \tag{7.131}$$

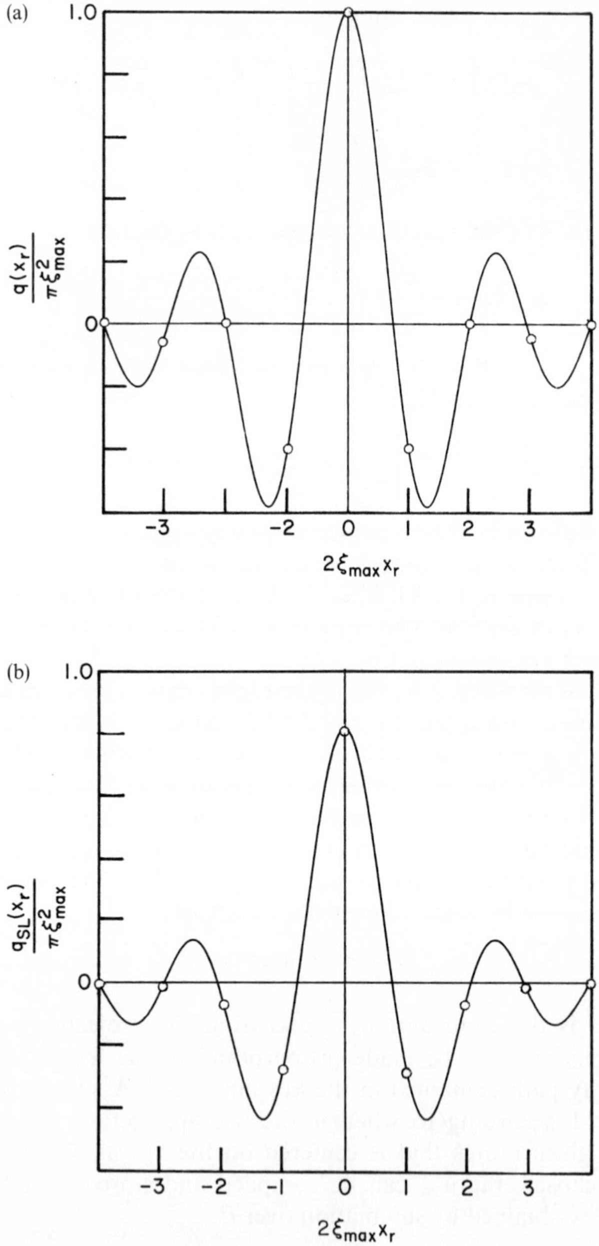

Fig. 7.25 (a) Solid line shows continuous form of the Ramachandran–Lakshminarayanan filter. Open circles show the points at which the filter is sampled for digital filtering methods. (b) As in (a) but for the Shepp and Logan filter. (c) Frequency response of the filters.

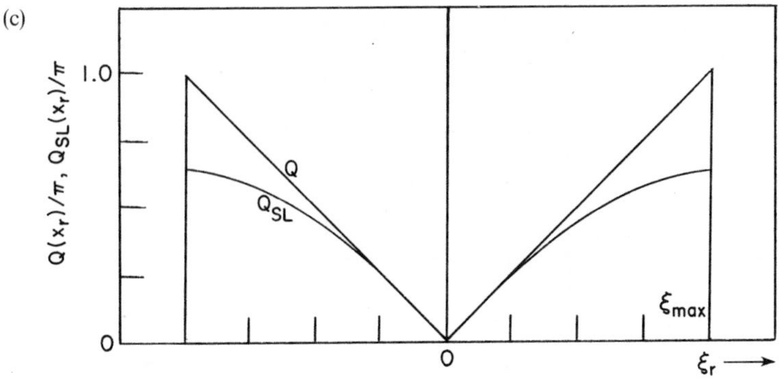

Fig. 7.25 (*continued*)

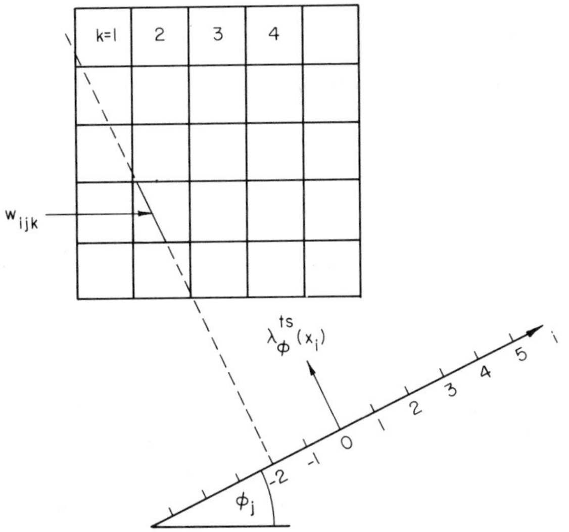

Fig. 7.26 Object is reconstructed on a grid of K pixels. The contribution to the kth pixel from the ith filtered projection point at the jth projection angle is weighted by w_{ijk}. In this example w_{ijk} is proportional to the length of the back-projected ray in the pixel area.

The second method interpolates the filtered projection data to find the value appropriate to the ray that passes exactly through the center of the kth image cell. This approach avoids the computational expense of storing the predetermined weights (see Fig. 7.27). If the ray is located at x_i', then

$$\hat{\mu}_j(k) = \lambda_j^{\dagger}(x_i'), \tag{7.132}$$

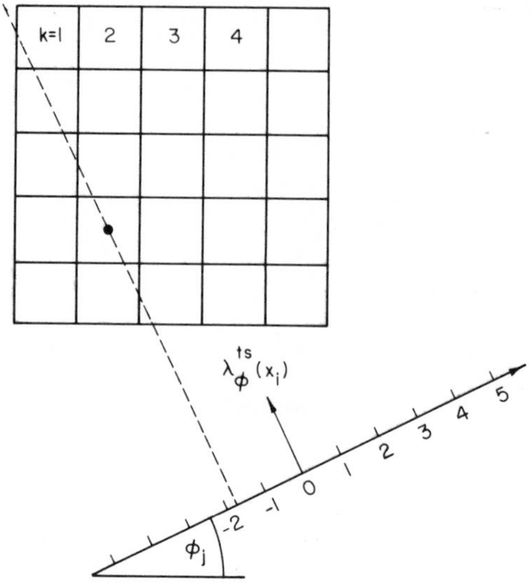

Fig. 7.27 Alternative to the scheme of Fig. 7.26 is to project the center of each pixel onto the filtered projection and assign to the pixel the value obtained by interpolation.

where $\lambda_j^\dagger(x_i')$ is found by interpolation. The simplest scheme is nearest-neighbor interpolation, i.e., simply assigning the value $\lambda_j^{\dagger s}(x_i)$, where x_i is the nearest sample abscissa to x_i'. Linear interpolation is better and is frequently used. The final image is obtained by summing as previously described in (7.131).

7.3.4 Fan-Beam Algorithms

High-speed data gathering requires a fan-beam geometry (see Fig. 7.20), so that a single source can be used to obtain multiple, simultaneous measures of the projection data. However, the projections are no longer parallel-beam projections, and the processing algorithms described so far are not directly applicable for reconstructing the object cross section. There are several ways to deal with this problem. We shall discuss three of them:

(i) reordering the data into parallel-beam arrays;
(ii) back-projection and summation followed by two-dimensional filtering of the summation image;
(iii) filtering each projection in real space or Fourier space, followed by back-projection and summation.

Iterative techniques discussed in Section 7.3.5 can also be used.

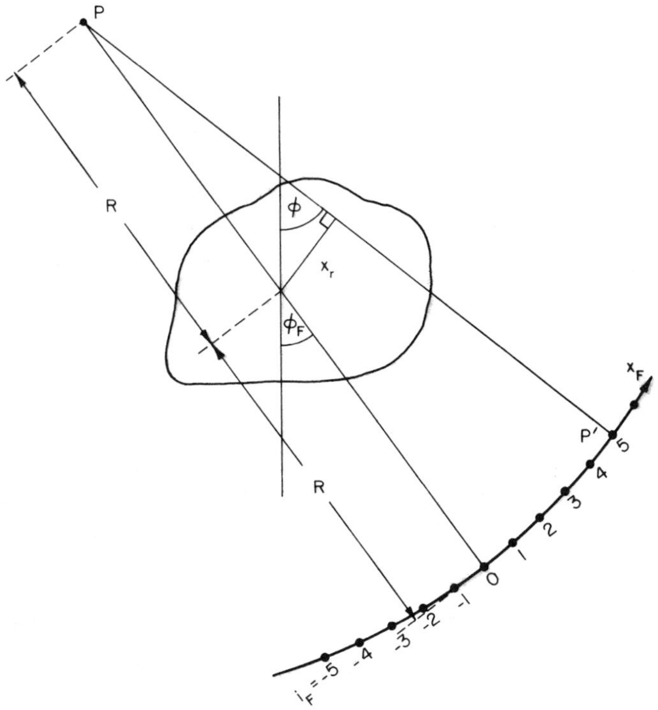

Fig. 7.28 With fan-beam geometry, a particular projection such as PP' can be specified by x_F and ϕ_F (i.e., data-space coordinates) or by x_r and ϕ, the corresponding parallel-beam parameters.

In the reordering method, data are collected over consecutive fan-beam projections. Figure 7.28 shows the geometry. The angle of the central ray of the fan is ϕ_F, the curvilinear distance along the detector array is x_F. It is assumed that the source defines the center of curvature of the detector arc. Thus the geometries shown in Figs. 7.20b, c, and e can be analyzed with this model (and only slight changes are needed to handle the geometry of Fig. 7.20d).

The relationship between x_F and ϕ_F and the corresponding quantities x_r and ϕ in the required parallel-beam data set is

$$x_r = R\sin(x_F/2R), \qquad (7.133)$$

$$\phi = \phi_F + x_F/2R, \qquad (7.134)$$

where $2R$ is the source-detector distance, and we have assumed that the gantry isocenter is at the source-detector midpoint.

The fan-beam projection data are represented by the elements of the discrete array $\lambda_F(i_F, j_F)$, where the detector positions $x_F(i_F)$ and central ray angles $\phi_F(j_F)$ are given by

$$x_F(i_F) = i_F\,\Delta x_F, \qquad i_F = 0, \pm 1, \pm 2, \ldots, \pm I_F, \tag{7.135a}$$

$$\phi_F(j_F) = j_F\,\Delta\phi_F, \qquad j_F = 1, 2, \ldots, J. \tag{7.135b}$$

This data set is to be reordered into a parallel-beam data set $\lambda(i, j)$, where integers i and j specify the detector positions $x_r(i)$ and projection angles $\phi(j)$ according to

$$x_r(i) = i\,\Delta x_r, \tag{7.136a}$$

$$\phi(j) = j\,\Delta\phi, \tag{7.136b}$$

where Δx_r and $\Delta\phi$ are free parameters.

The reordering is most conveniently done by two stages of interpolation. First, an intermediate array $\lambda^\dagger(i_F, j)$ is obtained by holding i_F constant and performing a one-dimensional interpolation over j_F in $\lambda_F(i_F, j_F)$:

$$\lambda^\dagger(i_F, j) = \tilde{\lambda}_F(i_F, j_F^*) \tag{7.137}$$

where the tilde denotes interpolation of the array to the noninteger value j_F^* given by

$$j_F^* = j\,\Delta\phi/\Delta\phi_F - i\,\Delta x_F/(2R\,\Delta\phi_F). \tag{7.138}$$

This value of j_F^* is obtained by substituting (7.135a), (7.135b), and (7.136b) into (7.134) and solving for the value of j_F. This intermediate array corresponds to parallel-beam data obtained at uniform angular intervals given by (7.136b) but with nonuniformly spaced detectors (see Fig. 7.29a).

The second stage of interpolation corrects for the nonuniform spacing (see Fig. 7.29b). This time j is held constant, and the desired array $\lambda(i, j)$ is given by

$$\lambda(i, j) = \tilde{\lambda}^\dagger(i_F^*, j) \tag{7.139}$$

where $\tilde{\lambda}^\dagger(i_F^*, j)$ is the interpolated value of $\lambda^\dagger(i_F, j)$ evaluated at

$$i_F^* = (2R/\Delta x_F)\sin^{-1}(i\,\Delta x_r/R). \tag{7.140}$$

This value of i_F^* is obtained from substituting (7.135a) and (7.136a) into (7.133).

It is not sufficient to collect data over the range $0 \leqslant \phi_F < \pi$ as in the parallel-beam case (see Fig. 7.30). The required range $0 \leqslant \phi_F < \phi_T$ is given by $\phi_T = \pi + \phi_A$, where ϕ_A, the fan angle, is given by

$$\phi_A = I_F\,\Delta x_F/R. \tag{7.141}$$

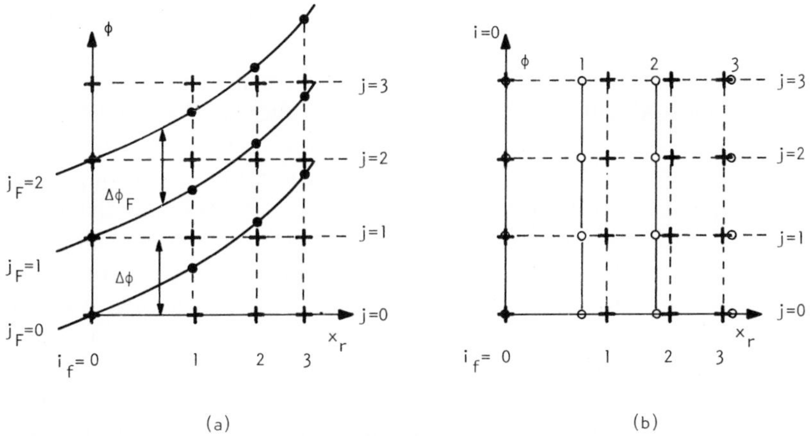

Fig. 7.29 (a) In sinogram space, the data from a fan-beam projection are distributed along a sine curve. The sine curve labeled $j_F = 0$ is for the projection $\phi_F = 0$. The first stage of interpolation (7.137) creates the intermediate array $\lambda^{\dagger}(i_F, j)$, denoted by crosses, from the fan-beam data array $\lambda_F(i_F, j_F)$, denoted by dots. The special case $\Delta\phi = \Delta\phi_F$ is illustrated. (b) The second stage of interpolation gives the parallel-beam array $\lambda(i, j)$, denoted by circles, from the intermediate array $\lambda^{\dagger}(i_F, j)$ denoted by crosses.

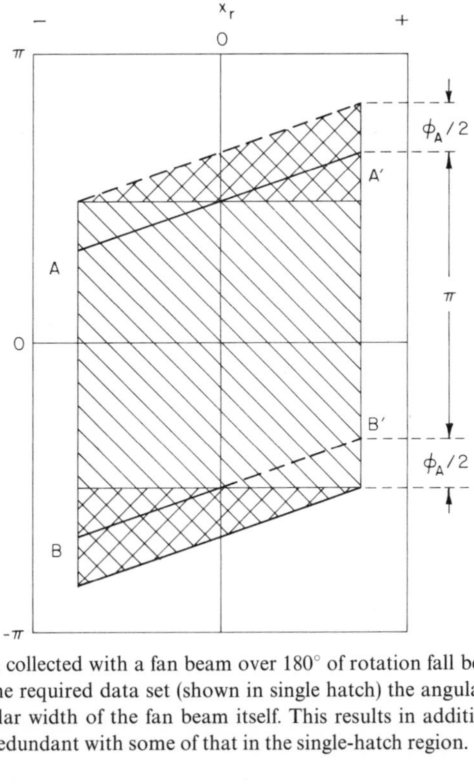

Fig. 7.30 Data collected with a fan beam over 180° of rotation fall between AA′ and BB′. In order to gather the required data set (shown in single hatch) the angular range must be expanded by the angular width of the fan beam itself. This results in additional data (shown in cross-hatch) that is redundant with some of that in the single-hatch region.

The second method of fan-beam reconstruction is back-projection followed by summation and two-dimensional filtering. We saw for parallel beams that the operation of back-projection and summation results in a $1/r$ position-invariant isotropic point spread function. For fan-beam geometry with a circular detector array, exactly the same result applies. (With fan-beam geometry, back-projection means smearing the projection back along a set of lines that converge on the x-ray source, i.e., along the direction of the x-ray beam that originally created the projection data.) Rather than give a formal proof of this assertion, we shall justify it with a geometrical illustration. Consider a single point object P as shown in Fig. 7.31. The dots on the circumference denote the positions of the x-ray source for N uniformly spaced consecutive projections. The lines passing through P represent the lines of the back-projections which automatically fall on the original source-point lines. A given angular range $\delta\phi$ will contain lines from both sides of the detector array, and the number of rays in $\delta\phi$ is given simply by the total number of detectors contained by both ends of the sector. Thus the angular density is given by

$$\frac{1}{\delta\phi}\left(\frac{N}{\pi d}\frac{\delta\phi}{\cos\theta}(a+b)\right)=\frac{N}{\pi}. \tag{7.142}$$

(See Fig. 7.31 for definition of a, b, and θ.) The angular density is independent of the location of P and of the direction chosen for the range $\delta\phi$. Thus the point spread function, which is given by the behavior of the spoke pattern

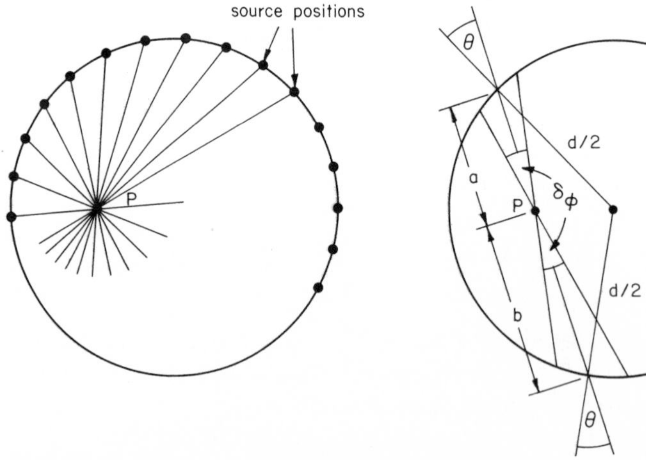

Fig. 7.31 For a single absorbing point P, the unfiltered back-projections would simply be line δ functions joining the point and the N positions of the source during exposure as seen on the left. On the right are the geometry and notation needed to calculate the angular density of the spokes in the back-projection pattern.

in the limit of continuous sampling, is position invariant and isotropic. The falloff in spoke density from P, which is proportional to $(\text{distance})^{-1}$, is the functional form of the PSF. (It is important to note that the full 360° rotation is needed for this result to hold. Projection data gathered over only 180° of rotation will not give either a space-invariant or isotropic point spread function.) It follows that any of the image processing methods alluded to in Section 7.2 can be used to undo the effects of the $1/r$ point spread function in the back-projected and summed image. Multiplicative frequency-domain filtering and convolutional filtering in the space domain are equally applicable.

Where speed of reconstruction is of the essence, this method is not preferred since all the data must be gathered before the filtering operation can begin. Other methods that allow the filtering to be performed on each projection before it is back-projected and summed are intrinsically faster. If the back-projection and summing are fast enough to keep up with the data gathering, then the reconstructed image is ready for viewing immediately after completion of the scan.

The third method illustrates one of these filtered back-projection algorithms. This method (Ramachandran and Lakshminarayanan, 1971) works with fan-beam data collected on a curved or straight detector array. The first data-processing step is to multiply the projection data by a weighting function of the form $(\cos\gamma)^{-1}$, where γ is the angle between the ray in question and the central ray of the fan. The next step is to filter the weighted convolution using a discrete filter function. Finally, each filtered, weighted projection is back-projected, and the summation image is formed. The back-projection operation also includes a weighting operation.

Figure 7.32 illustrates the geometry for a curved detector array. It is assumed that the detectors are evenly spaced along a circular arc with the source at the center of the circle. The angular separation between detectors, viewed from the source, is γ_0. The detectors are indexed $i = 0, \pm 1, \pm 2, \ldots, \pm I$, and the relative angle γ_i of the ith detector within the fan is $\gamma_i = i\gamma_0$.

Projection data are gathered at J discrete angular increments $\phi_{F,j}$:

$$\phi_{F,j} = 2\pi j/J, \qquad 1 \leqslant j \leqslant J, \tag{7.143}$$

where $\phi_{F,j}$ is the angle between the central beam in the fan and the y axis. We have dropped the subscript F on indices i and j. The data set can thus be described by a two-dimensional array of numbers $\lambda_F(i,j)$.

The first step is to apply the weighting function to yield $\lambda^*(i,j)$.

$$\lambda_F^*(i,j) = \lambda_F(i,j) \cdot p(i), \tag{7.144}$$

$$p(i) = [\cos(\gamma_i)]^{-1}. \tag{7.145}$$

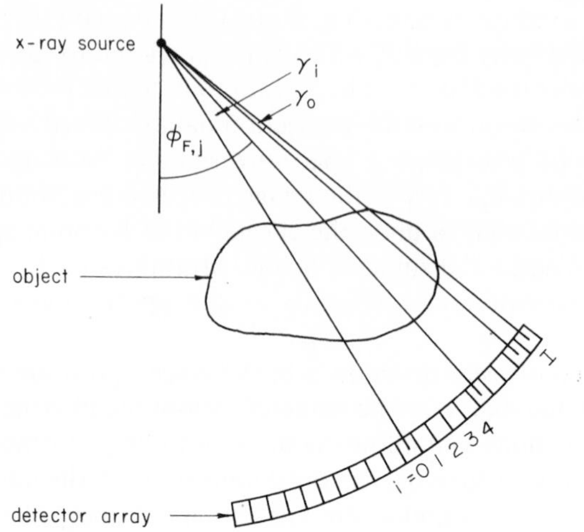

Fig. 7.32 Curved detector array geometry.

The filtered back-projection is given by

$$\lambda_F^\dagger(i, j) = \sum_{i'} \lambda_F^*(i - i', j) q(i'), \qquad (7.146)$$

with the elements of the discrete filter being given by

$$q(i) = \begin{cases} \pi/4, & i = 0 \\ -\dfrac{\gamma_0^2}{\pi \sin^2(\gamma_i)}, & i \text{ odd} \\ 0, & i \text{ even.} \end{cases} \qquad (7.147)$$

The reconstructed image is composed of K picture elements or image cells. The contribution of the jth projection to the kth image cell is given by the weighted summation

$$\hat{\mu}(j, k) = \sum_i f_{ijk} \lambda_F^\dagger(i, j), \qquad (7.148)$$

and the final image is given by summing over projections,

$$\hat{\mu}(k) = \sum_j \hat{\mu}(j, k). \qquad (7.149)$$

The weighting factor f_{ijk} consists of two components:

$$f_{ijk} = w_{ijk}/s_{jk}^2, \qquad (7.150)$$

where w_{ijk} is determined by the length of the ith ray of the jth projection that intersects the kth image cell (or some other equivalent algorithm) (see Fig. 7.26). Distance s_{jk} is the distance from the kth image cell to the source position in the jth projection. To make the algorithm expressed by (7.144)–(7.150) execute rapidly, quantities $\cos(\gamma_i)$, $q(i)$, and w_{ijk} should be precomputed, and the reconstruction algorithm then becomes simply a series of arithmetic operations. An alternative to (7.148) is

$$\hat{\mu}(j,k) = (1/s_{jk}^2)\tilde{\lambda}^{\dagger}(i^+, j), \tag{7.151}$$

where $\tilde{\lambda}^{\dagger}(i^+, j)$ is the interpolated value of $\lambda^{\dagger}(i,j)$, with i^+ (in general a noninteger) corresponding to the ray position that passes through the center of the kth cell at the jth projection. Nearest-neighbor interpolation can also be used, sometimes with negligible degradation in the final image.

There is an equivalent set of equations for the straight detector geometry shown in Fig. 7.33. The weight factors $p(i)$ used in the prefilter are the same as given by (7.145), although the γ_i no longer increment uniformly due to the change in geometry. The elements of the convolution filter (7.147), become

$$q(i) = \begin{cases} \pi/4, & i = 0 \\ -1/\pi i^2, & i \ \text{odd} \\ 0, & i \ \text{even}, \end{cases} \tag{7.152}$$

and the weights in the postfilter are given by

$$f_{ijk} = w_{ijk}/(s'_{jk})^2, \tag{7.153}$$

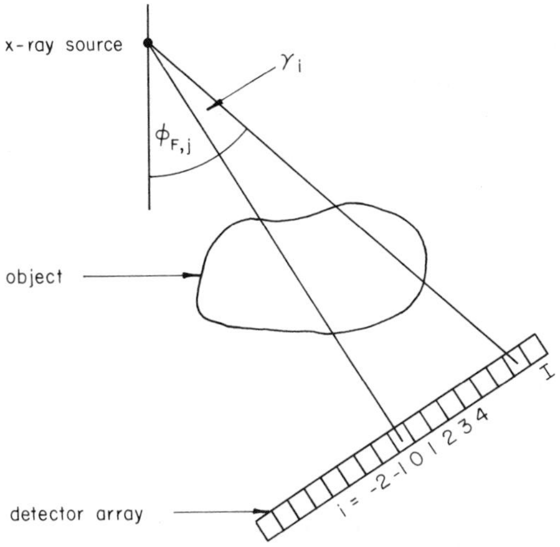

Fig. 7.33 Straight detector array geometry.

where s'_{jk} is the projection of the distance from the source to the image point onto the line from the source to the central detector.

Apart from the $(s_{jk})^2$ factor in the back-projection operation, these algorithms are very similar to those used for the parallel-beam case. The essential function of this factor is to convert the "back-projection to a point" operation into a "parallel back-projection" operation. In this way, the reconstruction point spread function is made effectively position invariant, as can be seen by considering the back-projection of the filter function itself. The asymptotic behavior in the wings of the filter is $1/x^2$. Thus, by boosting the amplitude by a factor $(s_{jk})^{-2}$, lines of constant amplitude in the wings of the back-projection of the filter lie on parallel, as opposed to converging, paths.

7.3.5 Iterative Methods

Statement of the Problem

We have an object $\mu(\mathbf{r})$, which is an unknown two-dimensional distribution of linear attenuation coefficient, and a limited set of experimentally determined projection measurements. The problem is to construct the "best" or "most realistic" representation of the object from this data. This representation is called the *estimate* of the object, or the *image*. In this section, the word "projection" will refer to a single data value obtained from a single detector output. Also, we shall change the subscript notation slightly. Subscript j $(1 \leqslant j \leqslant J)$ will run over all projections in the data set. Thus J of this section is equal to $J(2I + 1)$ of Section 7.3.4. Figure 7.34 shows the geometry that will be used in this discussion.

For simplicity, we assume parallel-beam geometry. Thus, a given object projection ${}_O\lambda_j$ $(1 < j < J)$ is obtained by performing a strip integration over $\mu(\mathbf{r})$, with the area of the strip defined by the jth ray. The total number of projections J is given by (7.110),

$$J = N_\phi N_s, \tag{7.155}$$

where N_ϕ is the number of projection angles and N_s is the number of projections measured at each angle.

The image is defined as a square $(n \times n)$ array of contiguous square pixels of side d. This image-space geometry, because of the computational convenience, is the most commonly used, although others are possible and have been used. The kth square $(1 < k < K,\ K = n \times n)$ is assigned an image value $\hat{\mu}_k$, and in a pictorial representation of the image, a brightness or gray level proportional to $\hat{\mu}_k$ would be displayed evenly over the kth pixel.

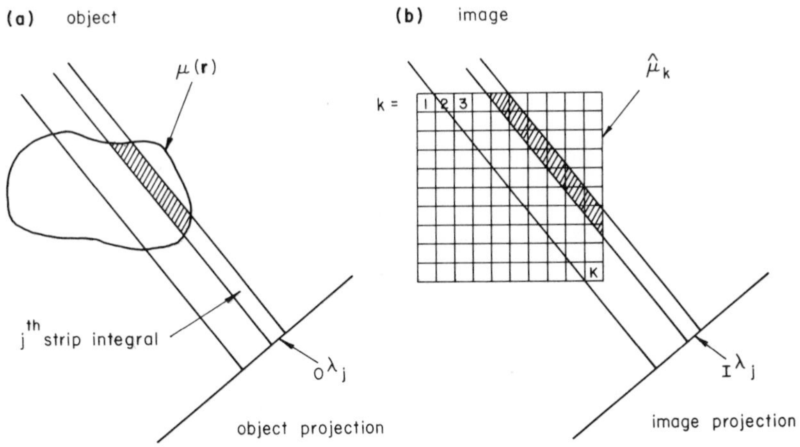

Fig. 7.34 (a) Object projection $_O\lambda_j$ is the strip integral of $\mu(\mathbf{r})$ over the area of the jth beam. (b) The image $\hat{\mu}_k$ is constructed as a discrete array of K pixels. Image projection $_I\lambda_j$ is the strip integral of $\hat{\mu}_k$ over the same domain as shown in (a).

Obviously, the image is only a representation or estimate of the real object. With only a finite number of object projection values, it is impossible to reconstruct the two-dimensional continuum $\mu(\mathbf{r})$. Ideally, one takes enough data points to ensure that the image has a sufficiently large number of independent pixels, thus allowing small object details to be represented in the image.

From Fig. 7.34, we see that image projections $_I\lambda_j$ can also be defined in an exactly analogous way to the definition of object projections, i.e., as a corresponding strip integral over the image. The reconstruction problem can now be stated more precisely. We seek the image set $\hat{\mu}_k$ $(1 < k < K)$, that makes the image projections most closely resemble the object projections $_O\lambda_j$. This image $\hat{\mu}_k$ is then regarded as the best estimate of $\mu(\mathbf{r})$ according to the criterion used in determining the resemblance. It should be noted that in practice there is generally no $\hat{\mu}_k$ that will give exact agreement between $_O\lambda_j$ and $_I\lambda_j$, because the image model is at best an approximation to the object and because the object data are experimental and thus contaminated by noise and artifacts discussed elsewhere in this chapter.

We now show how the image projection data are computed from the image. Consider first the attenuation of the jth x-ray beam (see Fig. 7.35). Using Beer's law and integrating over the width W of the ray, we find that the beam attenuation α_j is given by

$$\alpha_j = \frac{1}{W} \int_{x_{r,1}}^{x_{r,2}} \exp\left(-\sum_k \hat{\mu}_k l_{jk}(x_r) \right) dx_r, \tag{7.156}$$

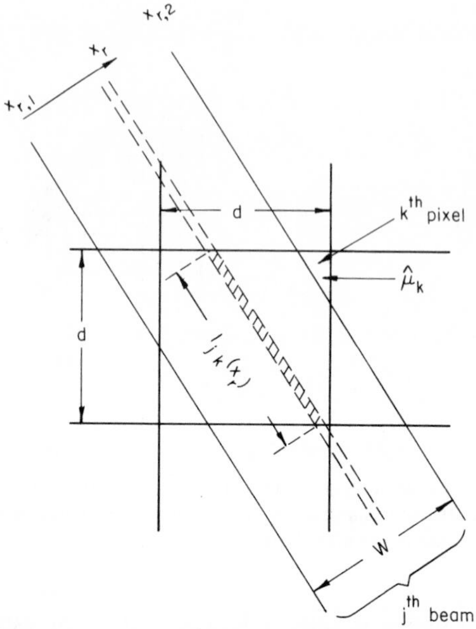

Fig. 7.35 Defining the quantities used in (7.156).

where $l_{jk}(x_r)$ is defined in Fig. 7.35 and $W = x_{r,2} - x_{r,1}$. The image projection is thus given by

$$_I\lambda_j = -\ln \alpha_j. \tag{7.157}$$

Only those pixels intersecting the beam need be considered in these equations.

The highly nonlinear relation expressed by (7.156) and (7.157) between $\hat{\mu}_k$ and $_I\lambda_j$ is virtually useless for computational purposes. The situation may be simplified by defining an average length,

$$\bar{l}_{jk} = \frac{1}{W}\int_{x_{r,1}}^{x_{r,2}} l_{jk}(x_r)\,dx_r = \frac{a_{jk}}{W}, \tag{7.158}$$

where a_{jk} is the area common to the jth beam and the kth pixel. The true length $l_{jk}(x_r)$ is given by

$$l_{jk}(x_r) = \bar{l}_{jk} + \Delta l_{jk}(x_r). \tag{7.159}$$

Now (7.156) can be written

$$\alpha_j = W^{-1}\exp\Big(-\sum_k \hat{\mu}_k \bar{l}_{jk}\Big)\int_{x_{r,1}}^{x_{r,2}} \exp\Big(-\sum_k \hat{\mu}_k\,\Delta l_{jk}(x_r)\Big)\,dx_r. \tag{7.160}$$

Since $\Delta l_{jk}(x_r)$ has both positive and negative values, the quantity $\sum_k \hat{\mu}_k\,\Delta l_{jk}(x_r)$ can be small compared to unity even if $\sum_k \hat{\mu}_k \bar{l}_{jk}$ is larger than unity. If this is the case, as it almost always will be in practice, we can write

$$\int_{x_{r,1}}^{x_{r,2}} \exp\left(-\sum_k \hat{\mu}_k \Delta l_{jk}(x_r)\right) dx_r = \int_{x_{r,1}}^{x_{r,2}} \left(1 - \sum_k \hat{\mu}_k \Delta l_{jk}(x_r) + \cdots\right) dx_r \approx W, \tag{7.161}$$

where we have used the fact that, by (7.158) and (7.159),

$$\int_{x_{r,1}}^{x_{r,2}} \Delta l_{jk}(x_r)\, dx_r = 0.$$

From (7.157), (7.160), and (7.161), it follows that

$${}_I\lambda_j \approx \sum_k \hat{\mu}_k \bar{l}_{jk} = W^{-1} \sum_k \hat{\mu}_k a_{jk}. \tag{7.162}$$

This is the required linear relationship between image elements $\hat{\mu}_k$ and the image projections ${}_I\lambda_j$.

We follow the common practice of making all components of the equation dimensionless by defining

$$w_{jk} = \text{fractional pixel area} = a_{jk}/d^2, \tag{7.163}$$

$$f_k = \hat{\mu}_k d^2/W, \tag{7.164}$$

where f_k is a dimensionless quantity that is directly proportional to the estimate of the linear attenuation coefficient. This yields

$${}_I\lambda_j = \sum_k w_{jk} f_k \tag{7.165}$$

as the fundamental equation that relates the image projection ${}_I\lambda_j$ to the image data f_k.

We can now formally state the problem. Given an object projection set ${}_O\lambda_j$, we seek solutions f_k to the equations

$${}_O\lambda_j = \sum_k w_{jk} f_k. \tag{7.166}$$

Since exact solutions will not in general exist, we seek f_k values that will maximize in some sense the similarity between ${}_I\lambda_j$ as given by (7.165) and ${}_O\lambda_j$. This image f_k is the required estimate of the object.

Direct Matrix Inversion

Equation (7.166) is an array of J simultaneous equations in K unknowns. A solution should be available by inverting the matrix w_{jk}, i.e.,

$$f_k = \sum_{j=1}^{J} (w^{-1})_{jk}\, {}_O\lambda_j. \tag{7.167}$$

There are several reasons that this particular method is not commonly used. These include:

(i) The number of elements in w_{jk} is prohibitively large.
(ii) A unique solution will not exist if the equations are under-determined.
(iii) No solution may exist because of noise or quantization errors in the data.

The iterative methods described next are ways of solving (7.166) without actually inverting the matrix.

Iterative Solutions

The iterative methods discussed below can all be described by the following set of operations:

(i) Assume an initial image f_k.
(ii) Compute the image projections ${}_I\lambda_J$.
(iii) Compare to the object projections ${}_O\lambda_j$.
(iv) Compute correction factors and update f_k values.
(v) When the f_k update is completed, repeat from (ii) with new iterations, or end with final image.

There are, however, several ways in which the comparisons can be made and several ways in which the correction factors can be applied. Thus several iterative methods have become popular, each apparently possessing the superior performance when given the appropriate experimental or test data. In the following sections, we present an outline of the methods that have been used in radiological applications

Algebraic Reconstruction Technique

The original method (Gordon *et al.*, 1970) has been modified into many versions. Here we describe the version called unconstrained *algebraic reconstruction technique* (ART) (Herman *et al.*, 1973).

In the course of one iteration, each of the J image projections ${}_I\lambda_j$ is addressed once. For each image pixel, a correction factor, ε_{jk}^l is computed by

$$\varepsilon_{jk}^l = w_{jk}({}_O\lambda_j - {}_I\lambda_j) \Big/ \sum_k w_{jk}^2, \qquad (7.168)$$

where l denotes the iteration number and ${}_I\lambda_j$ is the current value of the image projection. This correction is immediately applied to all the pixels in the image, but note that $\varepsilon_{jk}^l \equiv 0$ for image cells not intersected or contained in the jth projection. The corrected value is given by

$$f_k^l(j) = f_k^l(j-1) + \varepsilon_{jk}^l. \tag{7.169}$$

The $f_k^l(j)$ carries the temporary argument j to emphasize the fact that the image updates are made at the end of the ray-sum comparison, and the initial and final temporary values are assigned as follows:

$$f_k^l(1) = f_k^{l-1}, \qquad f_k^l = f_k^l(J), \tag{7.170}$$

where f_k^l is the image value at the end of the lth iteration.

An alternative to the additive correction method (7.169) is the multiplicative method:

$$f_k^l(j) = f_k^l(j-1)({}_O\lambda_j/{}_I\lambda_j). \tag{7.171}$$

With multiplicative methods, once a cell has been set to zero, it remains at zero; the silhouette of a convex object is precisely established after just the first iteration. ART is sometimes called the *ray-by-ray* reconstruction method.

Simultaneous Iterative Reconstruction Technique

In the simultaneous iterative reconstruction technique (SIRT) (Gilbert, 1972) it is the points in the image set that are addressed one at a time and corrected one at a time. Thus SIRT is sometimes called the *point-by-point* reconstruction method. For each point, all the image projections for rays passing through that point are calculated and summed. A correction factor, based on the discrepancy between this calculated sum of image projections and the sum of the actual object projections, is then applied immediately to that image point. The ${}_I\lambda_j$ are recalculated for every k and l. In unconstrained form, the additive algorithm is

$$f_k^l = f_k^{l-1} + \sum_{j=1}^{J} {}_O\lambda_j w_{jk} \Big/ \sum_{j=1}^{J} L_j w_{jk} - \sum_{j=1}^{J} {}_I\lambda_j w_{jk} \Big/ \sum_{j=1}^{J} N_j w_{jk}, \tag{7.172}$$

and the multiplicative form is

$$f_k^l = f_k^{l-1}\left(\sum_{j=1}^{J} {}_O\lambda_j w_{jk} \Big/ \sum_{j=1}^{J} L_j w_{jk}\right)\left(\sum_{j=1}^{J} N_j w_{jk} \Big/ \sum_{j=1}^{J} {}_I\lambda_j w_{jk}\right). \tag{7.173}$$

Length L_j is the actual length, in units of d^2/W (see Fig. 7.35) of the jth ray, and N_j is the number of pixel points contained in the jth ray. In the original version of this algorithm, the weighting factors w_{jk} were made 0 or 1, depending on whether or not the center of the kth image pixel lies outside or inside the jth ray, and were not explicitly included in the algorithm. We include them here to emphasize that the summations over j are meant to include only those projections that include the center of the kth pixel. With this restriction on w_{jk}, the term $\sum N_j w_{jk}$ is required because the number of points in an image projection can vary by a large amount for small displacements of the ray. Hence the calculated image projection, which is simply the sum of the image data at these points, is also subject to the same fluctuations. These fluctuations are stabilized by division of one sum by the other. The $\sum L_j w_{jk}$ term simply rescales the observed data ${}_O\lambda_j$ by the appropriate amount before the correction term is computed. It is emphasized that each image pixel is updated immediately after the correction term has been calculated. The updated value is used for computing subsequent image projections within the same iteration.

Iterative Least Squares Technique

This method (ILST) (Goitein, 1972) is similar to SIRT in that it is a point-by-point algorithm. However, updated values are stored separately and applied to the image only at the end of the iteration. Thus the order in which the pixels are addressed is immaterial. The image projections for rays that pass through the kth pixel are calculated, and the image value f_k is then adjusted to minimize, in a least-squares sense, the discrepancy between the image projections and the measured data. The minimization condition is

$$\sum_j \frac{({}_I\lambda_j^l - {}_O\lambda_j)^2}{\sigma_j^2} = \min, \tag{7.174}$$

where, as before, the sum includes only projections passing through pixel k. The quantity σ_j is the uncertainty (standard deviation) associated with the measurement ${}_O\lambda_j$. The correction factor is given by

$$\Delta f_k^l = \frac{\sum_{j=1}^{J} w_{jk}({}_O\lambda_j - \sum_{k=1}^{K} w_{jk} f_k^l)/\sigma_j^2}{\sum_{j=1}^{J} (w_{ij}/\sigma_j)^2}, \tag{7.175}$$

and at the end of the iteration the image is updated according to

$$f_k^{l+1} = f_k^l + \Delta f_k^l. \tag{7.176}$$

This algorithm gives f_k^l values that diverge in an oscillatory manner with increasing l. A multiplicative damping factor δ must be applied. A suitable damping factor is given by

$$\delta = \frac{\sum_{j=1}^{J} (c_j/\sigma_j^2)({}_O\lambda_j - {}_I\lambda_j)}{\sum_{j=1}^{J} (c_j^2/\sigma_j^2)},$$

where

$$c_j = \sum_{k=1}^{K} w_{jk} \Delta f_k^l. \tag{7.177}$$

After all the Δf_k^l values have been calculated using (7.175), δ is calculated and the image corrections are simultaneously incorporated at the end of the iteration according to

$$f_k^{l+1} = f_k^l + \delta\,\Delta f_k^l. \tag{7.178}$$

Further Considerations

We now look briefly at some topics that apply generally to iterative methods.

Initial Values The most popular choice of initial value is $f_k^0 = \bar{f}$, where $\bar{f}$ is the mean density of the object as determined by calculating the appropriate average of the object projections:

$$\bar{f} = \frac{1}{KN_\phi} \sum_{j=1}^{J} {}_O\lambda_j. \tag{7.179}$$

With additive algorithms, $f_k^0 = 0$ can also be used. Elaborate schemes may use a priori knowledge regarding the object.

Constraints Iterative methods are usually improved by restricting the range of image values. Most constraints are based on obvious physical arguments. It is commonly required that $f_k \geqslant 0$ at all times. If f_k is calculated to be less then zero it is immediately replaced by zero. Fully constrained algorithms also require $f_k < f_{\max}$ with similar replacement rules. Another constraint may be applied when the data set ${}_O\lambda_j$ is zero. In this case, all pixels contained by the ray path j are set to zero for all time. This is automatically achieved with algorithms such as (7.171) in which the corrections are applied multiplicatively.

Weighting Schemes The use of w_{jk} in some algorithms involves the calculation and storage of a large number of noninteger numbers. These algorithms can be greatly speeded up with little loss in accuracy by schemes such as the following (Gordon, 1974). The approximation is made that the projection data are given by

$${}_I\lambda_j = C_j \sum_k u_{jk} f_k, \tag{7.180}$$

where u_{jk} is 0 or 1 depending upon whether the kth pixel lies within the jth ray, and C_j is a constant that depends only on geometry and can be precomputed. Its function is to compensate for the fluctuations in the number of pixel centers per unit length of ray as the ray index changes. It is equivalent to the L/N term in the SIRT algorithm. If the object data set is prescaled according to

$${}_O\lambda'_j = {}_O\lambda_j / C_j, \tag{7.181}$$

then the equations to be solved are

$$_{O}\lambda'_j = \sum u_{jk} f_k. \qquad (7.182)$$

Since $u_{jk} = 0$ or 1, only the addition operation is required in computing the projections during iterations. Furthermore, if the data are appropriately scaled, integer arithmetic may be used. Algorithms can be greatly speeded up by eliminating the need for multiplication and floating-point operations.

Convergence Criteria Various methods for deciding when to stop iterating have been proposed. For example a measure of the entropy S^l given by

$$S^l = \frac{-1}{\ln K} \sum_{k=1}^{K} \frac{f_k^l}{\bar{f}} \ln\left(\frac{f_k^l}{\bar{f}}\right) \qquad (7.183)$$

may be used to stop the iterative process according to the outcome of a test such as

$$|S^{l+1} - S^l| < \alpha S^l, \qquad (7.184)$$

where α is the control parameter. The speed of convergence is also influenced strongly by the order in which consecutive corrections are made for those algorithms in which the corrections are immediately applied.

7.3.6 Beam-Hardening Artifacts

The Beam-Hardening Problem

To this point we have assumed that a beam of x rays is exponentially attenuated as it passes through matter. However, clinical x-ray sources emit polychromatic bremsstrahlung radiation, and we must now investigate how this affects the quality of the reconstructions. The problem is that lower-energy x rays are attenuated more strongly than those of higher energy, and as the beam propagates through the body, its spectral properties change. It becomes *harder* as the low-energy *softer* x rays are preferentially removed. Any attempt to reconstruct the image from the raw data without making appropriate corrections for the beam hardening will result in error. Such errors gives rise to *beam-hardening artifacts*, i.e., defects that are observable in the image. The magnitude of the error can be many times greater than the intrinsic noise level and, if unrecognized, beam-hardening artifacts could be misinterpreted as a serious clinical condition, so it is important to understand the cause of the problem and the ways in which it can be handled.

With no absorber in the x-ray path, the detector output is given by

$$I_{p,0} = k_D \int_0^{\mathscr{E}_{max}} S(\mathscr{E})\, d\mathscr{E}, \qquad (7.185)$$

where subscripts p and 0 denote polychromatic and no object, respectively, and k_D is a constant of proportionality. The source spectrum $S(\mathscr{E})$ is defined such that $S(\mathscr{E})\,d\mathscr{E}$ is the energy fluence in the energy range $\mathscr{E}$ to $\mathscr{E} + d\mathscr{E}$ reaching the detector, and the total energy fluence at the detector is thus

$$\Psi_0 = \int_0^{\mathscr{E}_{\max}} S(\mathscr{E})\,d\mathscr{E}. \tag{7.186}$$

In (7.185) and the following discussions we assume for simplicity that the detector responds linearly to the energy incident upon it, which is a good approximation for scintillation detectors. The expressions are readily modified for detectors that operate in a photon-counting mode.

To calculate the detector output with an absorbing object in the beam, Beer's law must be weighted with the energy spectrum and integrated:

$$I_{\mathrm{p}} = k_D \int_0^{\mathscr{E}_{\max}} S(\mathscr{E}) \exp\left(- \int_l \mu(\mathbf{r}, \mathscr{E})\,dl \right) d\mathscr{E}, \tag{7.187}$$

where l is the line-integral path between source and detector, and it is now necessary to take into account both the spatial and energy dependence of the linear attenuation coefficient $\mu(\mathbf{r}, \mathscr{E})$.

The projection values are

$$\begin{aligned} \lambda_{\mathrm{p}} &= -\ln\left(\frac{I_{\mathrm{p}}}{I_{\mathrm{p},0}}\right) \\ &= -\ln\left[\left(\frac{1}{\Psi_0}\right) \int_0^{\mathscr{E}_{\max}} S(\mathscr{E}) \exp\left(- \int_l \mu(\mathbf{r}, \mathscr{E})\,dl \right) d\mathscr{E}\right]. \end{aligned} \tag{7.188}$$

It is this *nonlinear* relationship between λ_{p} and $\mu(\mathbf{r}, \mathscr{E})$ that is the root of the problem. For monochromatic radiation, $S(\mathscr{E}) = \Psi_0\,\delta(\mathscr{E} - \mathscr{E}_0)$, (7.188) reduces to the previously used linear relationship (7.11).

$$\lambda_{\mathrm{m}} = \int_l \mu(\mathbf{r}, \mathscr{E}_0)\,dl. \tag{7.189}$$

We can define two distinct problems, and although both are present in most clinical situations, it is convenient to analyze them separately.

The first is caused by the different path lengths of tissue through which the projections are measured. Consider a uniform circular object made of water. Because proportionately more low-energy photons are absorbed as the path length increases, the projection data recorded for rays passing through the thicker parts are not as high as they should be (see Fig. 7.36). Compared to data derived with a monochromatic source, it appears that the center of the object is less dense than it actually is. Thus if the measured projections are used without correction, the reconstructed image will show

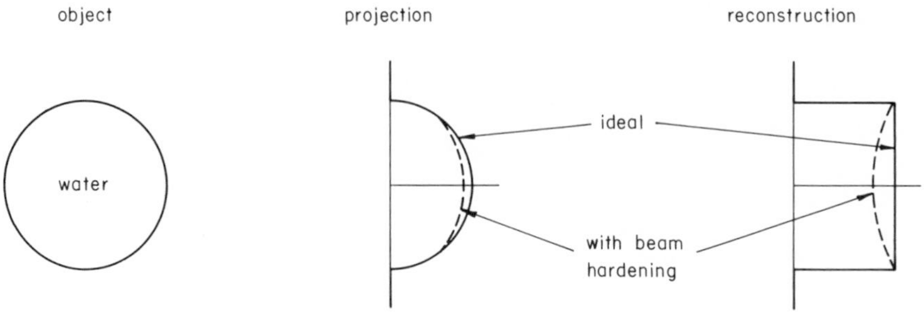

Fig. 7.36 Showing the effects of beam hardening.

a “dishing” or “cupping” artifact. The defect is caused by and depends upon the shape of the object.

The second problem is caused by the nonhomogeneous nature of the object being studied. The energy dependence of the linear attenuation coefficient varies according to the type of material—bone, water-equivalent tissue, fat, air, etc. This can introduce additional artifacts into the image. We now look at four ways by which these problems can be treated.

Single-Component Object

We can generalize the shape problem to include density variations, when it is assumed that all of the attenuating material has the same energy dependence of the mass attenuation coefficient $\mu_m(\mathscr{E})$. This would be the case, for example, where a study contains a large amount of lung ($\rho \approx 0.3$) and other water-equivalent soft tissue. The linear attenuation coefficient is separable:

$$\mu(\mathbf{r}, \mathscr{E}) = \rho(\mathbf{r})\mu_m(\mathscr{E}), \tag{7.190}$$

where $\mu_m(\mathscr{E})$ is the mass attenuation coefficient and $\rho(\mathbf{r})$ is the physical density of the object. Upon substituting (7.190) into (7.188), we obtain

$$\lambda_p = -\ln\left[\left(\frac{1}{\Psi_0}\right)\int_0^{\mathscr{E}_{max}} S(\mathscr{E})\exp\left(-\mu_m(\mathscr{E})\int_l \rho(\mathbf{r})\,dl\right)d\mathscr{E}\right]. \tag{7.191}$$

Again we have a nonlinear relationship. This time it is between the measured projection λ_p and the line integral of the physical density distribution $\rho(\mathbf{r})$. However, since $S(\mathscr{E})$ and $\mu_m(\mathscr{E})$ are presumed known, it is a simple matter to determine $\int\rho(\mathbf{r})\,dl$ given λ_p. By calculation or measurement, it can be shown that $\int\rho(\mathbf{r})\,dl$ and λ_p are almost linearly related, so it is convenient to define a corrected projection λ'_p that is linearly related to $\int\rho(\mathbf{r})\,dl$:

$$\lambda'_p = k_\lambda \int_l \rho(\mathbf{r})\,dl = f(\lambda_p). \tag{7.192}$$

We choose the constant k_λ so that $\lambda_p/\lambda'_p \to 1$ as $\int \rho(\mathbf{r})\,dl \to 0$. Thus λ'_p can be written

$$\lambda'_p = f(\lambda_p) = \lambda_p + \alpha\lambda_p^2 + \cdots. \tag{7.193}$$

For situations of clinical interest, α is typically in the range 0.01–0.03.

From (7.191), it is straightforward to show that

$$k_\lambda = \int_0^{\mathscr{E}_{\max}} \mu_m(\mathscr{E})S(\mathscr{E})\,d\mathscr{E} \bigg/ \int_0^{\mathscr{E}_{\max}} S(\mathscr{E})\,d\mathscr{E} = \bar{\mu}_m, \tag{7.194}$$

i.e., $\bar{\mu}_m$ is simply the average (over the source spectrum) of the mass attenuation coefficient.

It is apparent that $\bar{\mu}_m\rho(\mathbf{r})$ is just the average linear attenuation coefficient

$$\bar{\mu}(\mathbf{r}) = \bar{\mu}_m\rho(\mathbf{r}) = k_\lambda\rho(\mathbf{r}). \tag{7.195}$$

Thus the reconstruction algorithm is as follows: (1) The projection data λ_p are scaled using (7.193) to corrected values λ'_p. (2) According to (7.192) and (7.195), the λ'_p are the true line integrals of the (energy) averaged linear attenuation coefficient. These projections λ'_p are processed by any of the algorithms described previously.

Herman (1979) has shown that under some conditions beam-hardening artifacts can be substantially reduced even for multicomponent objects (water, lung, fat, and bone) by using polynomial approximations of the form,

$$\lambda'_p = \alpha_0 + \alpha_1\lambda_p + \alpha_2\lambda_p^2. \tag{7.196}$$

Water-Bath Compensation

Some commercial CT head scanners use water-bath techniques. The patient's head is surrounded by a water-filled bag arranged so that there is always a constant length L of absorber, either head or water, between the source and detector. Under these circumstances, we can write, using (7.187),

$$I_p = k_D \int_0^{\mathscr{E}_{\max}} S(\mathscr{E})\exp[-\mu_w(\mathscr{E})L]\exp\left(-\int_l [\mu(\mathbf{r},\mathscr{E}) - \mu_w(\mathscr{E})]\,dl\right)d\mathscr{E}, \tag{7.197}$$

where subscript w refers to the water. The factor $S(\mathscr{E})\exp[-\mu_w(\mathscr{E})L]$ can be replaced with $S_w(\mathscr{E})$, a modified system spectral response given by the product of $S(\mathscr{E})$ and a filter function corresponding to L cm of water:

$$I_p = k_D \int_0^{\mathscr{E}_{\max}} S_w(\mathscr{E})\exp\left(-\int_l [\mu(\mathbf{r},\mathscr{E}) - \mu_w(\mathscr{E})]\,dl\right)d\mathscr{E}. \tag{7.198}$$

To proceed further, we look at the value of the exponent. First, suppose that only soft tissue is in the beam, then $\mu(\mathbf{r},\mathscr{E}) - \mu_w(\mathscr{E})$ is typically 0.01 cm^{-1}.

(Most brain tissue has an attenuation coefficient within 5% of that of water, and $\mu_w \approx 0.2\ \mathrm{cm}^{-1}$.) For a typical value of 15 cm for a head diameter, the exponent in (7.198) is unlikely to exceed 0.15, and we can make use of the approximation $e^x \simeq 1 + x$. Large amounts of bone or air or adipose tissue will invalidate this argument, but small amounts are tolerable. Thus we can write

$$I_p \approx k_D \int_0^{\mathscr{E}_{max}} S_w(\mathscr{E}) \left(1 - \int_l [\mu(\mathbf{r}, \mathscr{E}) - \mu_w(\mathscr{E})]\, dl \right) d\mathscr{E}. \tag{7.199}$$

The signal received when the beam passes through only water is given by

$$I_w = k_D \int_0^{\mathscr{E}_{max}} S_w(\mathscr{E})\, d\mathscr{E}. \tag{7.200}$$

Thus we have

$$\frac{I_p}{I_w} \approx 1 - \left(\int_0^{\mathscr{E}_{max}} \int_l S_w(\mathscr{E})[\mu(\mathbf{r}, \mathscr{E}) - \mu_w(\mathscr{E})]\, dl\, d\mathscr{E} \Big/ \int S_w(\mathscr{E})\, d\mathscr{E} \right), \tag{7.201}$$

which is equivalent to

$$-\ln\left(\frac{I_p}{I_w}\right) = -\ln\left[1 - \int_l (\bar{\mu}(\mathbf{r}) - \bar{\mu}_w)\, dl\right] \approx \int_l (\bar{\mu}(\mathbf{r}) - \bar{\mu}_w)\, dl \tag{7.202}$$

In (7.202) we have simply defined $\bar{\mu}$ to be the average over the energy spectrum $S_w(\mathscr{E})$ of the corresponding μ. This time it is the *exit* spectrum, i.e., the source spectrum as filtered by length L of water, so that

$$\bar{\mu}(\mathbf{r}) = \int_0^{\mathscr{E}_{max}} S_w(\mathscr{E}) \mu(r, \mathscr{E})\, d\mathscr{E} \Big/ \int_0^{\mathscr{E}_{max}} S_w(\mathscr{E})\, d\mathscr{E}. \tag{7.203}$$

The constant $\bar{\mu}_w$ is a similarly defined quantity. Equation (7.203) is a linear relationship involving $\bar{\mu}(\mathbf{r})$ and the measured quantity I_p and thus forms the basis for the reconstruction algorithms. Thus, provided that the approximation used in deriving (7.199) is valid, the water bath method provides a solution to the beam-hardening problem. In practice, sufficient bone may be present that the approximation is not good enough and image artifacts will be visible.

Water baths are inconvenient except for head scanners. In some body scanners the water bath is replaced by one or more metal "dodgers" that are placed before and after the patient. Made of a low-atomic-number material such as aluminum so as to mimic water as closely as possible, these shaped metal sections provide a beam profile that in some average sense equalizes the line integral of attenuation for all beams. Results are often improved by using boluses of water-equivalent material packed around the patient in order to provide a roughly circular and hence symmetric cross section. Water baths and other dodging methods have the advantage of limiting the dynamic range requirements of the detector array. However, since some of the radiation that passes through the patient is scattered out of beam before reaching the detector, an unnecessarily high patient dose is delivered.

An Iterative Solution

When large amounts of bone are present in the section, the previous methods of correction are inadequate and deleterious image artifacts persist. The problem arises because bone has a different absorption spectrum from soft tissue. Low-energy x rays are more strongly absorbed because of photoelectric absorption by the calcium content. The iterative correction method simply determines those parts of the object that contain bone and then corrects the projections to account for the different spectral absorption properties in these regions. A preliminary reconstruction is made using the single-component algorithm (7.192)–(7.195). This eliminates gross shading and cupping artifacts. The resulting image is then subjected to a threshold or other test that identifies the areas of bone. The original projections can now be corrected for the presence of bone and an essentially artifact-free image reconstructed. Details of the method are described by Kijewski and Bjärngard (1978).

Dual-Energy Scanning

The absorption spectrum of a material depends upon its atomic composition, and thus there is additional information that may be put to good use. For x rays of diagnostic energy, attenuation takes place almost entirely by one of two processes: photoelectric absorption and Compton scattering. The energy dependences of these processes are known, and the linear attenuation coefficient can be separated into spatially varying and energy varying components as follows:

$$\mu(\mathbf{r}, \mathscr{E}) = a_{\mathrm{p}}(\mathbf{r})(1/\mathscr{E}^3) + a_{\mathrm{C}}(\mathbf{r}) f_{\mathrm{KN}}(\mathscr{E}), \tag{7.204}$$

where $a_{\mathrm{p}}(\mathbf{r})$ is a coefficient related to photoelectric absorption, given approximately by

$$a_{\mathrm{p}}(\mathbf{r}) = K \sum_i \frac{Z_i^4 \rho_i(\mathbf{r})}{A_i} \tag{7.205}$$

where Z_i, A_i, and $\rho_i(\mathbf{r})$ are the atomic number, atomic weight, and density distribution of the ith atomic species within the absorber [see (C.11)]. Similarly, $a_{\mathrm{C}}(r)$ is a coefficient related to Compton scattering, and given by

$$a_{\mathrm{C}}(\mathbf{r}) = \sigma^{\mathrm{C}} \sum_i \frac{N_0 Z_i}{A_i} \rho_i(\mathbf{r}), \tag{7.206}$$

and $f_{KN}(\mathscr{E})$ is the Klein–Nishina function [see (C.21) and (C.23)]. The general expression for the line integral can now be decomposed into two parts,

$$\int_l \mu(\mathbf{r}, \mathscr{E})\, dl = \frac{1}{\mathscr{E}^3} \int_l a_p(\mathbf{r})\, dl + f_{KN}(\mathscr{E}) \int_l a_C(\mathbf{r})\, dl$$

$$= A_p/\mathscr{E}^3 + A_c f_{KN}(\mathscr{E}), \tag{7.207}$$

where

$$A_p = \int_l a_p(\mathbf{r})\, dl, \qquad A_C = \int_l a_C(\mathbf{r})\, dl. \tag{7.208}$$

We are seeking a reconstruction of $\mu(\mathbf{r}, \mathscr{E})$, or rather its energy-independent components $a_p(\mathbf{r})$ and $a_C(\mathbf{r})$. To do this, we need to evaluate A_p and A_C for all projections through the object and then proceed using the methods described earlier. Two pieces of information are needed for each projection. These may be obtained by taking measurements with two different source spectra $S_1(\mathscr{E})$ and $S_2(\mathscr{E})$:

$$I_1 = k_D \int_0^{\mathscr{E}_{\max}} S_1(\mathscr{E}) \exp(-A_p/\mathscr{E}^3 - A_C f_{KN})\, d\mathscr{E},$$

$$I_2 = k_D \int_0^{\mathscr{E}_{\max}} S_2(\mathscr{E}) \exp(-A_p/\mathscr{E}^3 + A_C f_{KN})\, d\mathscr{E}. \tag{7.209}$$

These integral equations may be solved for A_p and A_C provided that the Jacobian,

$$J = \det \begin{vmatrix} \dfrac{\partial I_1}{\partial A_p} & \dfrac{\partial I_1}{\partial A_C} \\ \dfrac{\partial I_2}{\partial A_p} & \dfrac{\partial I_2}{\partial A_C} \end{vmatrix} \tag{7.210}$$

is nonzero, a condition that is not difficult to arrange in practice. The more dissimilar $S_1(\mathscr{E})$ and $S_2(\mathscr{E})$, the better conditioned the equations become.

A variation on this method is to expand the expression for the measurements (7.209) in the form

$$\begin{aligned} \ln I_1 &= b_0 + b_1 A_p + b_2 A_C + b_3 A_p^2 + b_4 A_C^2 + b_5 A_p A_C + b_6 A_p^3 + b_7 A_C^3, \\ \ln I_2 &= c_0 + c_1 A_p + c_2 A_C + c_3 A_p^2 + c_4 A_C^2 + c_5 A_p A_C + c_6 A_p^3 + c_7 A_C^3, \end{aligned} \tag{7.211}$$

where the coefficients $[b_i]$ and $[c_i]$ are determined by the source spectra. These simultaneous cubic equations may be solved for A_p and A_C, given I_1 and I_2 from measurements.

Decomposition methods like this are interesting because they permit the identification of actual tissue type (see Fig. 7.37). The soft-tissue discrimina-

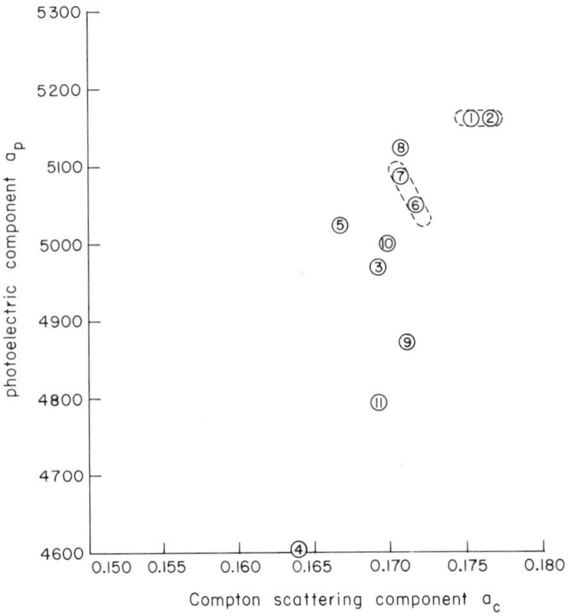

Fig. 7.37 Two-dimensional plot of the information available from energy spectral analysis. The values of the coefficients a_p and a_C are calculated from measurements of the attenuation coefficients of body materials at 16 energies in the diagnostic region. Each point represents the (a_p, a_C) values for a given body material:

1. Clotted blood
2. Clotted blood
3. Subdural haematoma
4. Water
5. Neuroma
6. Meningioma
7. Meningioma
8. Medullablastoma
9. Astrocytoma
10. Human grey matter
11. Human white matter

(From Alvarez and Macovski, 1976.)

tion is predominantly along the $a_p(\mathbf{r})$ axis due to the sensitivity of $a_p(\mathbf{r})$ to the (effective) atomic number of the material. For typical conditions, the error in determining A_p and hence $a_p(\mathbf{r})$ is substantially greater than that in determining A_C and hence $a_C(\mathbf{r})$ because the lower-energy photons, which interact mainly by the photoelectric effect, are strongly absorbed within the body. There are relatively few transmitted, and the statistical accuracy is reduced. This method was first described by Alvarez and Macovski (1976).

7.4 EMISSION COMPUTED TOMOGRAPHY

7.4.1 Introduction

Gamma rays emitted from a radioactive body organ are emitted with a uniform angular probability distribution. If we measure the distribution of only those gamma rays whose initial trajectories are contained within a specified flat slice, we have a situation quite analogous to x-ray transmission computed tomography. The difference is that with x rays we determine the sectional distribution of linear attenuation coefficient, whereas with gamma rays we determine the sectional distribution of radioactivity.

There are two methods used in emission tomography. The first one uses gamma-emitting radionuclides such as ^{99m}Tc that emit a single gamma ray in the nuclear disintegration. This gives rise to the single-photon-counting (SPC) method. The other method uses a positron-emitting radionuclide and *annihilation coincidence detection* (ACD). The emitted positron interacts by annihilation with an electron within a very small distance from the decaying nucleus to form two gamma rays traveling (almost) exactly in opposite directions. The annihilation gamma rays are identified by a coincidence detector and are used to form the sectional images. Noncoincident gamma events are ignored.

7.4.2 Single-Photon Counting

Collimator Considerations

An elementary system for data collection is shown in Fig. 7.38. A collimated detector makes a series of linear scans over the patient. After each scan, the detector gantry is rotated slightly. This scanning action defines a tomographic section within the patient, and the data set that is collected is related to the line integrals of the distribution of activity within that section.

The activity within the patient is described by a three-dimensional distribution of activity $f[x, y, z]$ (events per cubic centimeter per second), but in a single tomographic reconstruction no attempt is made to recover the variation of $f[x, y, z]$ in the z direction. Indeed, such variations are often deliberately suppressed by presuming that the distribution over the z direction is constant, so that the activity $f[x, y, z]$ can be written simply as $f[x, y]$ or, in the rotated frame, $f_r[x_r, y_r]$. This is the same assumption that is made for x-ray computed tomography, and emission tomography is susceptible to all of the partial-volume problems discussed in Section 7.3.1.

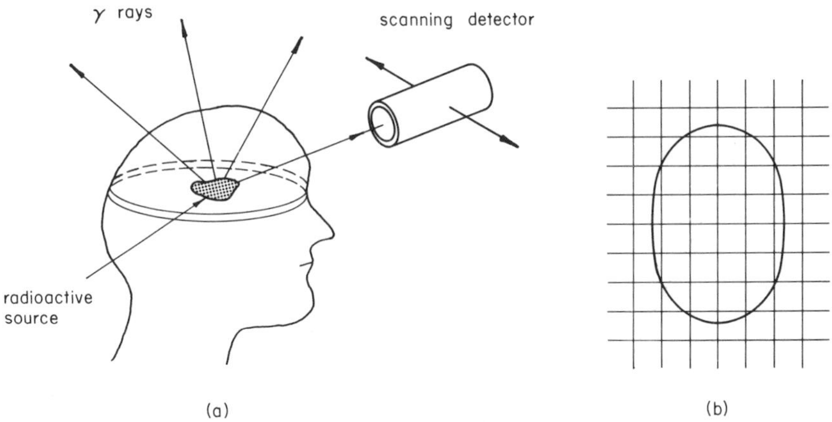

Fig. 7.38 (a) In its simplest form, single-photon emission tomography is performed with a single, collimated scanning detector. The complete data set consists of many parallel scans taken at a number of different angles within the plane. (b) The scans for just two of these directions are shown.

The response of the single-bore collimator is discussed in detail in Section 4.4.3, and the three-dimensional point spread function is given by (4.75). For the present purposes, a slight notational change is required since now the bore of the collimator is parallel to the y_r axis, whereas it was parallel to the z axis in Chapter 4. Thus, with the substitutions $\mathbf{r}_s \to (x_r, z)$, $z \to y_r$, (4.75) is applicable to the present problem. It is also useful to delete the factor of n_l/v_s from (4.75) since we are no longer discussing a raster scan.

The instantaneous count rate of the detector is given by

$$\text{count rate} = p_{sb}(x_r, y_r, z) *** f_r[x_r, y_r, z]. \tag{7.212}$$

This equation is a generalization of (4.94) to a three-dimensional object, but it neglects attenuation of the gamma rays by the object.

If the bore of the collimator is long and thin, $p_{sb}(x_r, y_r, z)$ is very compact in the x_r–z plane and may often be approximated by a two-dimensional delta function of suitable weight:

$$p_{sb}(x_r, y_r, z) \approx \delta(x_r)\,\delta(z) \int_\infty dx_r \int_\infty dz\, p_{sb}(x_r, y_r, z). \tag{7.213}$$

With the help of the discussion leading up to (4.98), this equation becomes

$$p_{sb}(x_r, y_r, z) \approx (\pi D_b^4/64L_b^2)\,\delta(x_r)\,\delta(z). \tag{7.214}$$

Note that (7.214) is independent of the depth dimension y_r.

It is valid to use the approximation (7.214) in (7.212) whenever $f_r[x_r, y_r, z]$ varies slowly compared to the width of the PSF in the x_r–z plane. Under

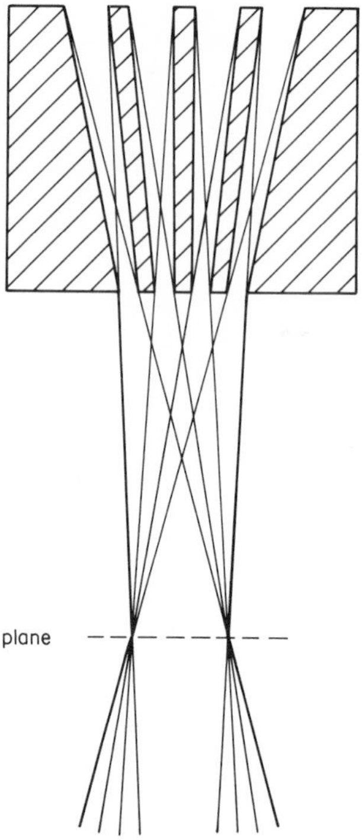

Fig. 7.39 Multihole focused collimator is suitable for single particle emission tomography because the response does not broaden significantly until the focal plane is reached.

those conditions, (7.212) becomes

$$\text{count rate} = \frac{\pi D_b^4}{64L_b^2}\int_\infty f_r[x_r, y_r, z]\,dy_r. \qquad (7.215)$$

We recognize the integral as the usual projection $\lambda_\phi(x_r)$, and can write

$$\text{count rate} = (\pi D_b^4/64L_b^2)\lambda_\phi(x_r). \qquad (7.216)$$

Thus the projection $\lambda_\phi(x_r)$ is directly measurable in this manner if attenuation is negligible.

The assumption that p_{sb} can be approximated by a delta function must be valid over the entire working depth range of the object if (7.216) is to hold. Single-bore collimators are not satisfactory in this respect because the penumbra increasingly widens the PSF with distance from the collimator face. The best type of collimator is a multihole focused collimator, designed to give a uniformly wide response out as far as the focal plane. After the focal plane, the PSF diverges rapidly with penumbra effects. Projection data from reasonably well-defined domains of integration can be obtained by

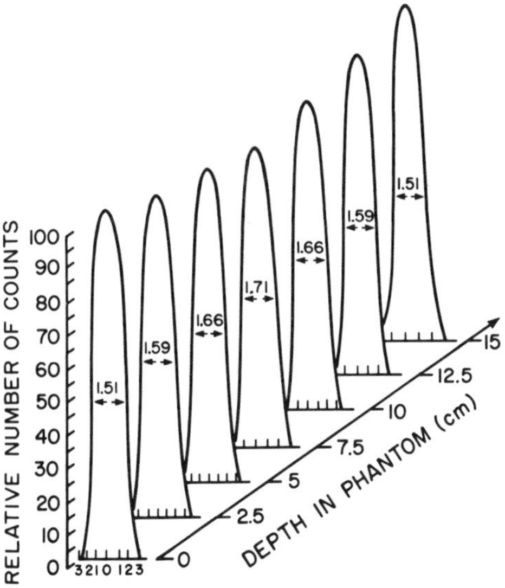

Fig. 7.40 Line spread function of a collimator optimized for single-photon emission tomography. Views from opposing directions have been combined and corrections for attenuation have been incorporated. (From Kircos *et al.*, 1978.)

combining data taken exactly along the same line but from opposite directions. Radiation originating from beyond the focal plane where collimation is poor is attenuated by scattering and absorption within the patient, and the deleterious effects of a broadening domain of integration are minimized (see Fig. 7.40).

Processing Algorithms

We showed above that the measured count rate is proportional to the projection $\lambda_\phi(x_r)$ if attenuation of the gamma rays in the patient's body is ignored. However, for the gamma-ray energies commonly encountered in nuclear medicine, attenuation cannot be ignored, and a weighting function $w(x_r, y_r, \phi)$ must be included. Denoting the count rate by $C_\phi(x_r)$, we can write

$$C_\phi(x_r) = k \int_\infty f_r[x_r, y_r] w(x_r, y_r, \phi)\, dy_r, \tag{7.217}$$

with $k = \pi D_b^4/64L_b^2$ and

$$w(x_r, y_r, \phi) = \exp\left(-\int_{(x_r, y_r)}^{D} \mu_r[x_r, y_r']\, dy_r'\right), \tag{7.218}$$

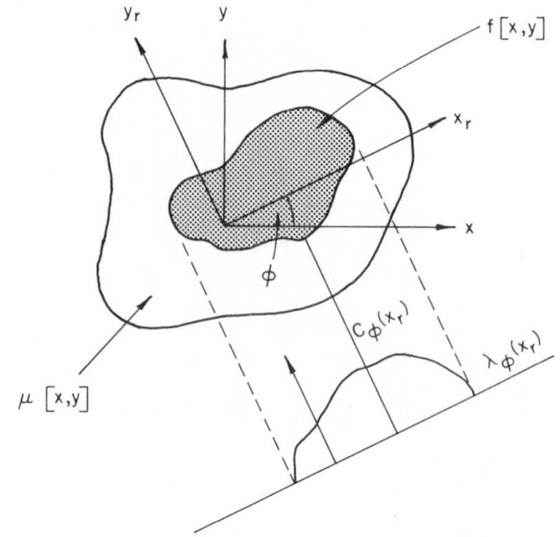

Fig. 7.41 In emission tomography there are two distributions to consider. $f[x, y]$ is the distribution of radioactivity and $\mu[x, y]$ is the linear attenuation coefficient of the body.

where as usual $\mu_r[x_r, y_r]$ is the linear attenuation coefficient in the rotated frame. We have here suppressed the uninteresting z dependence of both $\mu_r[\ ]$ and $f_r[\ ]$. The symbolic limits $(x_r, y_r) \to D$ denote that the integration is to be carried out between a given point of interest (x_r, y_r) and the detector D (see Fig. 7.41). The function $w(x_r, y_r, \phi)$ thus represents the attenuation in the flux of photons that are emitted from (x_r, y_r) and detected at projection position (x_r, ϕ). There is no known analytical solution for $f[x, y]$ in (7.217) except for trivial distributions of μ and f, so in practice iterative and approximate methods of solution are employed.

Two principal ways of handling the attenuation problem have evolved:

(1) The data are prefiltered; then techniques of x-ray CT reconstructions are used.

(2) Iterative methods using measured or assumed distributions of $\mu[x, y]$ are employed.

Prefiltering is more or less useful depending upon the structure of the object. Consider the object shown in Fig. 7.42 for which we assume that the radioactivity is confined to the small region (organ) and is uniformly distributed. We need data that will permit the reconstruction of the shape of the region and determine the activity therein. A collimated detector D_1 will generate a count rate C_1 given by

$$C_1 = k \int_{y_2}^{y_1} A \exp[-\mu(y - y_a)]\, dy, \qquad (7.219)$$

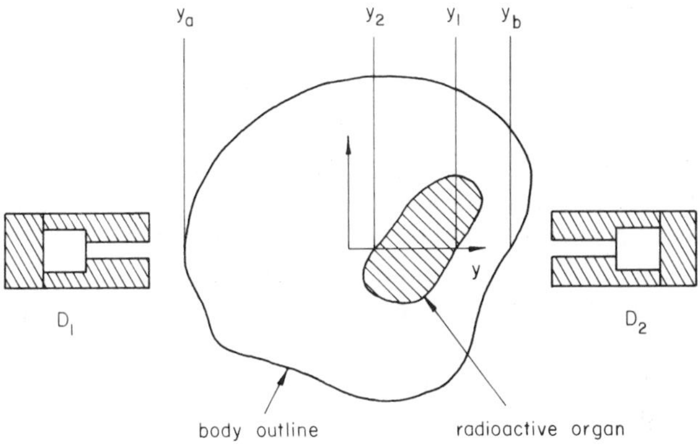

Fig. 7.42 Showing the geometry needed to derive the algorithm (7.223) which corrects the projection data for attenuation within the body.

where A is the activity, y_1 and y_2 define the organ edges, and y_a defines the body boundary nearest to D_1. If there were no attenuation, the desired line integral $A(y_1 - y_2)$ would be available immediately using $\mu = 0$ in (7.219):

$$C_1 = kA(y_1 - y_2). \tag{7.220}$$

It would then be straightforward to reconstruct the section using a set of such measured projections. However, for $\mu > 0$ we have

$$C_1 = (Ak/\mu)\exp(\mu y_a)[\exp(-\mu y_2) - \exp(-\mu y_1)]. \tag{7.221}$$

With the detector at D_2, i.e., exactly opposite the original position, the count rate will be

$$C_2 = (Ak/\mu)\exp(-\mu y_b)[\exp(\mu y_1) - \exp(\mu y_2)], \tag{7.222}$$

where y_b defines the edge of the object at D_2. For sufficiently small objects $(y_1 - y_2) \ll \mu^{-1}$, it is simple to show that

$$(C_1 C_2)^{1/2} = kA(y_1 - y_2)\exp(-\mu L/2). \tag{7.223}$$

This is a useful result. The overall length of the absorbing medium L $(= y_b - y_a)$ can always be obtained by measurement either directly or indirectly using transmission gamma rays. Thus we have a method for determining the required line integral [in this case $A(y_1 - y_2)$] for each projection, and the reconstruction follows at once. Because of the nonlinear nature of the algorithm, the method has limitations. For example, an activity distribution containing two small regions a distance Δ apart, each satisfying $\mu(y_1 - y_2) \ll 1$, will not yield a consistent data set when the $(C_1 C_2)^{1/2}$ algorithm is applied. It is straightforward to show that the line integral computed using (7.223) for the projection that passes through both regions will be higher than it should be. If the total activity at each site is the same, the fractional error is approximately $(\mu\Delta)^2/8$. Nevertheless, this prefiltering method, and others similar to it, have been used with considerable success.

The iterative solutions are similar to those discussed in Section 7.3.4. After an estimate of the object activity has been formed, the corresponding projections, corrected for attenuation, are computed. The difference between the results of this computation and the true projection data are then used for further iterations as necessary. The corrections for attenuation are based on assumed or measured body shape and distribution of attenuation coefficient. Reconstructions formed this way are generally more accurate than those obtained with prefiltering methods, but they are computationally much more expensive and require additional patient dose when x-ray or isotope transmission measurements are made to determine $\mu[x, y]$. Budinger and Gullberg (1977) give a detailed review of reconstruction algorithms for single-particle systems.

Typical Camera Systems

The Humongotron (Keyes *et al.*, 1977) uses a standard Anger camera head and collimator mounted so that it can rotate around the head of the patient (see Fig. 7.43). Each circular image (25 cm in diameter) is digitized into a 64×64 matrix and typically 60 views with 6° increments are used.

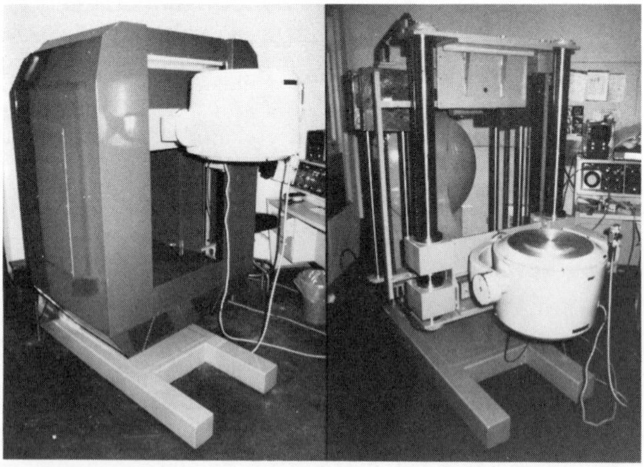

Fig. 7.43 The Humongotron, a single-photon emission tomography system using an Anger camera. (From Keyes *et al.*, 1977.)

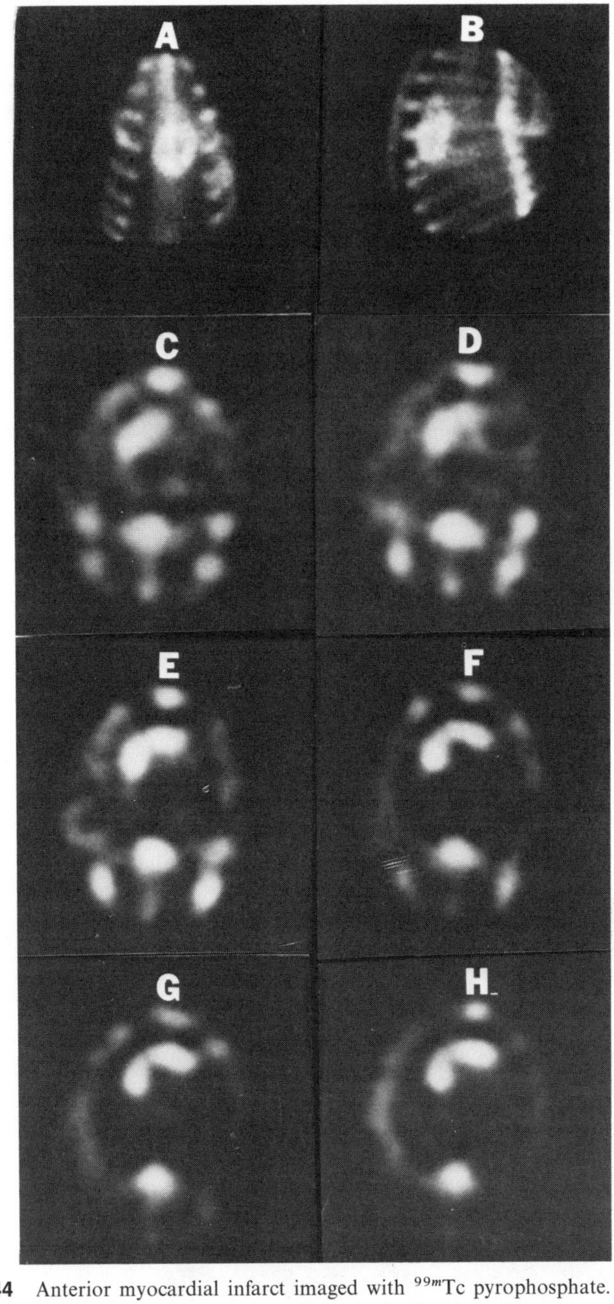

Fig. 7.44 Anterior myocardial infarct imaged with ^{99m}Tc pyrophosphate. A and B are conventional gamma camera images. C through H, obtained with the Humongotron, are successive tomographic sections beginning near the base (C) and progressing towards the apex (H). (From Keyes *et al.*, 1978.)

Having a two-dimensional detector means that projections of several (8–10) different sections may be recorded simultaneously. Apart from the non-standard mounting, the system is a conventional camera. Typical results are shown in Fig. 7.44.

The Mark IV Scanner (Kuhl *et al.*, 1976) is a system employing a four-sided arrangement of 32 independent detectors that rotate continuously as a unit, detecting, processing, and displaying the data while the study progresses (see Fig. 7.45). The only motion is rotation. Each bank of eight detecting crystals is tangentially offset by a small amount with respect to the others, creating 32 evenly spaced samples on each parallel projection. Data processing is by means of an ART type of algorithm using additive correction. The use of orthogonal projections provides rapid convergence. Mark IV images are shown in Fig. 7.46.

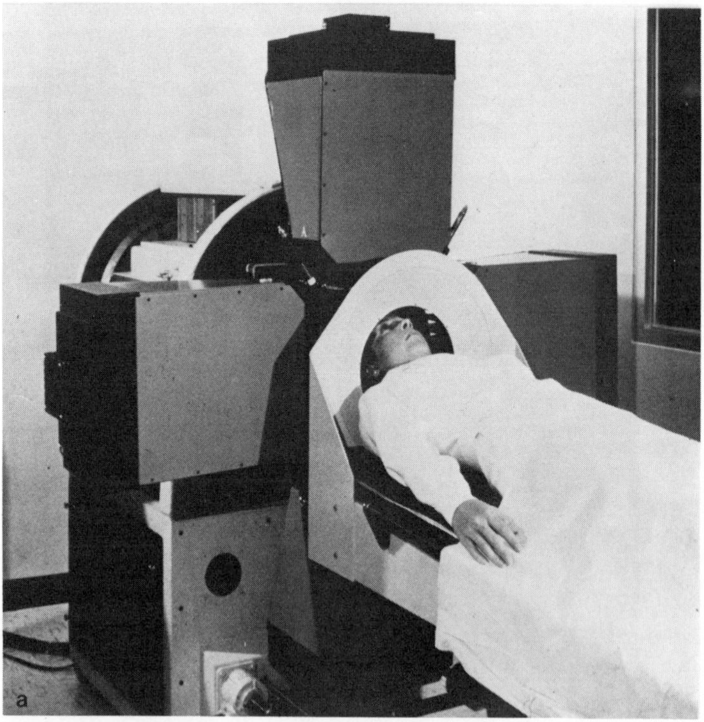

Fig. 7.45 Mark IV Scanner. A single-photon emission tomography system using 32 separate detectors arranged in 4 banks of 8. The detector banks rotate as a unit around the patient. (a) Equipment photograph. (b) Schematic diagram. (From Kuhl *et al.*, 1976.)

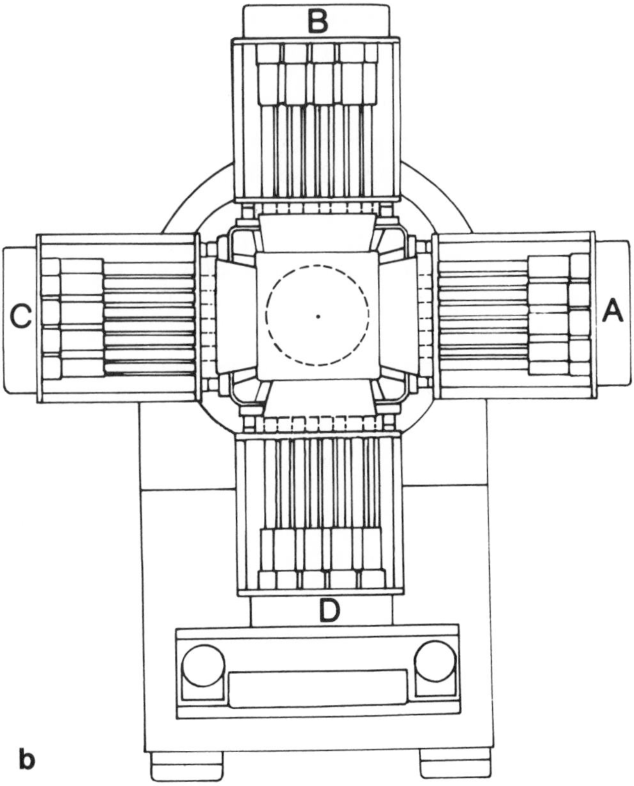

b

Fig. 7.45 *(continued)*

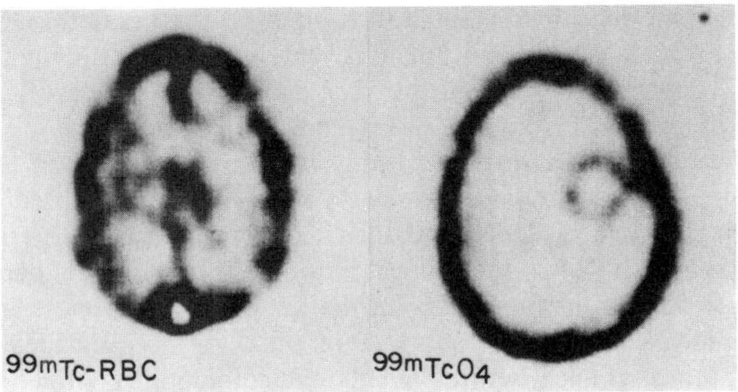

Fig. 7.46 Results from the Mark IV Scanner. Brain scans of a 17-year-old woman showing intracerebral hematoma. Left: image using ^{99m}Tc labeled red blood cells. Right: image using pertechnetate. (From Kuhl *et al.*, 1976.)

7.4.3 Annihilation Coincidence Detection

Principles of Operations

Several elements, including carbon, oxygen, and nitrogen, have isotopes that decay by positron emission. These elements are useful for nuclear imaging because they appear with great abundance in biological systems and pharmaceutical compounds, and there is the potential for developing tracer materials for investigating a wide range of physiological functions.

In water-equivalent material, the positron travels only a few millimeters before it annihilates with an electron, producing two oppositely directed 511-keV gamma rays in the process. Since these gamma rays originate close to the site of original decay, the distribution of radioactivity can be mapped. As we shall see, there are advantages from the imaging viewpoint to using a detection scheme that responds only when both gamma rays are detected in coincidence.

The major problem with ACD is that the more useful isotopes have a half-life of only a few minutes. It is necessary to have the isotope-producing facility (such as a cyclotron) in close proximity. Whether or not the improved images and potential for new studies can justify the cost of a cyclotron facility is a question that has not yet been resolved.

Superficially, SPC and ACD systems have similar appearances, with moving or stationary banks of gamma-ray detectors that encompass the subject, but the details of the collimators and detection circuitry are quite different.

Collimator Considerations

If we assume that the annihilation gamma rays are exactly collinear, it follows that when a true coincidence event is detected, the annihilation event must have taken place in the tube defined by the apertures of the detectors involved. This volume is very precisely defined, and the lack of physical barriers for in-plane collimation has given rise to the term *electronic collimation* (see Fig. 7.47). Since the detectors are not individually collimated, the counting efficiency is greatly enhanced; any given detector can register a coincidence with any other opposing detector in the array. Other parameters being equal, the count rate for coincidences using N detectors increases approximately as N^2, whereas the count rate for noncoincident events ("singles") increases linearly with N. Although collimators are not needed to define the volume in which the annihilation took place, they are needed to shield the detectors from radiation emitted or scattered from regions outside the tomographic plane.

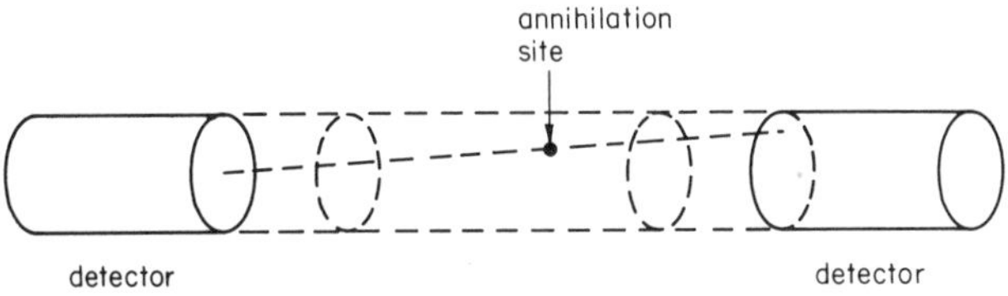

Fig. 7.47 When a true coincidence count is observed with appropriately directed gamma rays, the source event must lie in the volume defined by the detector faces.

Algorithms

The correction factor for attenuation of the gamma-ray pair is easy to determine. Consider a gamma-ray pair in air that creates a coincidence event on a pair of perfect detectors. With respect to this ideal situation, the relative probabilty that the coincidence would be detected with imperfect detectors and an attenuating medium is

$$p = [\eta \exp(-\mu l_1)][\eta \exp(-\mu l_2)], \tag{7.224}$$

where l_1 and l_2 are the path lengths in the attenuator for the two gamma rays, and η is the detector quantum efficiency. This probability is simply the product of the individual single-event probabilities. The total length of absorber L for any detector pair is simply given by $L = l_1 + l_2$, and the relative probability of detection is thus given by

$$p = \eta^2 \exp(-\mu L). \tag{7.225}$$

Thus the attenuation losses for a given detector pair can be exactly compensated by multiplying the coincidence count rate by a factor $e^{\mu L}$. Distance L can be determined from measurement or by using transmission tomography. Thus the data are modified by this factor and the activity distribution is then determined using any of the standard methods of tomographic reconstructions.

Count-Rate Considerations

In addition to the true coincidences, there are also false coincidences from an annihilation pair, one or both of which have been scattered prior to detection. Except for those scattering events that take place in the plane of the tomographic slice, these false counts can be reduced by careful screening. There are also false coincidences caused by independently produced gamma rays arriving at two detectors within the discrimination time set by the electronics. False coincidences increase in direct proportion to the

TABLE 7.1

High-Resolution Positron Ring Detector[a,b]

Quantity	Symbol	Units	Case I	Case II	Case III
Energy resolution (FWHM) at 511 keV	Γ	%	None	30	15
Energy threshold	E_p	KeV	100	410[c,d]	460[c,d]
Rate for true unscattered coincident events	C_1	events per sec	7100	1010	1010
Sensitivity	C_t/ρ	events per sec per [μCi/cm]	36	25	25
Coincidence rate for one-gamma scatter	C_1	events per sec	1840	270	220
Coincidence rate for two-gamma scatter	C_2	events per sec	1180	175	120
Singles rate for entire ring	C_s	10^5 events per sec	10.4	1.8	1.5
Accidental coincidence rate for entire ring	C_a	events per sec	1200	37	24
Total event rate $(C_t + C_1 + C_2 + C_a)$		events per sec	11 320	1529	1397
Background fraction $\dfrac{C_1 + C_2 + C_a}{C_t + C_1 + C_2 + C_a}$		%	37	34	28
Paralyzing deadtime	t_p	nsec	200	800	800
Fraction of events lost due to deadtime[d]	f_e	%	5[d]	23[d]	23[d]

[a] Adapted from Derenzo *et al.* (1977).

[b] Physical specification of assumed ring detector system are as follows: e: detector ring radius = 40 cm; s: shielding slit width = 2 cm; T: shielding slit depth = 20 cm; P_s: probability of scattering on emerging from the center of a 20-cm-diam cylinder of tissue = 63%; $f = 0.22$ (for 280 crystals, each would be in coincidence with the opposing 62 crystals); $\theta_j = 40^\circ$ maximum scattering angle imposed by coincidence requirement (approximate): ρ: activity density = 200 μCi per axial cm; t: time resolution = 10 nsec; dimension of crystals along gamma line of flight = 5 cm, dimension of crystals along ring axis = 3 cm, dimension of crystals transverse to ring axis = 0.8 cm; R = radius of uniform geometrical sensitivity = 14 cm; G = gross singles rate per segment = 1.3×10^5 counts per sec.

[c] Corresponds to a 7% photopeak loss, assuming that the photopeak has a Gaussian distribution.

[d] This event loss has not been included elsewhere in this table.

discrimination time. Single events, while not contributing to the image, outnumber the coincidence events by typically 100–1000, and since the ability of a detector to respond to a coincidence event is temporarily nulled following the receipt of a single event, it is important to reduce single events as much as possible by shielding. Typical paralysis and coincidence resolution times for NaI crystals and fast electronics are 1 μS and 10 nS, respectively. The paralysis time can be decreased if energy discrimination is not used.

The system can be made to reject scattered gamma rays whose energy is less than an adjustable threshold. This improves image quality by reducing background counts. Table 7.1 illustrates the effect of changing the energy threshold for a ring arrangement of detectors. Figure 7.48 shows the geometry of the array used in assembling Table 7.1. See also Derenzo *et al.* (1981) for a description of the imaging properties of a 280-detector positron ring camera.

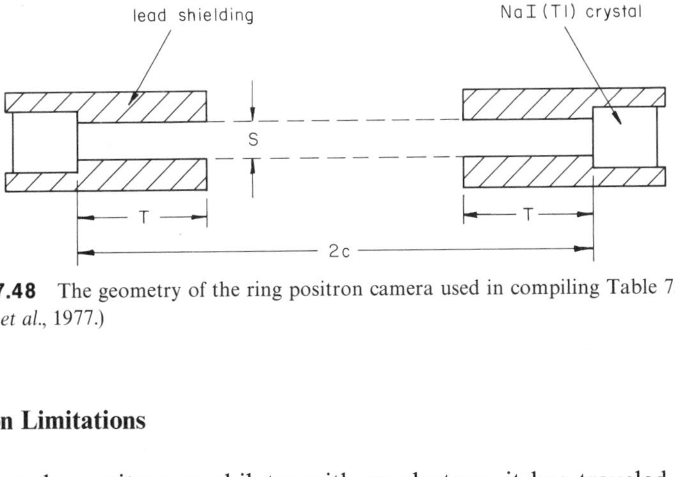

Fig. 7.48 The geometry of the ring positron camera used in compiling Table 7.1. (From Derenzo *et al.*, 1977.)

Positron Limitations

When the positron annhilates with an electron, it has traveled a short distance from the nucleus of origin. There is thus a contribution to the total image line spread function that is caused by the uncertainty in the location of the emitting nucleus. This contribution is difficult to calculate on theoretical grounds, but measurements indicate that it is in the range of 1–2 mm FMHM and 2–6 mm FWTM (full width at tenth-maximum). The FWHM due to positron range may be roughly estimated (Brownell *et al.*, 1978) by

$$\text{FWHM (mm)} = \frac{\mathscr{E}_{\max}\ (\text{meV})}{\rho\ (\text{gm cm}^{-3})}, \qquad (7.226)$$

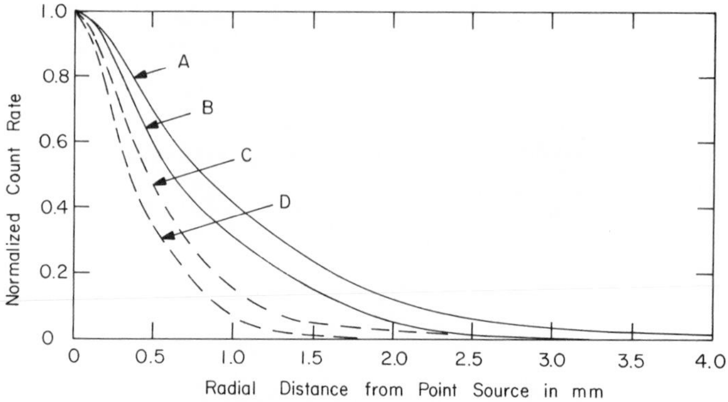

Fig. 7.49 Theoretical point spread function for positron imaging systems.

(a) ^{68}Ga source with 80 cm diameter ring.
(b) ^{11}C source with 80 cm diameter ring
(c) ^{68}Ga source with 40 cm diameter ring
(d) ^{11}C source with 40 cm diameter ring

(Courtesy J. A. McIntyre, private communication, 1981). These results include the effect of positron range and gamma ray angulation but do not include the effects of finite detector size.

where $\mathscr{E}_{max}$ is the maximum positron energy. In water-equivalent materials, this amounts to typically 2 mm of positional uncertainty.

Additionally, it has been assumed that the annihilation gamma rays are collinear. This would be true only if the positron had stopped moving completely prior to annihilation and if the negative electron were stationary. In fact, residual momentum must be imparted to the gamma rays, and there is a slight departure from exact collinearity. This again adds a small uncertainty to the exact location of the nucleus of origin. An angulation error of approximately 0.50° (FWHM) has been reported (Brownell *et al.*, 1978), and this error does not appear to be strongly influenced by the material density. In typical systems these limitations give rise to a total positional uncertainty of a few millimeters FWHM (see Fig. 7.49).

Positron Imaging Systems

Several systems have been developed or are now under development. They fall into two classes: those with opposing detector banks that require movement with respect to the object and those having a stationary circular detector array. To illustrate the diversity of approaches, we briefly describe one system from each category.

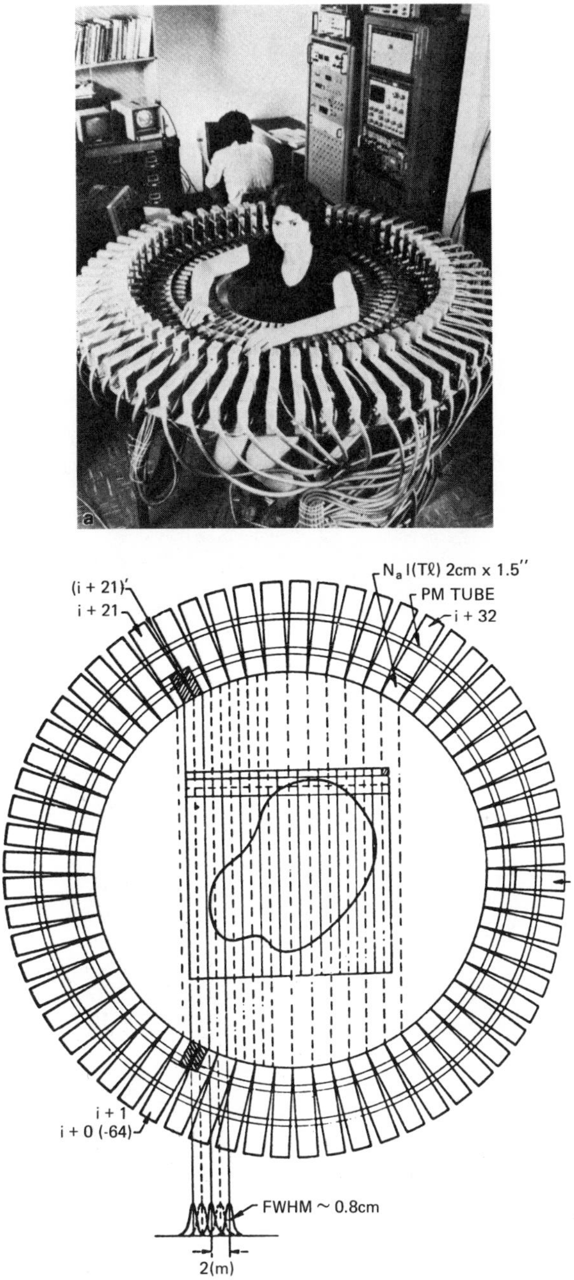

Fig. 7.50 The UCLA positron ring camera. (a) Photograph. (b) Detector layout. (From Cho *et al.*, 1977.)

Figure 7.50 shows the circular ring transverse axial camera located at the University of California at Los Angeles (Cho *et al.*, 1977). It consists of 64 separate 2-cm-diam detectors in a ring arrangement.

Coincidences between each detector and the opposing 41 detectors are counted. The measured spatial resolution is in the range 1.5–2.0 cm FWHM. Some phantom reconstructions are shown in Fig. 7.51.

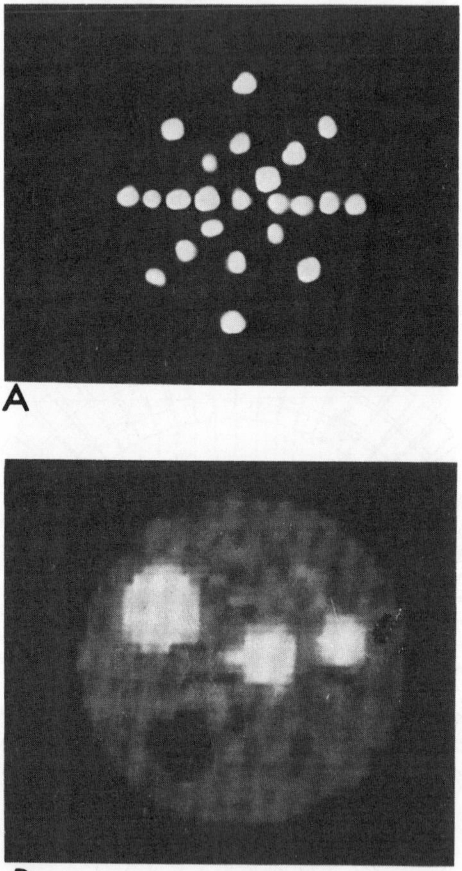

A

B

Fig. 7.51 Phantom studies made with UCLA ring camera: (a) Resolution test study with line sources of 2-mm diameter, distributed as shown. The smallest separation is 2 cm, and other lines are 3-, 4-, and 5-cm separations. (b) A structured phantom with three hot spots and one cold spot. Hot spots to background ratio is 3:1. Average resolution is 1.5–2 cm FWHM. (From Cho *et al.*, 1977.)

Figure 7.52 shows a system developed at Massachusetts General Hospital (Brownell and Burnham, 1974). There are two opposed arrays, each with 127 NaI(Tl) scintillation crystals. Each bank of crystals is viewed by a 9×8 array of photomultipliers using lucite light guides to distribute the optical flux. This multiplexing system simplifies the coincidence logic and reduces the cost of the required phototube array. Some results obtained with this system are shown in Fig. 7.53.

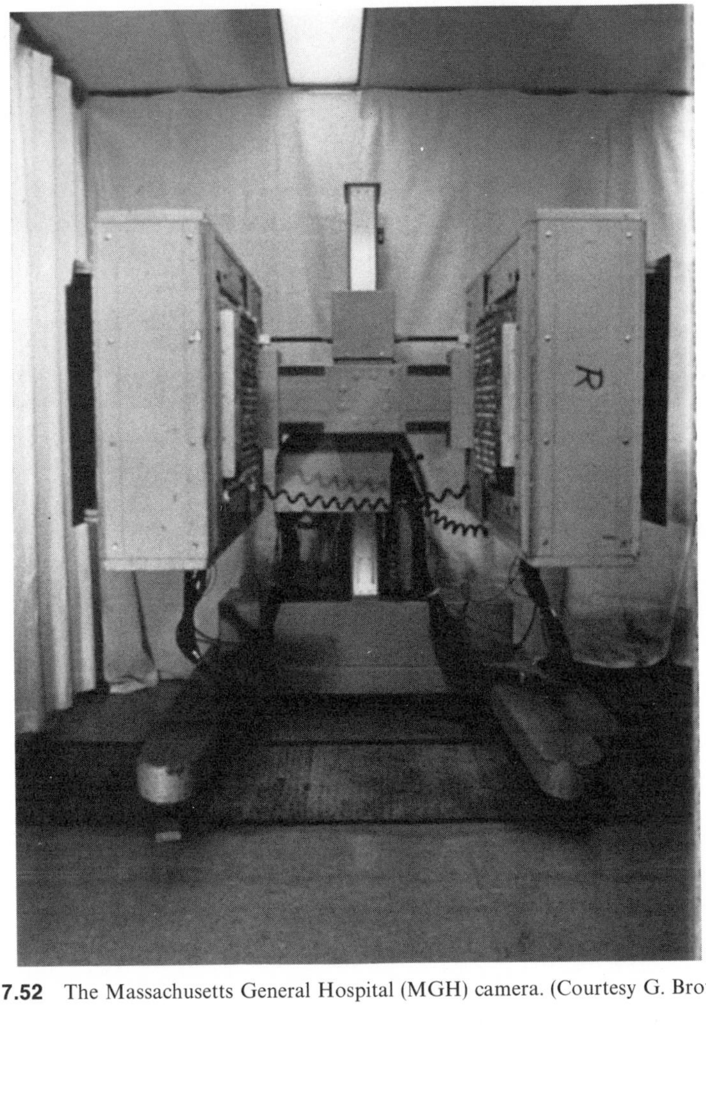

Fig. 7.52 The Massachusetts General Hospital (MGH) camera. (Courtesy G. Brownell.)

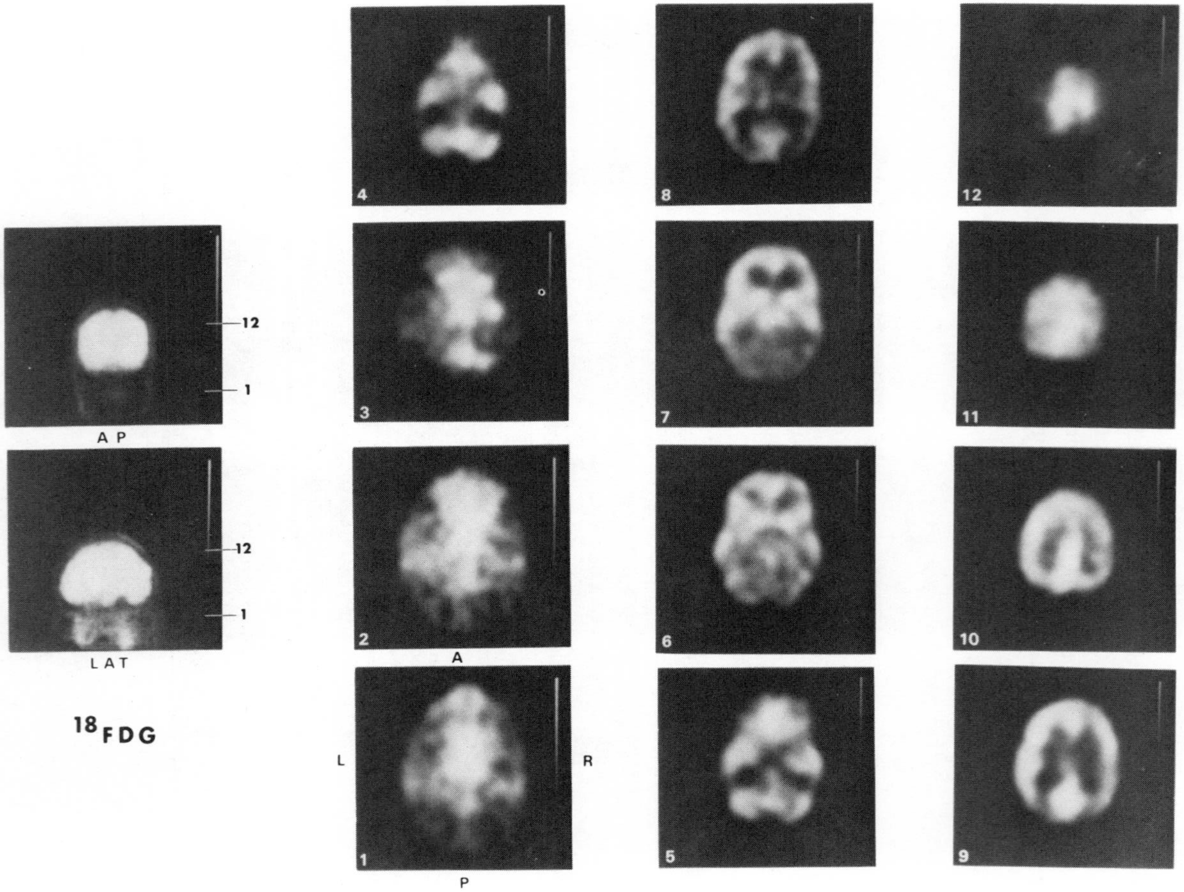

Fig. 7.53 Cerebral images obtained with ^{18}F-2-deoxyglucose on the MGH position camera. Standard anterior–posterior and lateral views are shown at left, while sections 1–12 are successive tomographic layers. (Courtesy G. Brownell.)

8

Multiplex Tomography

8.1 INTRODUCTION

8.1.1 The Coded-Aperture Concept

In the jargon of communication theory, the term *multiplexing* refers to the simultaneous transmission of more than one message over a single communication channel. An early example is *time-division multiplexing* in telegraphy. A telegraph cable is capable of transmitting frequencies up to a megahertz or so, but the signals from a manually operated telegraph key require only a few kilohertz. The messages from many keys can be sent over a single cable if a rapidly rotating commutator or rotary switch is used to switch from one key to another. A similar, synchronously rotating switch at the other end of the cable is used to *demultiplex* the incoming signals and route them to separate receiving stations. So long as the switching speed is high enough and synchronism is maintained, no information is lost.

More modern examples of multiplexing come from the commercial broadcast field. An FM stereo station uses *frequency-division* multiplexing to transmit two separate audio signals. One signal is transmitted as the frequency modulation of the main radio-frequency carrier, while the other is on a subcarrier displaced 38 kHz from the main carrier. Similarly, broadcast television uses a frequency-modulated subcarrier to transmit audio information and a phase-modulated subcarrier to convey color information.

The general concept of multiplexing has been carried over into other fields as well. An important example is *multiplex spectroscopy* in which the "message" of interest is the wavelength spectrum of some emitting source or absorbing medium. Conventional prism or grating spectrometers measure one small wavelength region at a time, using a slit to reject unwanted wavelengths. Multiplex spectrometers, such as the widely used Fourier-transform and Hadamard-transform instruments, measure the spectrum at many wavelengths simultaneously, often with important improvements in measurement accuracy or reduced observation time.

There are several ways in which the idea of multiplexing can be applied to images. One approach is to consider a complete image as one "message." Various schemes can then be devised to send several messages over the same channel. The encoding or multiplexing parameter can, for example, be time, wavelength, polarization, or propagation direction of the radiation. Appropriate techniques are then required to sort out or demultiplex the individual images at the system output.

A different viewpoint is to divide the input object into resolution cells or pixels, and to think of the object radiance in each pixel as a separate message.

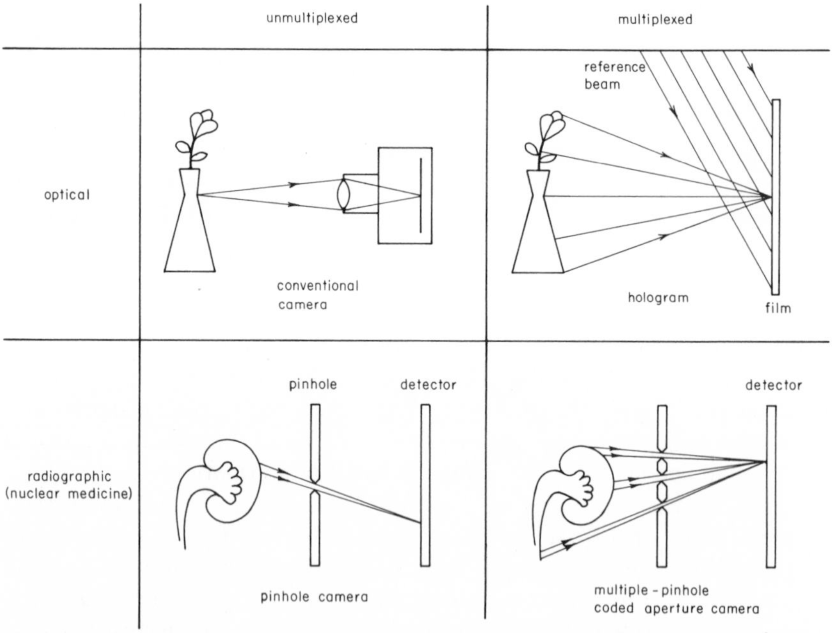

Fig. 8.1 Examples of multiplexed and unmultiplexed imaging systems. In all cases, the radiation paths to a single detector point are shown. The optical hologram and the radiographic coded image are multiplexed because each point in the detector plane receives radiation from many distinct, resolvable points on the object. In both cases a demultiplexing or decoding operation is required in order to obtain a recognizable image.

The detector is similarly divided into pixels, not necessarily the same size as the object pixels. Each detector pixel can then be thought of as a separate communication channel. If each detector pixel receives radiation predominantly from one pixel in the input, then we have no multiplexing. If, on the other hand, each detector pixel receives radiation from many input pixels, then we are dealing with multiplex imaging. There is an inherent vagueness in this definition since the boundaries of the pixels are not distinct; the finite width of the point spread function produces "crosstalk" between the channels. This is different from deliberate multiplexing, however, because we have no reasonable expectation of demultiplexing the output image to recover information about object points less than δ apart, where δ is the system resolution distance. Optical and radiographic examples of multiplexed and unmultiplexed imaging systems are shown in Fig. 8.1.

The multiplexed imaging systems that are the main concern of this chapter are better known in the literature as *coded-aperture* systems. This approach to radiographic imaging originated in the field of x-ray astronomy with the early work of Mertz and Young (1961) and Dicke (1968). The basic idea, as applied to astronomical objects, is illustrated in Fig. 8.2. The x-ray star being imaged may be thought of as a point source at infinity. The goal of the measurement is to locate the star (for example, by specifying its angular altitude and azimuth) and to determine the x-ray source strength

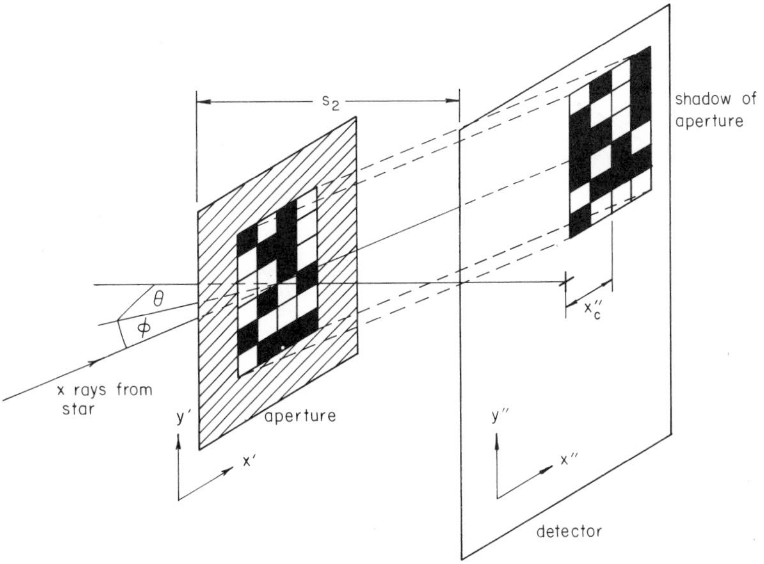

Fig. 8.2 Coded-aperture system for x-ray astronomy. The coordinates of the center of the shadow, x_c'' and y_c'', are related to the angular coordinates of the x-ray star by $\tan\theta = x_c''/s_2$ and $\tan\phi = y_c''/s_2$.

(emitted x rays per second). X-ray astronomy is thus analogous to nuclear medicine, except that the latter is concerned with nearby continuous objects rather than point sources at infinity.

From Fig. 8.2 we see that the x-ray star casts a shadow of the aperture onto the detector. The lateral coordinates of the center of the shadow (x_c'', y_c'') are sufficient to determine the angular coordinates (θ, ϕ) of the star, while the total number of detected photons is proportional to the source strength. If there are two stars within the field of view, two (possibly overlapping) shadows of the aperture will be cast on the detector plane. The data processing must then be capable of determining the coordinates of the centers of each shadow and of estimating what fraction of the total number of detected photons was contributed by each star. As we shall see in later sections of this chapter, these data-processing tasks can indeed be carried out successfully if the aperture pattern is judiciously chosen.

When the source point is a finite distance s_1 from the aperture as in Fig. 8.3, a *magnified* shadow of the aperture is cast onto the detector. In principle, the shadow now contains even more information. Its lateral coordinates still give the lateral $(x\text{–}y)$ coordinates of the source, and the total number of detected photons is still proportional to the source strength, but now the

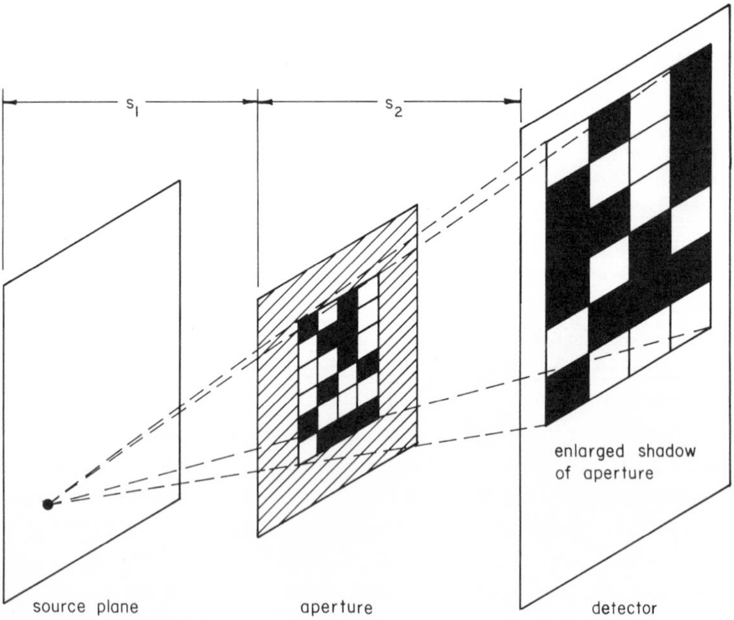

Fig. 8.3 Modification of Fig. 8.2 when the source point is not at infinity. The shadow magnification m_s can be used to determine the distance s_1 to the source plane since $m_s = (s_1 + s_2)/s_1$.

size of the shadow can also be used to determine the longitudinal coordinate (z or s_1) of the source. The data processing is correspondingly more difficult, and in general it is not possible to unambiguously extract all of this information for each point of a complicated object. Nevertheless, a great deal of useful information can be gleaned from the shadow if the aperture code and the data-processing algorithm are suitably chosen.

It must be emphasized that coded-aperture imaging is a two-step process. The first step—encoding or multiplexing—is just geometrical shadowcasting (as, indeed, is all of radiographic imaging). The second step, referred to variously as decoding, demultiplexing, or reconstruction, is carried out by some sort of computer. We are using the term "computer" here in a very broad sense to encompass digital or analog electronic systems, coherent or incoherent optical systems, and even mechanical or electromechanical devices, but whatever the incarnation of the data-processing computer, its presence is essential to the operation of the coded-aperture system. It is not merely an optional image-enhancement device since no recognizable image is obtained without it.

8.1.2 Terminology

In addition to the coded-aperture systems introduced above, there is another type of multiplexed radiographic imaging, which we shall designate as *coded source*. As illustrated in Fig. 8.4, this term applies to transmission imaging or diagnostic radiology, while coded-aperture imaging applies to emission imaging or nuclear medicine.

In both coded-aperture and coded-source systems as described so far, the multiplexing is based on different object points producing different *spatial* patterns of detected radiation, but it is also possible to make good use of the *temporal* variable. It is often desirable to use a sequence of different coded apertures or to use a single aperture with some sort of temporal modulation of its transmission. This procedure is sometimes called *multicoding*. Important examples to be discussed in this chapter include the use of sequences of zone-plate apertures, the rotating slit aperture, and the time-modulated pseudorandom pinhole array.

Coded apertures and coded sources may be either *filled* or *dilute*. A filled aperture has approximately half of its area transmissive to the radiation; examples include the zone plate (Section 8.3), the uniformly redundant pinhole array (Section 8.4.3), and the stochastic aperture (Section 8.5.2). Dilute apertures, such as the annulus (Section 8.2), rotating slit (Section 8.5.1), and nonredundant pinhole arrays (Section 8.4.2) are opaque over most of their area. A coded source is filled if about half of its area actively

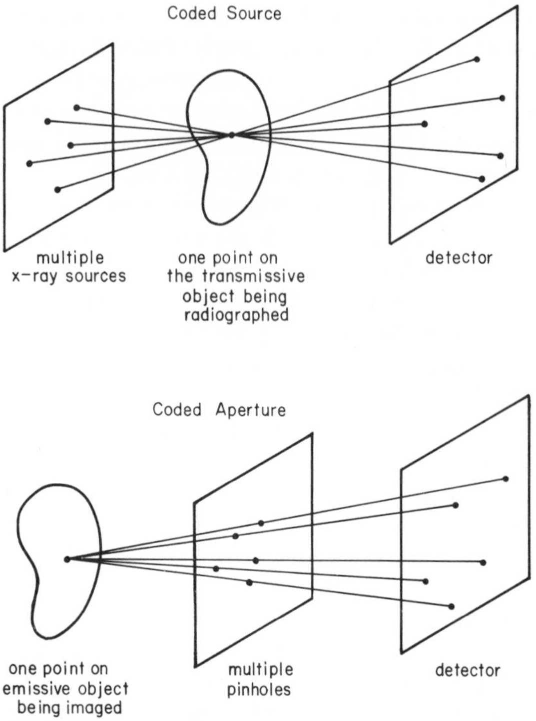

Fig. 8.4 Illustration of the distinction between coded-source transmission imaging and coded-aperture emission imaging.

emits radiation and is dilute if the emissive area is much less than half the total area.

Multiplex radiographic systems are almost always tomographic in nature, and therefore may be classified in the same way as other tomographic systems (see Chapter 6). Coded-aperture and coded-source systems almost always provide *longitudinal* tomographic sections. They are multiplanar in the sense that many different object planes can be reconstructed in focus from a single coded image. However, the tomography is less than ideal since the unwanted planes are *blurred* rather than completely eliminated.

8.1.3 Advantages and Disadvantages of Coding

Much of the early impetus for research into coded apertures arose from the large increase in geometrical collection efficiency that they afford. As noted in Chapter 4, a pinhole or collimator has a rather low efficiency, $(\Omega/4\pi) \sim 10^{-4}$. This number may be larger by a factor of 100 or more for a coded aperture. For a single point source such as an isolated x-ray star, this means that the exposure time can be reduced by the same factor without loss of signal-to-noise ratio (SNR). Alternatively, the exposure time may be left the same and the SNR will be increased by the square root of the collection-efficiency gain.

Unfortunately, the object to be imaged is seldom as simple as an x-ray star, and the SNR situation is much less favorable for a collection of point sources or an extended object. A full treatment is given in Chapter 10, but the reader should be aware of this limitation of coded apertures from the outset. As more points are added to the object scene, each detected photon conveys less information because of the difficulty in determining with which of the overlapping aperture shadows it is associated. The result is that the SNR in the decoded image will be less than it would be if the same object were imaged with the same number of detected photons by a pinhole or collimator. Stated differently, coded apertures collect more photons than conventional apertures, but also require more for the same SNR. As the object size increases from a single point, the advantage of the coded aperture progressively decreases. There may even be a net disadvantage to coded apertures for imaging broad continuous objects that fill the field of view, or for imaging weakly emitting areas near much stronger areas. Thus coded apertures are not panaceas and are not indicated for every imaging situation.

Even when there is little or no SNR advantage for coded apertures, the tomographic capability may still be useful. One advantage of coded-aperture tomography over most of the methods discussed in the last two chapters is that no mechanical motion is required; multiplane tomographic sections can be obtained from a single exposure with a single coded aperture. A corresponding disadvantage is that the out-of-focus behavior of the reconstruction can be quite complex. The out-of-focus planes do not necessarily blur smoothly and continuously, but can exhibit sharp structure and even negative values. These tomographic artifacts can seriously confuse the diagnostic process and must therefore be thoroughly understood and, if possible, minimized or eliminated before coded-aperture systems are used clinically.

The use of a coded aperture in a radiographic imaging system has consequences for other system components as well. In particular, the specifications on the detector are different when conventional apertures are used. The detector count-rate capability must be greater with coded apertures since more counts are required in the image. On the other hand, detector nonuniformities are less important since the coding process spreads the counts from one object point over a large area of the detector. Furthermore, if the detector itself contributes excess noise (that is, if the detective quantum efficiency is less than the quantum efficiency), then there can be a large SNR advantage to the use of coded apertures. More generally, if a component of the noise is independent of the signal, then the SNR can be increased by collecting more photons and hence increasing the signal. This consideration is of little importance in medical radiography since the detectors used there are usually quantum-limited, but it may apply to other radiographic imaging tasks.

Of course, coded images must be decoded by some sort of computer, possibly increasing the complexity and cost of the system. Some attempts to ameliorate this problem by the use of optical computers are described below.

8.2 THE ANNULUS

We begin our discussion of specific coded apertures with the annulus, an aperture originally proposed by Walton (1973) and later studied in detail by Simpson (1978). This selection was made not because the annulus is necessarily the aperture of choice in any particular application, but rather because it is a convenient vehicle for introducing a number of important mathematical techniques. In particular, explicit forms can be given for the PSF and MTF in the decoded image, the uses and limitations of matched filtering can be shown, a close similarity to the methods of transaxial tomography can be exploited, and the advantage of multicoding can be demonstrated.

8.2.1 Formation of the Coded Image

The mathematical formalism necessary to describe the formation of a coded image was developed in Chapter 4. We showed there that a planar source with emission function $f(\mathbf{r})$ and a planar aperture of transmission $g(\mathbf{r}')$ give rise to a mean density of detected photons $h(\mathbf{r}'')$ specified by (4.13):

$$h(\mathbf{r}'') = C \int_{\text{source}} d^2r\, f(\mathbf{r})g(a\mathbf{r}'' + b\mathbf{r}), \tag{8.1}$$

$$a = s_1/(s_1 + s_2), \tag{8.2}$$

$$b = s_2/(s_1 + s_2), \tag{8.3}$$

$$C = T/4\pi(s_1 + s_2)^2, \tag{8.4}$$

where T is the exposure time.

The formalism for coded apertures differs from that for a pinhole only in that a different aperture transmission $g(\mathbf{r}')$ is required. The ideal pinhole was transmissive over a circular region of diameter d'_{ph} in the $\mathbf{r}'$ plane, and opaque elsewhere. Therefore $g(\mathbf{r}')$ was the function $\text{circ}(2r'/d'_{\text{ph}})$. The annulus is transmissive over an annular region of mean radius $\bar{r}'$ and width $\Delta r'$, both measured in the $\mathbf{r}'$ plane. The inner and outer boundaries of this region are circles of radius $\bar{r}' - \frac{1}{2}\Delta r'$ and $\bar{r}' + \frac{1}{2}\Delta r'$, respectively (see Fig. 8.5). We may therefore write

$$g_{\text{ann}}(\mathbf{r}') = \text{circ}\left(\frac{r'}{\bar{r}' + \frac{1}{2}\Delta r'}\right) - \text{circ}\left(\frac{r'}{\bar{r}' - \frac{1}{2}\Delta r'}\right)$$
$$= \begin{cases} 1 & \text{if } \bar{r}' - \frac{1}{2}\Delta r' < r' < \bar{r}' + \frac{1}{2}\Delta r' \\ 0 & \text{otherwise,} \end{cases} \tag{8.5}$$

where, as usual, $r' = |\mathbf{r}'|$.

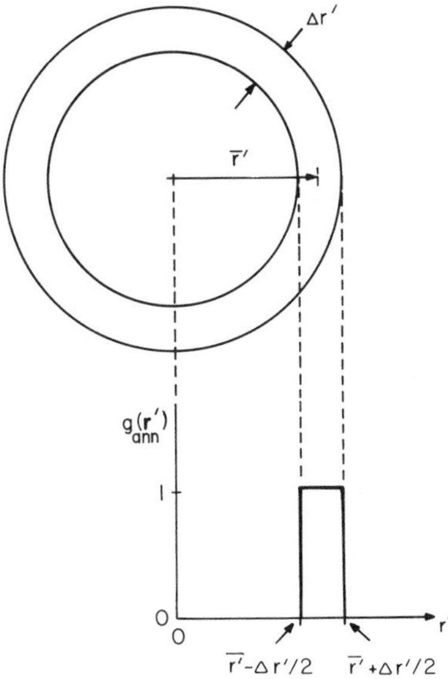

Fig. 8.5 Annulus and its transmission function.

For many calculations it will be useful to assume that $\Delta r' \ll \bar{r}'$ so that $g_{\text{ann}}(\mathbf{r}')$ may be approximated by a delta function:

$$g_{\text{ann}}(\mathbf{r}') \approx \Delta r'\, \delta(r' - \bar{r}'). \tag{8.6}$$

Note carefully that this is a *one-dimensional* delta function in the scalar variable r'; the argument is *not* the difference between two vectors. Therefore $\delta(r' - \bar{r}')$, sometimes called a *ring delta function*, can be used to perform only the radial part of a two-dimensional integral. To visualize the two-dimensional function $g_{\text{ann}}(\mathbf{r}')$ given by (8.6), we should think of a function that is infinite on a circle of radius $\bar{r}$ and zero elsewhere.

To illustrate the use of the ring delta function, let us verify the constant in (8.6) by finding the area of $g_{\mathrm{ann}}(\mathbf{r}')$. A two-dimensional integral of (8.6) in polar (r', θ') coordinates is

$$\int_\infty d^2r'\, g_{\mathrm{ann}}(\mathbf{r}') \approx \int_0^{2\pi} d\theta' \int_0^\infty r'\, dr'\, \Delta r'\, \delta(r' - \bar{r}'). \tag{8.7}$$

The integrand is independent of θ', so the integral over θ' simply yields a factor of 2π. The remaining integral over r' is performed by use of the sifting property of delta functions, with the result

$$\int_\infty d^2r'\, g_{\mathrm{ann}}(\mathbf{r}') \approx 2\pi r'\, \Delta r'. \tag{8.8}$$

The exact expression for $g_{\mathrm{ann}}(\mathbf{r}')$, (8.4), gives

$$\int_\infty d^2r'\, g_{\mathrm{ann}}(\mathbf{r}') = \pi(\bar{r}' + \tfrac{1}{2}\Delta r')^2 - \pi(\bar{r}' - \tfrac{1}{2}\Delta r')^2 = 2\pi\bar{r}'\,\Delta r', \tag{8.9}$$

in agreement with (8.8).

Regardless of whether (8.5) or (8.6) is used for $g_{\mathrm{ann}}(\mathbf{r}')$, (8.1) still describes the count density in the coded image. For the special case of a unit point source located at $\mathbf{r} = \mathbf{r}_s$, we may write

$$f^\delta(\mathbf{r}) = \delta(\mathbf{r} - \mathbf{r}_s), \tag{8.10}$$

so that (8.1) becomes

$$\begin{aligned} h^\delta(\mathbf{r}'') &= C g_{\mathrm{ann}}(a\mathbf{r}'' + b\mathbf{r}_s) \\ &= C g_{\mathrm{ann}}\{a[\mathbf{r}'' + (b/a)\mathbf{r}_s]\}. \end{aligned} \tag{8.11}$$

In other words, the coded image is, not unexpectedly, a shifted and scaled replica of the aperture transmission function. The scale factor a in the argument of (8.11) shows that the aperture shadow is enlarged by a factor of $1/a$ or $(s_1 + s_2)/s_1$. The center of the shadow is at $\mathbf{r}'' = -(b/a)\mathbf{r}_s'$ so the quantity $-b/a$ (or $-s_2/s_1$) is the system magnification, just as in the pinhole case.

For more general objects, we may rewrite (8.1) in terms of the scaled functions $\tilde{g}_{\mathrm{ann}}$ and $\tilde{f}$ defined, as in Section 4.1, by

$$\tilde{g}_{\mathrm{ann}}(\mathbf{r}'') = g_{\mathrm{ann}}(a\mathbf{r}''), \tag{8.12}$$

$$\tilde{f}(\mathbf{r}'') = f(-a\mathbf{r}''/b), \tag{8.13}$$

so that (8.1) becomes [cf. (4.18)]

$$h(\mathbf{r}'') = (a/b)^2 C \tilde{f}(\mathbf{r}'') ** \tilde{g}_{\mathrm{ann}}(\mathbf{r}''). \tag{8.14}$$

Thus, apart from the scale factors, the coded image is a convolution of the planar object with the aperture transmission function.

The frequency-domain counterpart of (8.14) is also very useful. By analogy to (4.22), we have

$$H(\boldsymbol{\rho}'') = (C/a^2)F(-b\boldsymbol{\rho}''/a)G_{\text{ann}}(\boldsymbol{\rho}''/a)$$
$$= C(a/b)^2\tilde{F}(\boldsymbol{\rho}'')\tilde{G}_{\text{ann}}(\boldsymbol{\rho}''). \tag{8.15}$$

To find G_{ann}, we must Fourier-transform (8.5). From (B.114), the transform of circ$(\mathbf{r}/R)$ is $\pi R^2[2J_1(2\pi\rho R)/2\pi\rho R]$. Therefore (8.5) transforms to

$$G_{\text{ann}}(\boldsymbol{\rho}') = \pi R_1^2 \frac{2J_1(2\pi\rho' R_1)}{2\pi\rho' R_1} - \pi R_2^2 \frac{2J_1(2\pi\rho' R_2)}{2\pi\rho' R_2}, \tag{8.16}$$

where

$$R_1 = \bar{r}' + \tfrac{1}{2}\Delta r', \qquad R_2 = \bar{r}' - \tfrac{1}{2}\Delta r'. \tag{8.17}$$

An approximate expression for G_{ann} may be found by transforming (8.6). Since g_{ann} is circularly symmetric, the two-dimensional Fourier transform becomes a Hankel transform (see Section B.8 in Appendix B) of the form

$$G_{\text{ann}}(\boldsymbol{\rho}') \approx 2\pi\,\Delta r' \int_0^\infty r'\,dr'\,\delta(r' - \bar{r}')J_0(2\pi\rho' r'). \tag{8.18}$$

The delta function allows the integral to be performed, with the result

$$G_{\text{ann}}(\boldsymbol{\rho}') \approx 2\pi\bar{r}'\,\Delta r'\,J_0(2\pi\rho'\bar{r}'). \tag{8.19}$$

The reader may wish to verify that (8.19) is the first term in a Taylor-series expansion of (8.16) in powers of Δr. {It is necessary to know that $(d/dx)\cdot[xJ_1(x)] = xJ_0(x)$.}

8.2.2 Correlation Decoding

The mathematics of Section 8.2.1 may be summarized by saying that in the encoding process each point on the object is transformed into an annular shadow. The decoding process must transform annular shadows back to points as nearly as possible. One approach to this task, an approach called correlation decoding or matched filtering, is the subject of this section.

Matched filtering (see Section 3.5.3) is the same as correlating the noisy signal with the known signal we are trying to detect. For two-dimensional signals, matched filtering may be conveniently thought of as template matching. To detect an annular shadow (or, more precisely, the recorded gamma-ray photons that define the shadow), a cutout or template in the form of an annulus of suitable scale is laid over the coded image. The number of photons visible through the template is recorded and the template is moved to a new location. The process is repeated systematically until the entire coded image has been scanned by the template. If the scale of the annular template is the same as the scale of the recorded annular shadows, all of the detected photons in a particular shadow will be seen when the template is exactly in register with the shadow, and some smaller number of photons will be seen when the template is shifted so that it only partially overlaps that shadow.

The procedure just described is mechanically cumbersome, but the same result can be achieved without mechanical motion with the incoherent optical correlator shown in Fig. 8.6. The mechanical scanning is replaced by optical parallax in this system. The light reaching each point on the viewing screen comes from a certain annular region on the transilluminated coded image; different points on the output correspond to different annular regions on the input. Furthermore, moving the template along the axis of the system changes the scale of the annular region being viewed, thereby accommodating different scales of the annular shadows in the coded image. Indeed, the optical correlator is nothing more than another coded-aperture system, identical to the one used to form the original coded image, except that optical photons are substituted for gamma rays. We have already shown

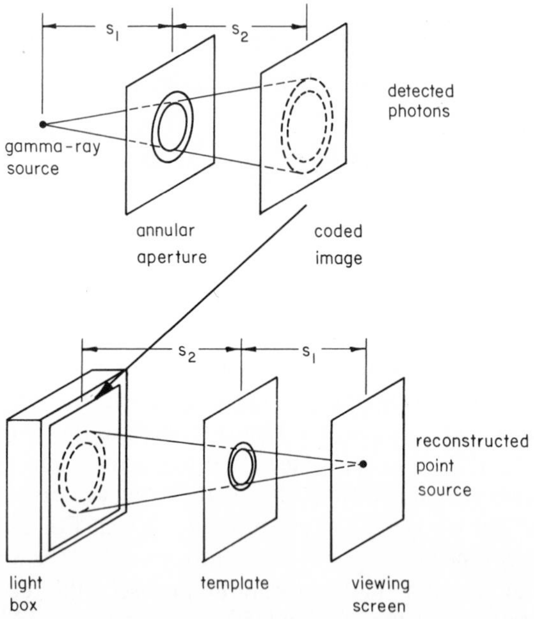

Fig. 8.6 Incoherent optical computer for correlation decoding of annular coded-aperture images. For simplicity, imagine that the gamma-ray image is detected on a positive film so that each gamma ray produces a small transmissive region, while the rest of the film is opaque after development. The film is then placed in the optical correlator at the bottom. The irradiance on the viewing screen is proportional to the correlation of the coded image with the annular template, with scale factors depending on the axial position of the template.

that the coded image is, apart from scale factors, the convolution of the source density with the aperture transmission. The same reasoning shows that the irradiance on the viewing screen in the optical correlator is the convolution (or correlation—the distinction is unimportant since the annulus is an even function) of the coded image on the light box with the annular template.

In mathematical terms, the correlation-decoded image is the original image $h(\mathbf{r}'')$ correlated with an annular filter function $q_{\text{ann}}(\mathbf{r}'')$:

$$h^{\dagger}(\mathbf{r}'') = h(\mathbf{r}'') \star\star\, q_{\text{ann}}(\mathbf{r}''), \tag{8.20}$$

where $h^{\dagger}(\mathbf{r}'')$ is a filtered version of $h(\mathbf{r}'')$. The filter function is assumed to be an annulus identical in scale and width to $\tilde{g}_{\text{ann}}(\mathbf{r}'')$. However, it is convenient to normalize $q_{\text{ann}}(\mathbf{r}'')$ to unit area, so we write

$$q_{\text{ann}}(\mathbf{r}'') = (2\pi\bar{r}'\,\Delta r'/a^2)^{-1}\tilde{g}_{\text{ann}}(\mathbf{r}''). \tag{8.21}$$

With this normalization, $\int_{\infty} q_{\text{ann}}(\mathbf{r}'')\,d^2r'' = 1$.

Using (8.14) we have

$$h^{\dagger}(\mathbf{r}'') = (a/b)^2 C\tilde{f}(\mathbf{r}'') ** [\tilde{g}_{\text{ann}}(\mathbf{r}'') \star\star\, q_{\text{ann}}(\mathbf{r}'')]. \tag{8.22}$$

In other words, the combined effect of imaging the object $f(\mathbf{r})$ through an annular coded aperture and then correlating with another annulus for decoding is the same, apart from scale factors, as convolving the object with a filter function equal to the autocorrelation function of an annulus. This autocorrelation function is evidently the system point spread function.

To get the scale factors right, we shall follow the convention of Chapter 4 and refer everything back to the scale of the original object. By analogy to (4.36) we define

$$\begin{aligned} \hat{f}(\mathbf{r}) &\equiv (b/a)^2[h^{\dagger}(\mathbf{r}'')]_{\mathbf{r}''=-(b/a)\mathbf{r}} \\ &= C[\tilde{f}(\mathbf{r}'') ** \tilde{g}_{\text{ann}}(\mathbf{r}'') \star\star\, q_{\text{ann}}(\mathbf{r}'')]_{\mathbf{r}''=-(b/a)\mathbf{r}}, \end{aligned} \tag{8.23}$$

where $\hat{f}(\mathbf{r})$ is the reconstructed *estimate* of $f(\mathbf{r})$.* In order to identify the PSF, we must recast (8.23) in the form

$$\hat{f}(\mathbf{r}) = f(\mathbf{r}) ** p_{\text{cda}}(\mathbf{r}). \tag{8.24}$$

(The subscript cda denotes a *c*orrelation-*d*ecoded *a*nnular-aperture PSF.) For this purpose, let

$$\tilde{p}_{\text{cda}}(\mathbf{r}'') \equiv C\tilde{g}_{\text{ann}}(\mathbf{r}'') \star\star\, q_{\text{ann}}(\mathbf{r}''). \tag{8.25}$$

* Even for a perfect imaging system, $\hat{f}(\mathbf{r})$ differs from $f(\mathbf{r})$ by a constant of proportionality since (8.23) takes no account of the exposure time. A factor of T^{-1} should be included to make $\hat{f}$ and f dimensionally equivalent, but this is unimportant if $\hat{f}$ is to be displayed on a CRT or other analog display.

Then (8.23) becomes

$$\hat{f}(\mathbf{r}) = [\tilde{f}(\mathbf{r}'') ** \tilde{p}_{\text{cda}}(\mathbf{r}'')]_{\mathbf{r}''=-(b/a)\mathbf{r}}$$
$$= \int_\infty d^2r_0'' \tilde{f}[-(b\mathbf{r}/a) - \mathbf{r}_0'']\tilde{p}_{\text{cda}}(\mathbf{r}_0''). \tag{8.26}$$

The change of variables, $\mathbf{r}_0 = -(a/b)\mathbf{r}_0''$, and the use of (8.13) then lead to

$$\hat{f}(r) = \left(\frac{b}{a}\right)^2 \int_\infty d^2r_0 f(\mathbf{r} - \mathbf{r}_0)\tilde{p}_{\text{cda}}(-b\mathbf{r}_0/a). \tag{8.27}$$

Comparison of (8.24) and (8.27) shows that

$$p_{\text{cda}}(\mathbf{r}) = (b/a)^2\tilde{p}_{\text{cda}}(-b\mathbf{r}/a)$$
$$= (b/a)^2 C[\tilde{g}_{\text{ann}}(\mathbf{r}'') \star\star\ q_{\text{ann}}(\mathbf{r}'')]_{\mathbf{r}''=-(b/a)\mathbf{r}}$$
$$= C(2\pi\bar{r}'\,\Delta r'/b^2)^{-1}[\tilde{g}_{\text{ann}}(\mathbf{r}'') \star\star\ \tilde{g}_{\text{ann}}(\mathbf{r}'')]_{\mathbf{r}''=-(b/a)\mathbf{r}}. \tag{8.28}$$

The minus sign in the argument of $\tilde{p}_{\text{cda}}(-b\mathbf{r}/a)$ is unimportant since an autocorrelation must be an even function.

To interpret the scale factors in (8.28), recall that $\tilde{g}_{\text{ann}}(\mathbf{r}'')$ is just the aperture function projected from a point in the object plane to the detector plane. The substitution $\mathbf{r}'' = -(b/a)\mathbf{r}$ corresponds to then projecting it through a point in the aperture plane back to the object plane.

More important than the scale factors, however, is the general shape of $p_{\text{cda}}(\mathbf{r})$, plotted in Fig. 8.7. At first blush it might seem to be a rather respectable PSF, having a pronounced peak at $\mathbf{r} = 0$ and relatively low values

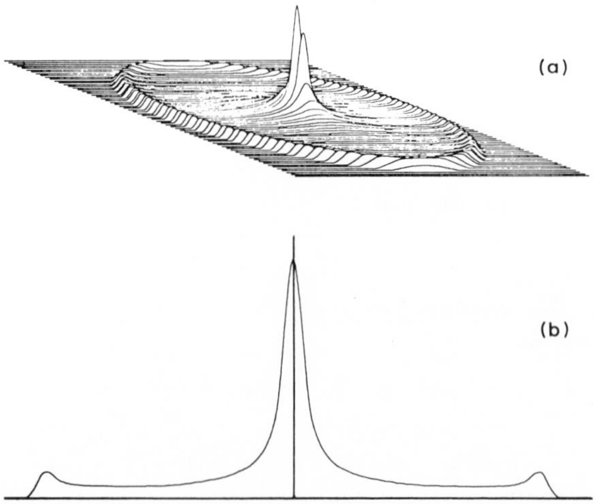

Fig. 8.7 PSF for an annular coded-aperture system with correlation decoding. (a) Isometric plot; (b) profile. (From Simpson, 1978.)

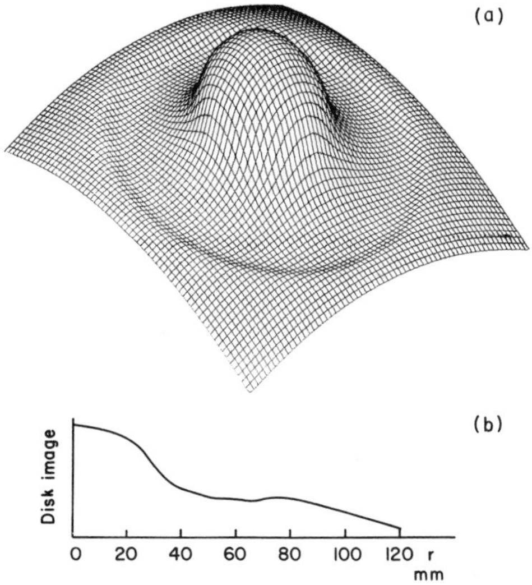

Fig. 8.8 Reconstruction of a uniform disk object. (a) Isometric plot (b) profile. The coded image was formed with an annular aperture, and decoding was carried out by correlation with an annulus. Note that the edges are quite indistinct. The poor quality of this image is a direct result of the low-amplitude tails on the PSF as shown in Fig. 8.7. (From Simpson *et al.*, 1977.)

elsewhere. However, the low-amplitude tails can be quite serious when extended objects are imaged, as shown in Fig. 8.8.

To understand why the apparently innocuous tails on $p_{\text{cda}}(\mathbf{r})$ are so troublesome, it is useful to return to the ring-delta-function approximation to $g_{\text{ann}}(\mathbf{r}')$ as given by (8.6). If we think of the ring delta function as a two-dimensional function, denoted temporarily by

$$u(\mathbf{r}) = \delta(r - \bar{r}) = \delta(|\mathbf{r}| - \bar{r}), \tag{8.29}$$

then its two-dimensional autocorrelation, as derived in Appendix A [see (A.46)], is

$$u(\mathbf{r}) \star\star\, u(\mathbf{r}) = \int_\infty d^2r_0\, \delta(r_0 - \bar{r})\, \delta(|\mathbf{r} + \mathbf{r}_0| - \bar{r}) = \frac{4\bar{r}^2}{r(4\bar{r}^2 - r^2)^{1/2}}. \tag{8.30}$$

This function, plotted in Fig. 8.9, has singularities at $r = 0$ and $r = 2\bar{r}$. The latter singularity corresponds to the little bump at the end of the autocorrelation of a finite-width annulus as seen in Fig. 8.7. It occurs when the two annuli being correlated are displaced by their common diameter $2\bar{r}$ and are therefore just tangent to each other. Since this singularity will come up often in subsequent discussions, it is useful to give it a name. Following Simpson (1978), we shall call it the "glitch."

Of more interest at the moment, however, is the $1/r$ factor in (8.30). Near the origin, the factor $(4\bar{r}^2 - r^2)^{1/2}$ is nearly constant and the PSF, in

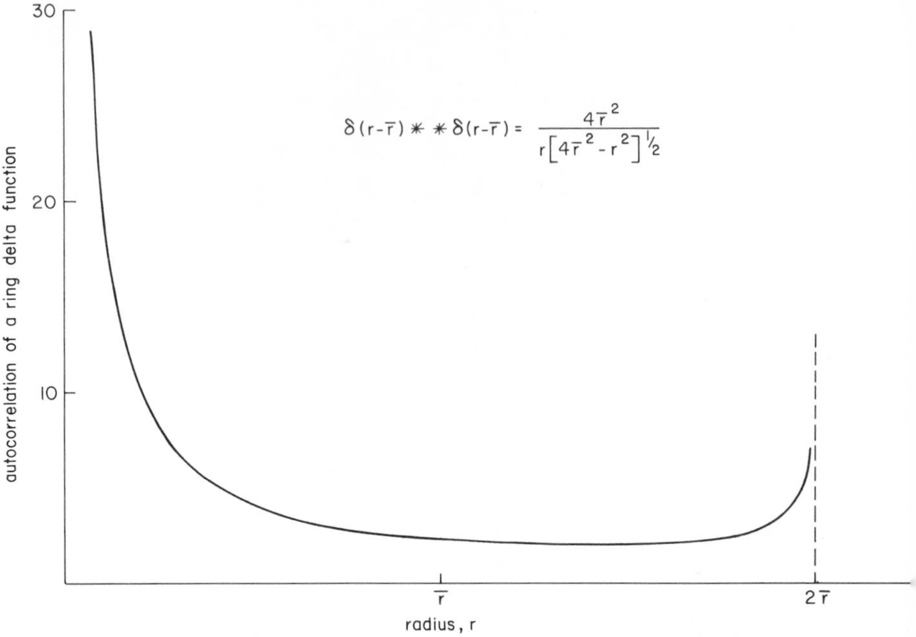

Fig. 8.9 Plot of the autocorrelation of a ring-delta function as given by (8.30).

the ring-delta-function approximation, behaves as $1/r$. Nearly the same behavior is observed in the exact PSF, Fig. 8.7, except that it does not actually go to infinity.

A $1/r$ PSF figured prominently in the discussion of transaxial tomography in Chapter 7, where it was the result of unfiltered back projection. The graphical construction of Fig. 8.10 is analogous to the spoke pattern in Fig. 7.9, so it is not surprising that both problems should exhibit a PSF that

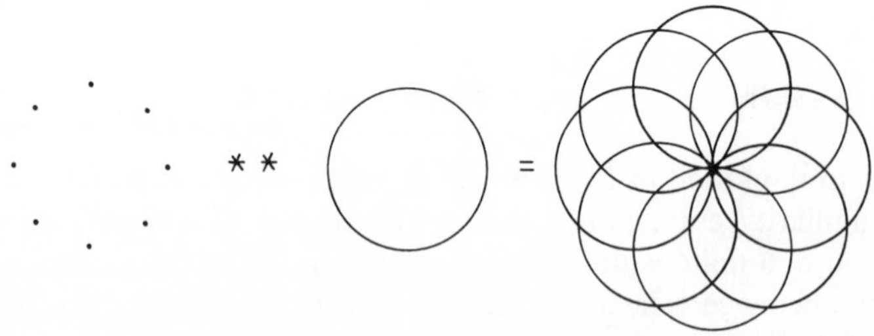

Fig. 8.10 Graphical construction to illustrate the autocorrelation of a ring-delta function. The correlation operation consists of replacing each point on one ring with a ring of the same diameter. If one of the two rings is treated as a finite number of points, a rosette pattern is formed. If the number of points in the ring goes to infinity, the density of lines in the rosette approaches the exact autocorrelation in Fig. 8.9.

varies as $1/r$. By the same token, both unfiltered back projection in transaxial tomography and correlation decoding of annular-aperture images give very poor renditions of the original object.

8.2.3 Spatial Filtering

The mathematical similarity to the transaxial tomography problem suggests that spatial filtering—in particular, ρ filtering—will be useful in the annular-aperture problem as well.

After correlation decoding, the system PSF is given by (8.28). Its Fourier transform, the system transfer function, is

$$\begin{aligned} P_{\mathrm{cda}}(\boldsymbol{\rho}) &= \mathscr{F}_2\{p_{\mathrm{cda}}(\mathbf{r})\} = (a/b)^2[2\pi\bar{r}'\,\Delta r'/b^2]^{-1}C|\tilde{G}_{\mathrm{ann}}(-a\boldsymbol{\rho}/b)|^2 \\ &= C[2\pi\bar{r}'\,\Delta r' a^2]^{-1}|G_{\mathrm{ann}}(-\boldsymbol{\rho}/b)|^2, \end{aligned} \tag{8.31}$$

where the scaling law for Fourier transforms, (B.94), has been used twice.

The quantity $|G_{\mathrm{ann}}(-\boldsymbol{\rho}/b)|^2$ can be calculated from (8.16), but more insight is obtained if we use the approximate form (8.19). We then have

$$P_{\mathrm{cda}}(\boldsymbol{\rho}) \approx (C/a^2)(2\pi\bar{r}'\,\Delta r')[J_0(2\pi\rho\bar{r}'/b)]^2. \tag{8.32}$$

Apart from constants, $P_{\mathrm{cda}}(\boldsymbol{\rho})$ is thus the square of a J_0 Bessel function, as plotted in Fig. 8.11. The first zero of $J_0(x)$ is at $x = 2.44$. For values of x greater than 2.44, an excellent approximation to $J_0(x)$ is

$$J_0(x) \approx \sqrt{2/\pi x}\cos(x - \pi/4). \tag{8.33}$$

Therefore

$$\left[J_0\!\left(\frac{2\pi\rho\bar{r}'}{b}\right)\right]^2 \approx \frac{b}{\pi^2\rho\bar{r}'}\cos^2\!\left[\frac{2\pi\rho\bar{r}'}{b} - \frac{\pi}{4}\right]. \tag{8.34}$$

In other words, $P_{\mathrm{cda}}(\boldsymbol{\rho})$ consists of a cosine-squared oscillatory factor and a $1/\rho$ envelope. Roughly speaking, the cosine-squared factor produces the glitch in the PSF at $r = 2\bar{r} = 2\bar{r}'/b$, while the $1/\rho$ envelope produces the $1/r$ behavior near the origin. (Recall that $\mathscr{F}_2\{1/\rho\} = 1/r$.)

To remove the $1/r$ tails in $p_{\mathrm{cda}}(\mathbf{r})$, we can perform a ρ-filtering operation just as in transaxial tomography. The correlation-decoded image in the frequency domain, $H^{\dagger}(\boldsymbol{\rho}'')$, is multiplied by $\rho'' A(\rho'')$, where $A(\rho'')$ is a slowly

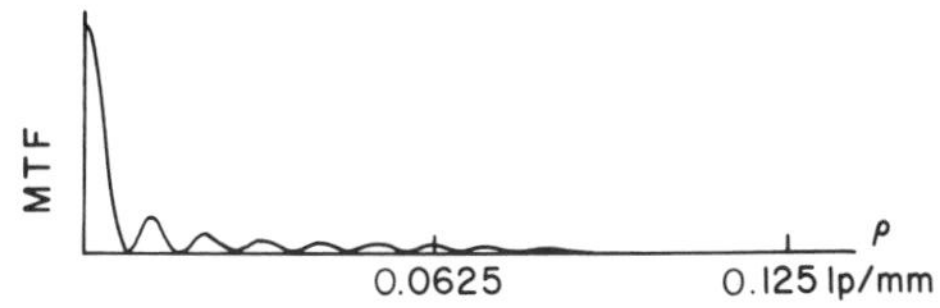

Fig. 8.11 Plot of the MTF of the annular aperture system with correlation decoding [see (8.32)]. (From Simpson, 1978.)

varying apodizing function. This operation yields a new filtered image which we shall denote by $H^{\dagger\dagger}(\boldsymbol{\rho}'')$, the double dagger indicating that two separate filtering operations have been performed. We now have

$$H^{\dagger\dagger}(\boldsymbol{\rho}'') = H^{\dagger}(\boldsymbol{\rho}'')\rho'' A(\rho'') = (a/b)^2 C\tilde{F}(\boldsymbol{\rho}'')\tilde{G}_{\text{ann}}(\boldsymbol{\rho}'')Q_{\text{ann}}(\boldsymbol{\rho}'')\rho'' A(\rho''). \quad (8.35)$$

The final estimate of the object Fourier transform is found by scaling $H^{\dagger\dagger}(\boldsymbol{\rho}'')$ back to the object plane. The result is

$$\begin{aligned}\hat{F}(\boldsymbol{\rho}) &= H^{\dagger\dagger}(-a\boldsymbol{\rho}/b) \\ &= CF(\boldsymbol{\rho})G_{\text{ann}}(-\boldsymbol{\rho}/b)Q_{\text{ann}}(-a\boldsymbol{\rho}/b)(a\rho/b)A(-a\rho/b), \quad (8.36)\end{aligned}$$

where (4.20) has been used to relate $\tilde{F}$ to F. The coefficient of $F(\boldsymbol{\rho})$ in this equation is the new net transfer function, which we shall denote by $P_{\text{rfa}}(\boldsymbol{\rho})$ (where rfa stands for "*r*ho-*f*iltered *a*nnulus"). It is given by

$$P_{\text{rfa}}(\boldsymbol{\rho}) = C(a/b)(2\pi\bar{r}'\,\Delta r')^{-1}\rho|G_{\text{ann}}(-\boldsymbol{\rho}/b)|^2 A(-a\rho/b). \quad (8.37)$$

This transfer function is plotted in Fig. 8.12 for a Gaussian apodization, while its transform, the PSF, is shown in Fig. 8.13. Neither of these functions is yet ideal. The transfer function goes to zero at a number of frequencies,

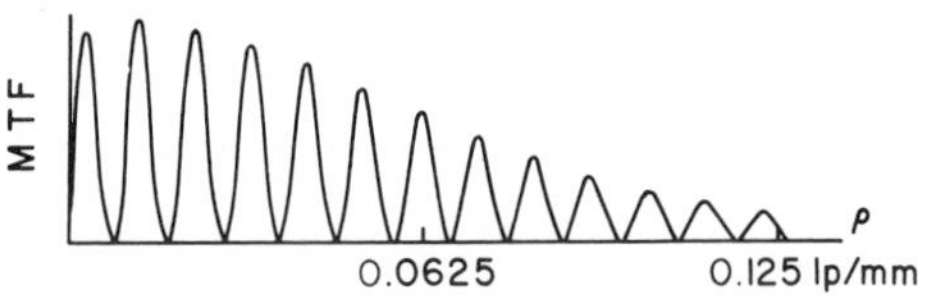

Fig. 8.12 MTF for annular coded-aperture imaging with correlation decoding and ρ filtering. (From Simpson, 1978.)

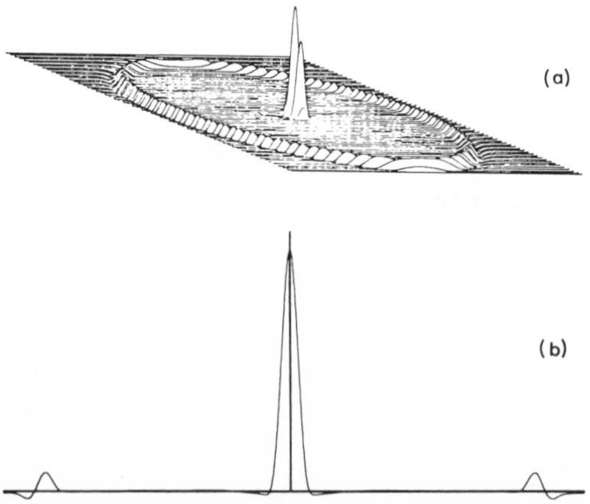

Fig. 8.13 Point-spread function for annular coded-aperture imaging with correlation decoding and ρ filtering. This figure is the Fourier transform of Fig. 8.12. (a) Isometric plot; (b) profile. (From Simpson, 1978.)

indicating that no information at all about the object is present in $\hat{F}(\boldsymbol{\rho})$ at these frequencies. By the same token, the PSF is deficient because of the glitch at $r = 2\bar{r}$. The glitch has changed character as a result of ρ filtering—it now goes both positive and negative—but it has not been eliminated.

The glitch in the PSF and the zeros in the transfer function are closely related, as we shall show in Section 8.2.4. Basically, both problems arise because the Fourier transform of the aperture function $G_{\text{ann}}(\boldsymbol{\rho}')$ is zero at certain frequencies. Object information at these frequencies was not present in the coded image in the first place, and no amount of linear filtering can recover it.

Nevertheless, the annulus is still a useful aperture when used with correlation decoding and ρ filtering, provided the object is not too large. Indeed, if $r < 2\bar{r}$ (where $\bar{r} = \bar{r}'/b$), the PSF has a nearly ideal behavior. It is sharply peaked in the center and essentially zero elsewhere. If the object lies entirely within a circle of radius $\bar{r}'/b$, the glitch will not overlap the usable part of the reconstruction and may thus be ignored. The glitch is no detriment at all to imaging small objects, but rather serves to limit the object size. A reconstruction of a disk object, with the glitch artifact entirely outside the reconstruction field, is shown in Fig. 8.14. Comparison with Fig. 8.8 should make it apparent that the ρ filter effected a great improvement over correlation decoding alone.

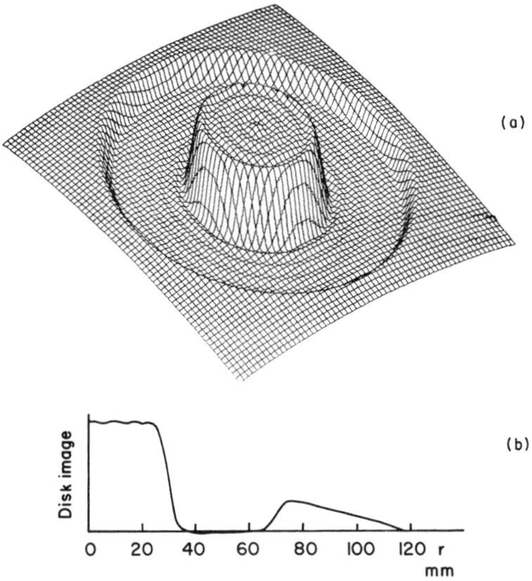

Fig. 8.14 Reconstruction of a disk object imaged with an annular coded aperture (computer simulation). Decoding consisted of correlation with an annulus and ρ filtering. This figure is thus the convolution of the disk with the PSF of Fig. 8.13. (a) Isometric plot; (b) profile. (From Simpson *et al.*, 1977.)

8.2.4 Two Annuli

Perhaps the easiest way to understand the origin of the glitch is to use the approximations of (8.32)–(8.34). Recall that (8.32) for $P_{\text{cda}}(\boldsymbol{\rho})$ resulted from the ring delta-function approximation to $g_{\text{ann}}(\mathbf{r}')$, and that a further approximation of replacing the J_0 Bessel function by a cosine led to (8.34). Use of this double approximation, which is still quite reasonable, in (8.37) yields the following behavior for the transfer function after ρ filtering:

$$P_{\text{rfa}}(\boldsymbol{\rho}) \propto A(\rho)\cos^2\left(\frac{2\pi\rho\bar{r}'}{b} - \frac{\pi}{4}\right). \tag{8.38}$$

A familiar trigonometric identity then leads to

$$P_{\text{rfa}}(\boldsymbol{\rho}) \propto \tfrac{1}{2}A(\rho) + \tfrac{1}{2}A(\rho)\sin(4\pi\rho\bar{r}'/b). \tag{8.39}$$

The first term is the desirable one; $A(\rho)$ is a broad structureless function that transforms to a sharply peaked function approximating a delta function. The second term in (8.39) produces the glitch. If we were dealing with a one-dimensional function, we could say that $\sin(2\pi x_0\xi)$ transforms to delta functions at $x = \pm x_0$. We cannot, however, say that $\sin(2\pi r_0\rho)$ transforms two dimensionally to delta functions at $r = \pm r_0$, although qualitatively the effect is similar. The term $\sin(4\pi\rho\bar{r}'/b)$ in (8.38) produces a disturbance in the vicinity of $r = 2\bar{r}'/b$ that we are calling the glitch.

Fundamentally, the glitch arises because we have not collected information about the object at all spatial frequencies. The transform of the annular transmission function goes to zero at a set of more or less regularly spaced

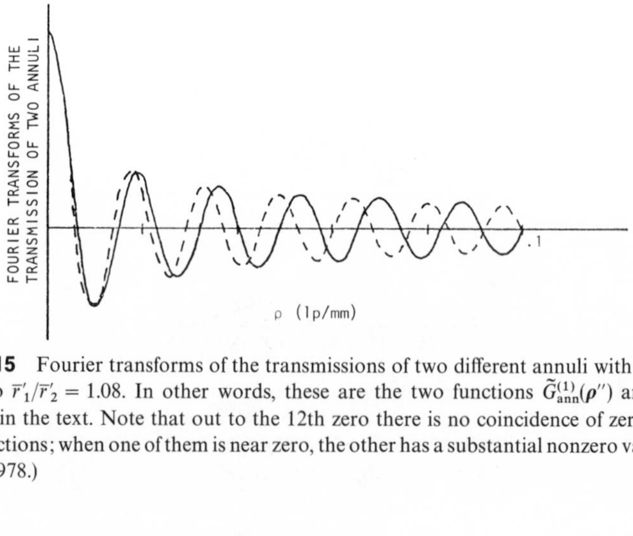

Fig. 8.15 Fourier transforms of the transmissions of two different annuli with mean radii in the ratio $\bar{r}'_1/\bar{r}'_2 = 1.08$. In other words, these are the two functions $\tilde{G}^{(1)}_{\text{ann}}(\boldsymbol{\rho}'')$ and $\tilde{G}^{(2)}_{\text{ann}}(\boldsymbol{\rho}'')$ referred to in the text. Note that out to the 12th zero there is no coincidence of zeros between the two functions; when one of them is near zero, the other has a substantial nonzero value. (From Simpson, 1978.)

radial frequencies. The only effective solution to this problem is to collect more information. One way to do this is to form two separate coded images with two annuli of different mean radius $\bar{r}'$. Since this parameter determines the scale of the undesirable sine term in (8.39), it can be arranged that when the transform of one annulus goes to zero, the transform of the other one is nonzero. In this way object information at all frequencies is present in at least one of the coded images. The situation is illustrated in Fig. 8.15.

Having collected a complete data set, all that remains is to make proper use of it in the decoding operation. Basically, the idea is to linearly combine the two coded images in the frequency domain in such a way that the resulting transfer function is broad and smooth. The following algorithm, devised by Simpson (1978), achieves this goal. Let the scaled transmissions of the two annuli be $\tilde{g}^{(1)}_{\text{ann}}(\mathbf{r}'')$ and $\tilde{g}^{(2)}_{\text{ann}}(\mathbf{r}'')$, with Fourier transforms of $\tilde{G}^{(1)}_{\text{ann}}(\boldsymbol{\rho}'')$ and $\tilde{G}^{(2)}_{\text{ann}}(\boldsymbol{\rho}'')$, respectively. Then for each frequency $\boldsymbol{\rho}''$ we calculate two weighting factors $W_1(\boldsymbol{\rho}'')$ and $W_2(\boldsymbol{\rho}'')$ which satisfy the simultaneous equations,

$$W_1(\boldsymbol{\rho}'')\tilde{G}^{(1)}_{\text{ann}}(\boldsymbol{\rho}'') + W_2(\boldsymbol{\rho}'')\tilde{G}^{(2)}_{\text{ann}}(\boldsymbol{\rho}'') = A(\rho), \tag{8.40}$$

$$\tilde{G}^{(1)}_{\text{ann}}(\boldsymbol{\rho}'')/\tilde{G}^{(2)}_{\text{ann}}(\boldsymbol{\rho}'') = W_1(\boldsymbol{\rho}'')/W_2(\boldsymbol{\rho}''), \tag{8.41}$$

where $A(\rho)$ is the desired broad, smooth function. These weighting factors are then used to combine the transforms of the two coded images, $H_1(\boldsymbol{\rho}'')$ and $H_2(\boldsymbol{\rho}'')$, frequency by frequency, forming the quantity

$$H^{\dagger}(\boldsymbol{\rho}'') = W_1(\boldsymbol{\rho}'')H_1(\boldsymbol{\rho}'') + W_2(\boldsymbol{\rho}'')H_2(\boldsymbol{\rho}''). \tag{8.42}$$

By analogy to (8.15), the coded images are given by

$$H_i(\boldsymbol{\rho}'') = C(a/b)^2\tilde{F}(\boldsymbol{\rho}'')\tilde{G}^{(i)}_{\text{ann}}(\boldsymbol{\rho}''), \qquad i = 1 \text{ or } 2. \tag{8.43}$$

Equations (8.40), (8.42), and (8.43) can be combined to give

$$H^{\dagger}(\boldsymbol{\rho}'') = C(a/b)^2\tilde{F}(\boldsymbol{\rho}'')A(\rho''). \tag{8.44}$$

Scaling this result back to the object plane as usual, we have an estimate of the object Fourier transform given by [cf. (8.36)]

$$\hat{F}(\boldsymbol{\rho}) = H^{\dagger}(-a\boldsymbol{\rho}/b) = CA(-a\rho/b)F(\boldsymbol{\rho}). \tag{8.45}$$

The transfer function with this algorithm is thus

$$P_{\text{ta}}(\boldsymbol{\rho}) = CA(-a\rho/b), \tag{8.46}$$

where the subscript ta stands for "two annuli." The glitch has now been eliminated.

Several comments about this algorithm are in order. First, it should be noted that we did not explicitly carry out correlation and ρ-filtering operations, but achieved much the same effect anyway. To understand this result, consider the structure of the weighting factors in both the frequency domain (Fig. 8.16) and the space domain (Fig. 8.17). That this algorithm succeeds in boosting high frequencies is evident from the frequency-domain plots since the peak values of $W_1(\rho'')$ and $W_2(\rho'')$ generally increase with frequency. Similarly, the correlation operation is implicit in the algorithm since both $w_1(\mathbf{r})$ and $w_2(\mathbf{r})$ cluster around a specific radius (Fig. 8.17) and therefore have a generally annular appearance.

It should also be noted that in the derivation leading to (8.45), the condition (8.41) was not used. The transfer function is determined fully by (8.40), and any of a whole family of weighting functions satisfying this equation could be used. Equation (8.41) is included in the algorithm for noise reasons. It says that if one of the two functions $\tilde{G}^{(i)}_{\text{ann}}(\rho'')$ is near zero at some particular frequency, then the corresponding coded image conveys very little information at that frequency and should have a very small weighting factor.

Some practical results obtained with the two-annulus algorithm are shown in Figs. 8.18 and 8.19.

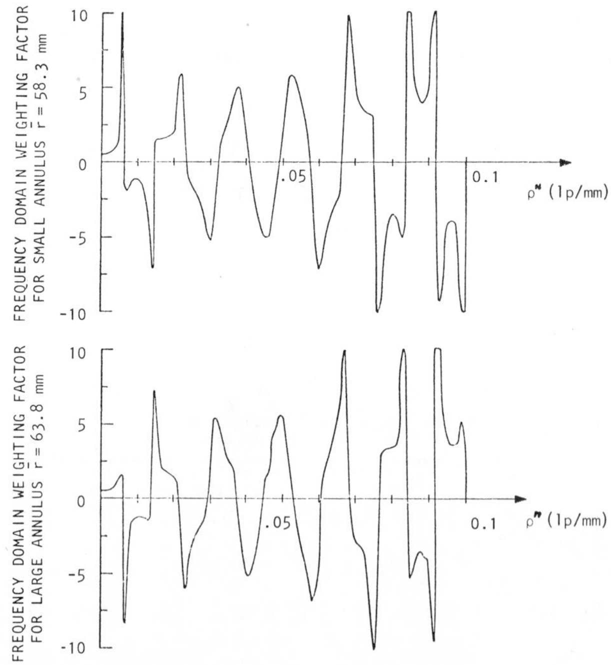

Fig. 8.16 Set of weighting functions $W_1(\rho'')$ and $W_2(\rho'')$ used in the two-annulus reconstruction algorithm. Note that the peak values grow approximately as $\sqrt{\rho''}$, offsetting the falloff in $G^{(i)}_{\text{ann}}(\rho'')$ which varies as $1/\sqrt{\rho''}$ [see (8.32) and (8.33)]. (From Simpson, 1978.)

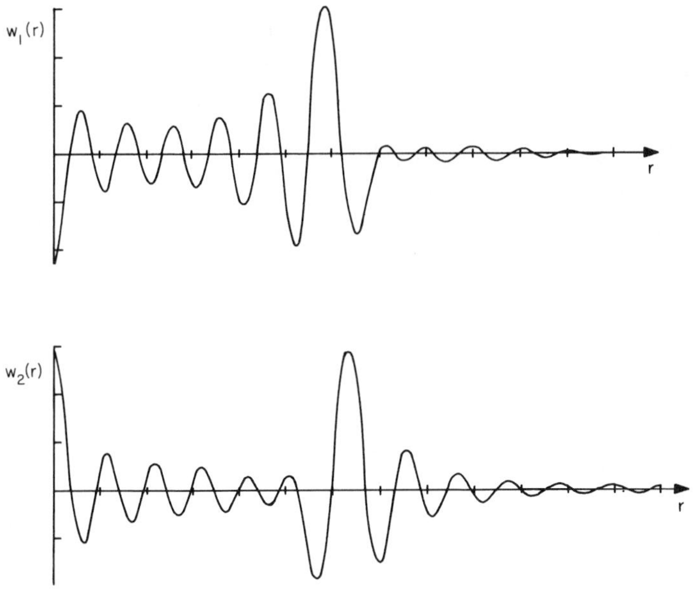

Fig. 8.17 Functions $w_1(\mathbf{r})$ and $w_2(\mathbf{r})$, the space-domain counterparts of the functions shown in Fig. 8.16. Note that these decoding functions are basically annuli with negative sidelobes to produce image sharpening. (From Simpson, 1978.)

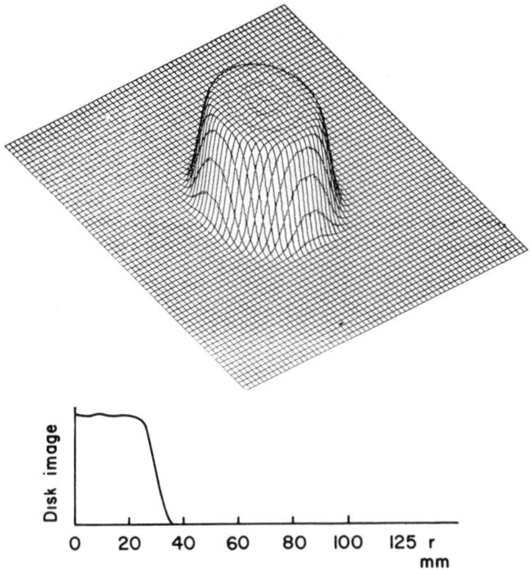

Fig. 8.18 Reconstruction of a disk object with the two-annulus algorithm (computer simulation). Note that the glitch is now absent. (a) Isometric plot; (b) profile. (From Simpson *et al.*, 1977.)

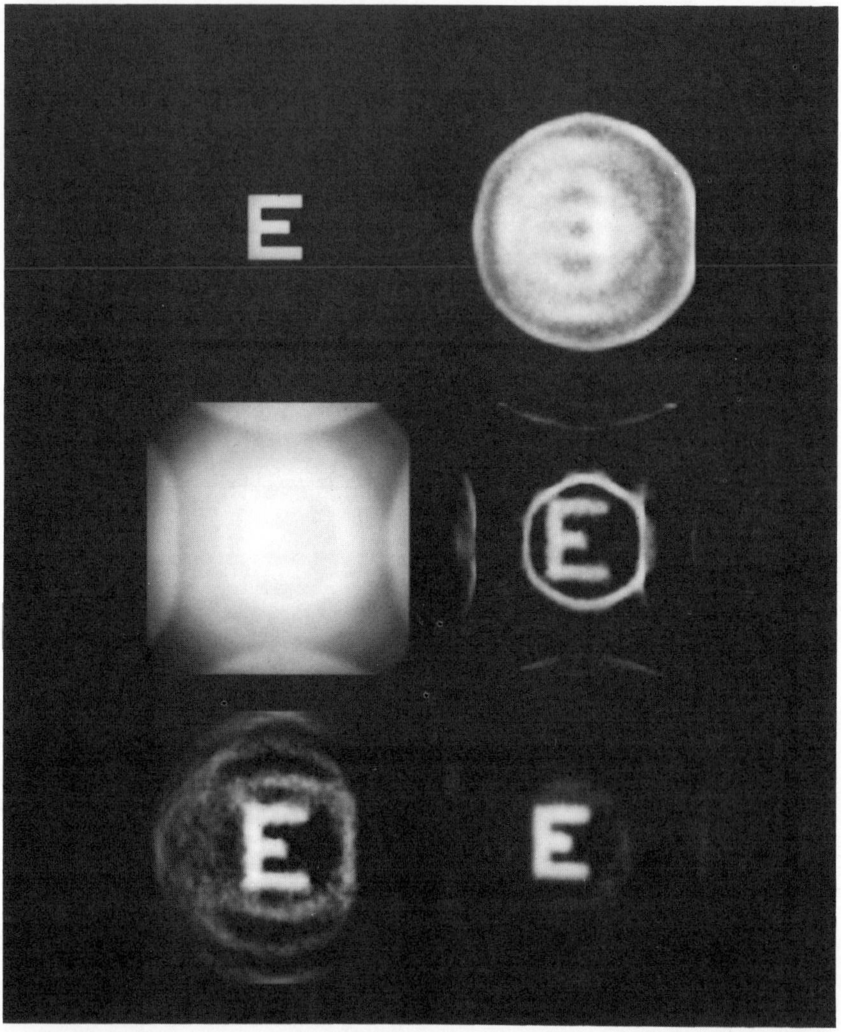

Fig. 8.19 Examples of imagery obtained by Simpson (1978) with annular aperture systems. Top left: The original object, a radioactive letter E 10-cm high with 2 cm bars. Top right: coded image recorded with an Anger camera. Center left: Correlation-decoded image. Note the severe blurring caused by the $1/r$ PSF. Center right: Image obtained by correlation decoding and ρ filtering. The circle is an artifact caused by the abrupt edge of the coded image. Bottom left: Same as center right, except that a trimming algorithm has been used to suppress the edge artifact. (For details, see Simpson, 1978.) The remaining background artifacts are due to the glitch. Bottom right: Image obtained with the two-annulus system, now essentially artifact-free.

8.2.5 Three-Dimensional Behavior

The entire discussion of annular coded apertures to this point has been based on a planar model for the object $f(\mathbf{r})$. Furthermore, we have assumed, quite unrealistically, that we know the object-aperture distance s_1 and can adjust the scale of our decoding function accordingly.

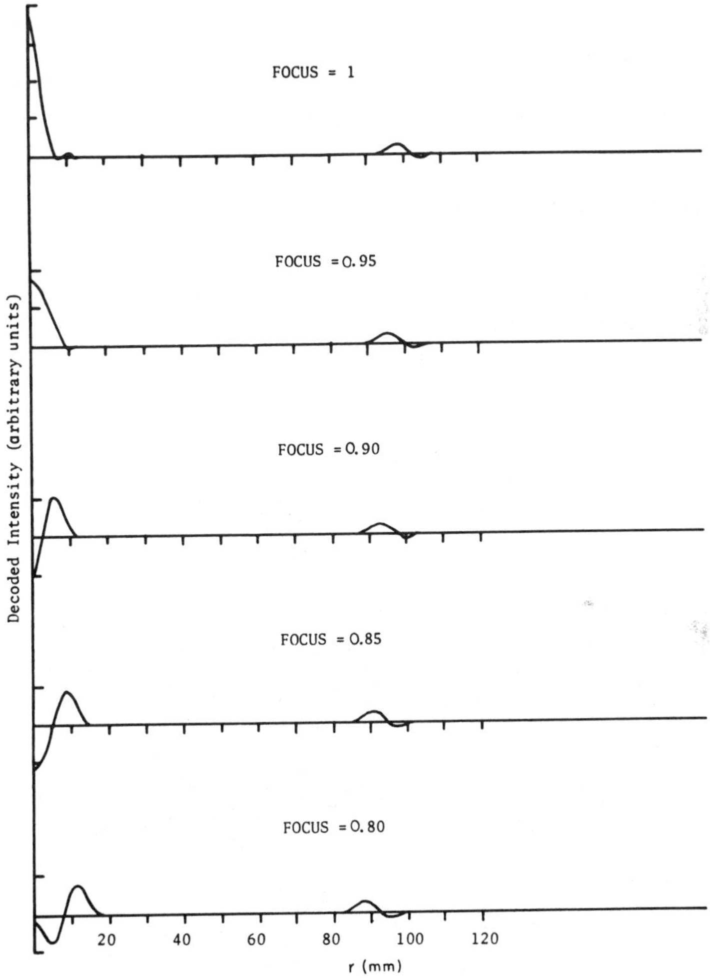

Fig. 8.20 Behavior of the PSF for an annular aperture system with correlation decoding and ρ filtering when the scale of the correlating annulus does not match the scale of the recorded annular shadows. The parameter FOCUS is the ratio of these two scales. This figure may be regarded as depicting the *three-dimensional* PSF of the annular-aperture system. (From Simpson, 1978.)

One way to investigate the three-dimensional behavior of this system is to assume we do *not* know s_1, but must decode by correlating the coded image with a sequence of filter functions of different scales. When the scale of the decoding function happens to match the scale of the annular shadows produced by points in some particular plane, then that plane will be sharply imaged and all other planes will be blurred in some manner.

The out-of-focus PSF is illustrated in Fig. 8.20. Ideally, this figure should show a sharp peak for the plane in focus and no response at all to other planes. Second best would be for the out-of-focus planes to blur smoothly and continuously without sharp structures or negative values. Neither of these desirable behaviors is actually obtained.

8.3 THE FRESNEL ZONE PLATE

The Fresnel zone plate, shown in Fig. 8.21, has been used as a coded aperture in nuclear medicine, x-ray astronomy, laser fusion studies, and nuclear reactor safety research. Long before its use in radiography, however,

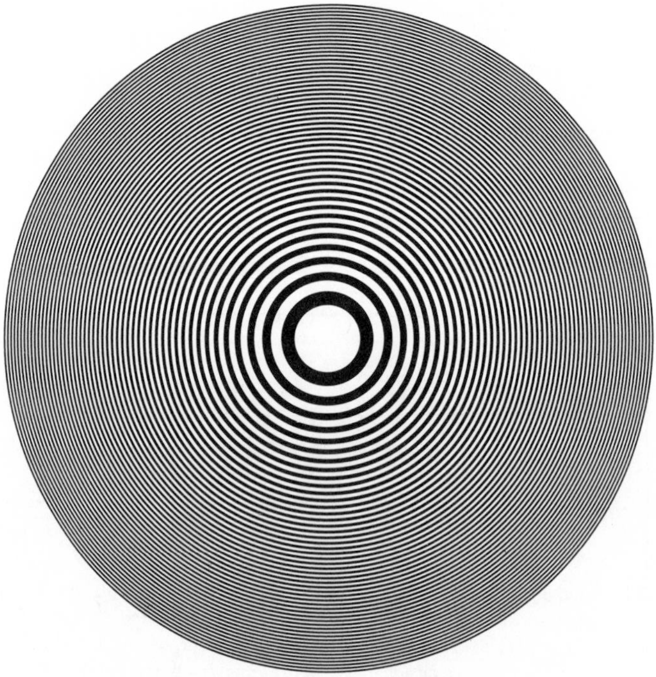

Fig. 8.21 Fresnel zone plate.

the zone plate was well known in optics. Indeed, most of its radiographic applications either use optical reconstruction methods or exploit the analogy between radiography and optics. Therefore, before describing the use of the zone plate as a coded aperture, we digress briefly to discuss its role in optics. Some knowledge of diffraction theory is presumed in this discussion; suitable reviews are given by Goodman (1968) and Gaskill (1978).

8.3.1 The Zone Plate in Optics

The Fresnel zone plate is a pattern of alternately transparent and opaque annular zones. The edge of the nth zone occurs at a radius of

$$r_n = r_1\sqrt{n}, \qquad n = 1, 2, 3, \ldots, N, \tag{8.47}$$

where r_1 is the radius of the first zone. It is easy to demonstrate from this formula that all zones have the same area.

The optical amplitude transmittance of the zone plate is given by

$$t_{zp}(\mathbf{r}) = \begin{cases} 1 & \text{if} \quad \sin(\pi r^2/r_1^2) > 0 \\ 0 & \text{if} \quad \sin(\pi r^2/r_1^2) < 0. \end{cases} \tag{8.48}$$

This function may be expanded as (Shulman, 1970)

$$t_{zp}(\mathbf{r}) = \tfrac{1}{2} + (2/\pi)\sin(\pi r^2/r_1^2) + (2/3\pi)\sin(3\pi r^2/r_1^2) + \cdots, \tag{8.49}$$

or, using the usual exponential representation for the sines,

$$t_{zp}(\mathbf{r}) = \frac{1}{2} + \frac{1}{\pi i} \sum_{\substack{j=-\infty \\ \text{odd values only}}}^{\infty} (1/j)\exp(-i\pi j r^2/r_1^2). \tag{8.50}$$

Each term in this sum is a pure phase factor. If a plane wave of light of wavelength λ is incident on the zone plate, each phase factor will alter the phase of the wave by an amount proportional to r^2. Precisely this behavior occurs when a plane wave passes through a lens, as demonstrated by Goodman (1968). The amplitude transmittance of a thin lens is given by

$$t_l(\mathbf{r}) = \exp(-i\pi r^2/\lambda f_l). \tag{8.51}$$

where f_l is the focal length of the lens.

Comparison of (8.50) and (8.51) shows that the zone plate behaves as whole series of lenses at once. For a normally incident plane wave, the wave that emerges from the zone plate is a superposition of spherical waves, one for each term in the sum, plus the undiffracted plane wave corresponding to the $\frac{1}{2}$ in (8.50). This latter term is frequently referred to, in optical jargon, as *the dc term.*

As shown in Fig. 8.22, the converging spherical waves, corresponding to positive j in (8.50), come to a focus after propagating a distance f_j given by

$$f_j = r_1^2/\lambda j, \qquad j \text{ odd}, \tag{8.52}$$

while the diverging spherical waves (negative j) appear to emanate from virtual foci located behind the zone plate at distances f_j also given by (8.52). The foci are the points where the light waves from all points on all transparent zones add up in phase. Light from the opaque zones would arrive at the focal points out of phase with that from the transparent zones, but is prevented from doing so because, by definition, the opaque zones transmit no light.

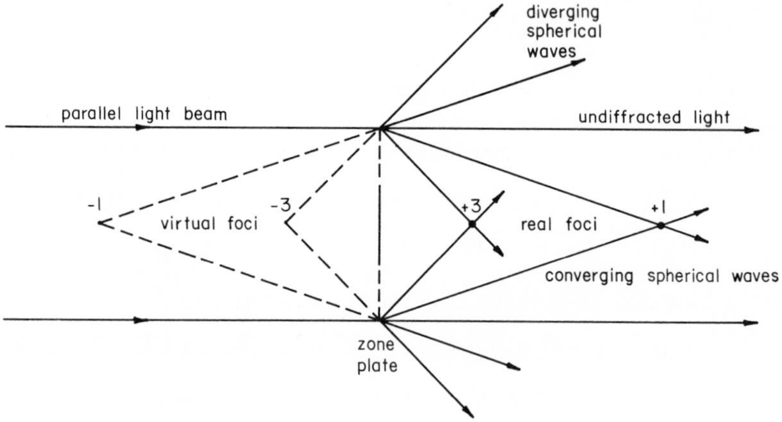

Fig. 8.22 Illustration of the focusing properties of a zone plate when illuminated with a plane wave of wavelength λ.

An important variation on the basic Fresnel zone plate is the off-axis zone plate depicted in Fig. 8.23. Constructed by taking an off-axis section from a larger, on-axis zone plate, the off-axis plate has somewhat different focusing properties as shown in Fig. 8.24. The important point is that with the off-axis zone plate, the various diffracted waves can be spatially separated. One of the terms in a sum like (8.50) can be observed in its focal plane without interference from the other terms.

One reason for the interest in the Fresnel zone plate in optics is that it arises quite naturally as the interference pattern between a plane wave and a spherical wave. Isaac Newton first observed such a pattern, which we now call Newton's rings, when a spherical glass surface was placed near a flat one. The spherical surface reflected a spherical wave and the flat reflected a plane wave when a plane wave was incident. The zone plate described by (8.48) is just a binary (black and white) version of Newton's rings.

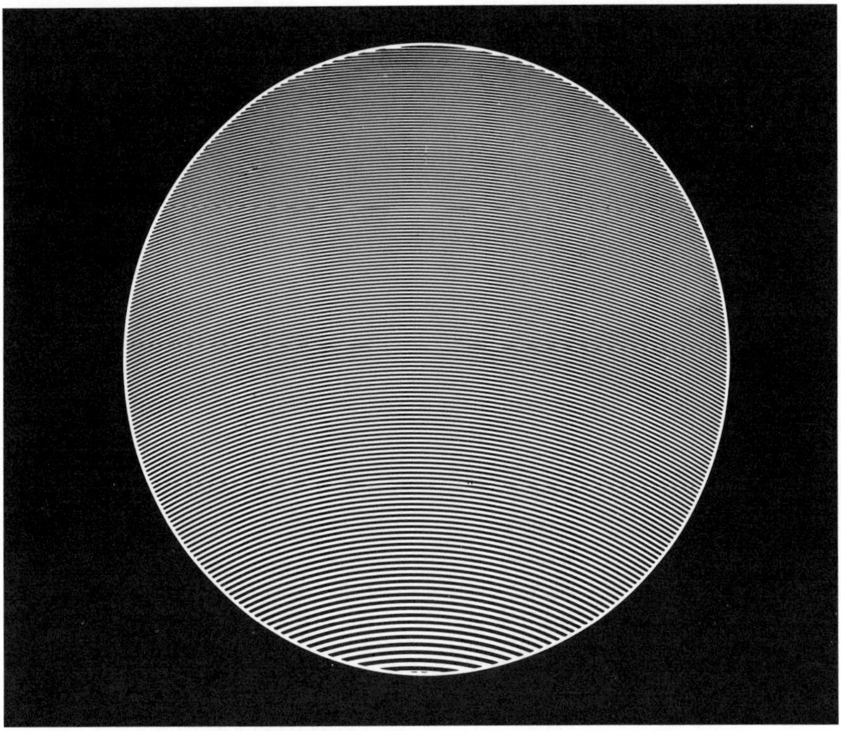

Fig. 8.23 Off-axis zone plate.

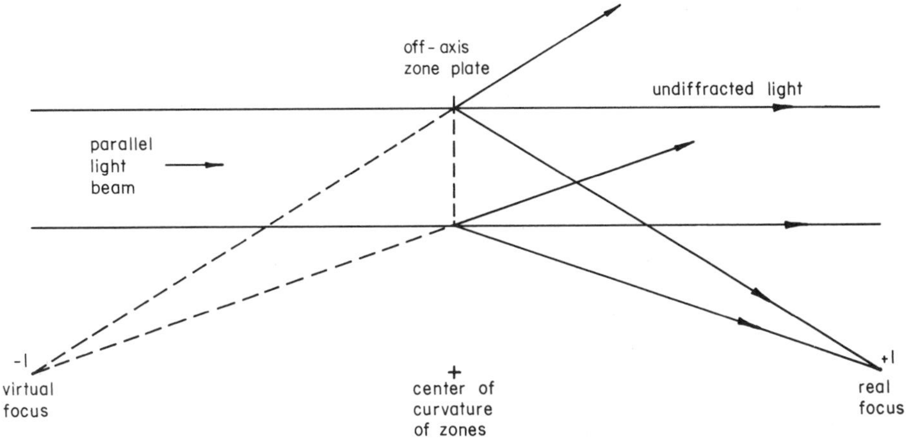

Fig. 8.24 Illustration of the focusing properties of an off-axis zone plate.

The zone plate comes up also in holography. Consider the simple holographic setup shown in Fig. 8.25. We assume that the incident wave ψ_i is a unit-amplitude plane wave traveling parallel to the z axis, i.e.,

$$\psi_i = \exp(ikz), \tag{8.53}$$

where $k = \omega/c = 2\pi/\lambda$, with ω being the radian frequency of the light wave. The wave scattered by a point scatterer is a diverging spherical wave. In the Fresnel approximation (see Goodman, 1968; Gaskill, 1978), the scattered wave may be written

$$\psi_s = \alpha \frac{\exp(ikz)}{i\lambda z} \exp\left[\left(\frac{ik}{2z}\right) r^2\right], \tag{8.54}$$

where α is related to the scattering cross section, and $r^2 = x^2 + y^2$. (For simplicity, we are assuming that the scatterer is located at the origin of coordinates.)

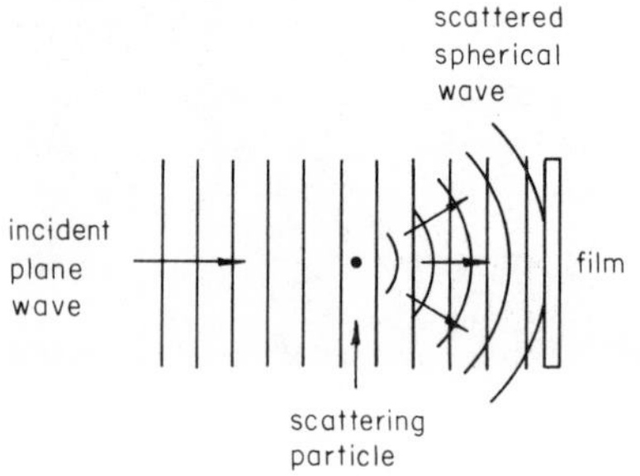

Fig. 8.25 Arrangement for producing a Gabor hologram. A plane wave is scattered by a dust particle or other small object and produces a diverging spherical wave. The spherical wave interferes with the original plane wave so that the film exposure is essentially a zone plate. The developed film is called a hologram.

If α is small, very little energy is scattered out of the incident wave, and the total wave amplitude on the film in plane z is

$$\psi_z(x, y) = \psi_s + \psi_i. \tag{8.55}$$

The film does not respond directly to the complex wave amplitude, but rather to the energy flux which is given by

$$|\psi_z(x, y)|^2 = |\psi_s + \psi_i|^2 = 1 + (\alpha/\lambda z)^2 + (2\alpha/\lambda z)\sin(kr^2/2z). \tag{8.56}$$

It is possible to develop the film in such a way that its final *amplitude* transmittance is proportional to the exposing *energy* flux,

$$\begin{aligned} t_H(x, y) &= \text{const} \cdot |\psi_z(x, y)|^2 \\ &= \text{const} \cdot \{1 + (\alpha/\lambda z)^2 + (\alpha/i\lambda z)\exp(ikr^2/2z) - (\alpha/i\lambda z)\exp(-ikr^2/2z)\}, \end{aligned} \tag{8.57}$$

where the subscript H stands for hologram. (More specifically, holograms recorded in this configuration are called Gabor holograms.)

There is a strong similarity between t_H and t_{zp} [cf. (8.50)]. The main difference is that t_{H} has only two quadratic phase terms, while t_{zp} has an infinite series, but this is just a consequence of the assumption that t_{H} is linearly related to the exposure. If we use a very high-contrast film, the hologram of a point scatterer is almost exactly a zone plate with a large number of orders [j values in (8.50)] present. Indeed, it is then only the finite resolution of the film that prevents the sum from going to infinity. Since the analysis is much simpler if we assume film linearity, we shall continue to do so.

If we place the developed hologram back in its original location and reilluminate it with ψ_{i}, the wave that emerges is given by

$$\psi_{\text{i}} t_{\text{H}}(x, y) = \text{const} \cdot \exp(ikz)\{1 + (\alpha/\lambda z)^2 + (\alpha/i\lambda z)\exp(ikr^2/2z) - (\alpha/i\lambda z)\exp(-ikr^2/2z)\}. \quad (8.58)$$

The various terms in (8.58) all have simple physical interpretations. The first two terms, $1 + (\alpha/\lambda z)^2$, correspond to a transmitted plane wave still traveling parallel to the z axis. The term proportional to $\exp(ikr^2/2z)$ is exactly a continuation of ψ_{s}, even though the scatterer is no longer present. In other words, the hologram, when illuminated with one of the two exposing waves, launches a wave that is an exact replica of the other exposing wave. An observer looking through the hologram sees a virtual image of the scatterer just as if it were still there.

The final term in (8.58), proportional to $\exp(-ikr^2/2z)$, represents a converging spherical wave that comes to a focus a distance z beyond the hologram. This focus may be regarded as another image of the point scatterer, this time a real image that can be viewed with a ground glass. It is often called the *twin image*.

Although couched in terms of a single point scatterer, the above discussion can be extended to more complicated objects by invoking the principle of linear superposition. Each point on the object independently sends out a spherical wave that interferes with the incident wave. Each object point is therefore encoded as a zone plate interference pattern. When reilluminated, each zone plate pattern behaves as a lens independently and produces a focal spot that serves as a reconstructed image of the object point.

However, as the object becomes larger and more complex, the undiffracted plane-wave and twin-image terms become more bothersome, until eventually the Gabor hologram configuration is no longer usable. A solution to this problem was devised by Leith and Upatnieks (1962) who used the configuration shown in Fig. 8.26. In this case the original coherent light beam is split into two parts, one of which falls directly on the photographic film while the other illuminates the object. The total wave amplitude at the film plane is thus the wave scattered by the object, plus an obliquely incident

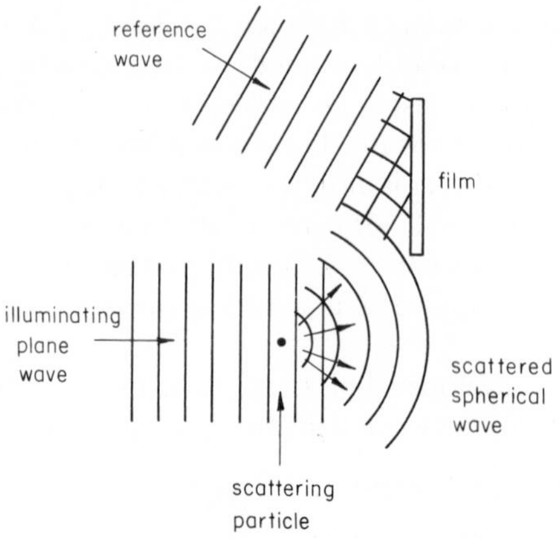

Fig. 8.26 Arrangement for producing a Leith and Upatnieks hologram. A separate reference wave is now used, and each object point is encoded as an off-axis zone plate interference pattern.

plane wave called the reference wave. The latter is described by

$$\psi_r = \exp(i\mathbf{k}_r \cdot \mathbf{r}) = \exp(ikz\cos\theta_r + ikx\sin\theta_r), \tag{8.59}$$

where for simplicity we have set its magnitude to unity and assumed that it propagates in the x–z plane at an angle θ_r to the z axis.

Consider again a point scatterer at the origin of coordinates. The scattered wave is again given by (8.54), but now the total film exposure is proportional to

$$|\psi_z(x, y)|^2 = |\psi_s + \psi_r|^2 = 1 + (\alpha/\lambda z)^2 + (2\alpha/\lambda z)\sin[(kr^2/2z) - kx\sin\theta_r + kz(1 - \cos\theta_r)]. \tag{8.60}$$

To aid in the interpretation of this equation, we define

$$x_0 = z\sin\theta_r, \qquad \phi = kz(1 - \cos\theta_r) - (kx_0^2/2z). \tag{8.61}$$

In terms of these quantities, (8.60) becomes

$$|\psi_z(x, y)|^2 = 1 + (\alpha/\lambda z)^2 + (2\alpha/\lambda z)\sin[(k/2z)(x - x_0)^2 + (ky^2/2z) + \phi]. \tag{8.62}$$

Note that z, and hence x_0 and ϕ, are constant over the film plane, Therefore the argument of the sine in (8.62) has the same quadratic phase structure as in t_{zp}.

As before, we assume that the film is developed so that its amplitude transmittance is proportional to the exposing energy flux. If we reilluminate the hologram with a plane wave traveling parallel to the z axis, the emerging wave is

$$\exp(ikz)t_{\mathrm{H}}(x, y) = \text{const} \cdot \exp(ikz) \cdot \{1 + (\alpha/\lambda z)^2 + (\alpha/i\lambda z)\exp[(ik/2z)(x - x_0)^2 + (iky^2/2z)] - (\alpha/i\lambda z)\exp[(-ik/2z)(x - x_0)^2 - (iky^2/2z)]\}. \quad (8.63)$$

The physical interpretation of the various terms is the same as in the Gabor hologram case: there is a plane wave, a diverging spherical wave, and a converging spherical wave. The important difference, however, is that the focal points of the two spherical waves are displaced off the z axis by an amount x_0. If the width of the hologram in the x direction is substantially less than $2x_0$, then the plane wave does not overlap either focal spot (cf. Fig. 8.24) and a clean reconstruction of the point scatterer is observed. There is now no difficulty in extending this argument to large, complex objects. So long as there is no overlap of the desired focus (real or virtual) and the unwanted waves, then a system that works for a single point object will work for an arbitrary superposition of points.

The three-dimensional aspect of holography is implicit in the formalism developed above. Recall that we started with a point scatterer a distance z from the film, and ended up with terms in t_{H} that vary as $\exp(\pm ikr^2/2z)$. Since a lens has an amplitude transmittance that varies as $\exp(-ikr^2/2f)$, where f is the focal length [see (8.51)], we see that the focal length of the recorded zone plate is $\pm z$. In other words, object points farther from the film in the recording process produce foci farther from the hologram during reconstruction—a three-dimensional image is formed. Another way to say the same thing is to repeat that the hologram launches a wave that is identical to the original object wave. An observer therefore perceives the reconstruction just the way he would perceive the actual object, with depth cues such as parallax and accommodation intact.

To summarize, zone plates are important in optics because they behave as lenses, but with diffraction rather than refraction serving to bring the light to a focus, and also because they arise naturally from the interference between plane waves and spherical waves. In forming a hologram, each object point launches a spherical wave that interferes with a reference wave to produce a zone plate pattern on film. When reilluminated, each elemental zone plate produces a real and a virtual focus, either of which may be regarded as a reconstruction of the object point that produced the zone plate in the first place. In the Gabor configuration, Fig. 8.25, there is a confusion of overlapping beams in the reconstruction process, but this problem is eliminated by going to the configuration of Fig. 8.26, where the elemental patterns are off-axis zone plates.

It should be emphasized that holography, like coded-aperture imaging, is a two-step process. The intermediate record—hologram or coded image—is generally not recognizable or usable without reconstruction.

8.3.2 The On-Axis Zone Plate in Radiography

The concepts of holography can be applied to radiography by using a Fresnel zone plate as a coded aperture as first suggested by Mertz and Young (1961) and Young (1963) (see Fig. 8.27). They proposed the use of a zone plate, with the opaque zones made of lead, for imaging x-ray stars. Because the zones were to be rather coarse ($r_1 \sim 1$–10 mm) and the wavelengths of interest were very short ($\lambda < 100$ Å), the diffraction properties of the zone plate were quite negligible. For example, $r_1 = 10$ mm and $\lambda = 100$ Å $= 10^{-5}$ mm gives a primary focal length r_1^2/λ of 10^7 mm or 10 km. Since the aperture-to-detector distance s_2 is probably less than a meter, it is a good approximation to treat the coded image as a geometric shadow rather than as a

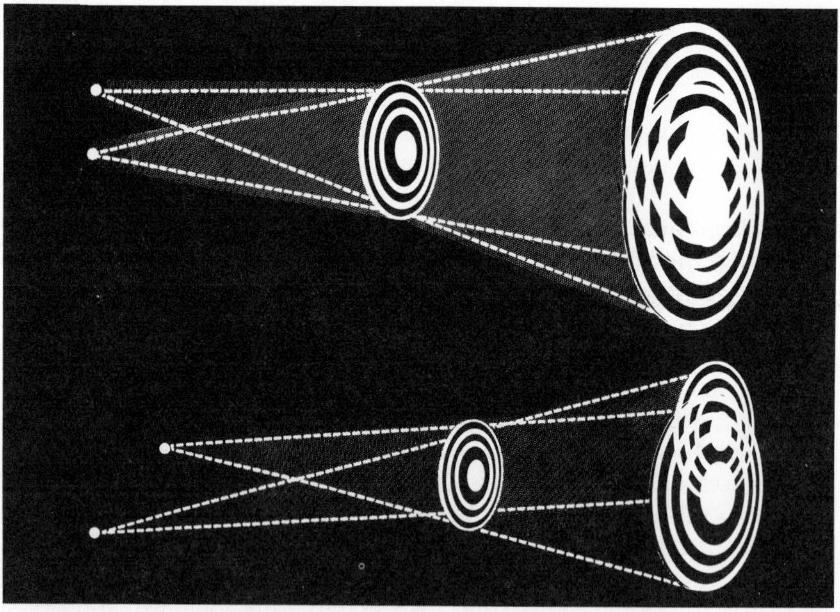

Fig. 8.27 Illustration of the use of an on-axis zone plate as a coded aperture. In general, each object point casts an enlarged shadow of the zone plate onto the detector plane. For x-ray astronomy the points are at infinity and there is no enlargement. The coded image bears a close formal resemblance to a Gabor hologram, even though the elemental zone-plate patterns are formed by shadowcasting rather than by interference.

diffraction pattern. Nevertheless the result is the same as in holography—each object point (x-ray star) is encoded as a zone-plate pattern. The coded image is essentially a hologram.

Parenthetically, we should mention that zone plates have on occasion been used as true focusing elements for soft x rays. Since the focal length scales as r_1^2, a tiny zone plate with $r_1 = 0.1$ mm has $f = 1$ m for $\lambda = 100$ Å, making it a marginally useful imaging device at this wavelength. However, in medical imaging, we are interested in $\lambda < 1$ Å where there is no hope at all of using a zone plate as a focusing element. Thus we shall ignore diffraction of x rays by the zone plate.

On the other hand, diffraction plays a crucial role in the reconstruction process suggested by Mertz and Young. The focal lengths of the recorded zone plates can be brought down to a manageable scale by either reducing r_1 or increasing λ. The first option can be exercised by making a photographic reduction of the coded image, while the second, an increased λ, comes about automatically if we use visible light in the reconstruction step. To repeat the earlier example, if the coded image which originally had $r_1 = 10$ mm is reduced $20\times$ and reconstructed with green light, $\lambda = 5000$ Å, the pertinent focal length becomes $(10/20)^2/(5 \times 10^{-4}) = 500$ mm $= 0.5$ m, a very practical number. Thus when the reduced coded image is illuminated with visible light each elemental zone plate produces a bright focal spot that can be regarded as the reconstruction of the x-ray or gamma-ray point source that was responsible for that particular zone plate shadow. The parallel with true optical holography is a close one, the primary difference being that the zone plates are produced by shadowcasting in the coded-aperture case and by interference in the hologram case. In both cases, however, reconstruction involves the diffraction of light.

Although the parallel with holography is an appealing one, it is also instructive to treat zone plate coded apertures by the same formalism we use for other radiographic systems. To do so, we assume that a zone plate can be constructed with zones that are alternately perfectly transmissive and perfectly opaque to the high-energy radiation of interest. Then the aperture transmission function $g_{zp}(\mathbf{r}')$ has the same functional form as the optical amplitude transmittance $t_{zp}(\mathbf{r}')$, as expressed in infinite-series form in (8.50). For simplicity, we shall assume that we can concentrate on just one term in the expansion and ignore all others; methods for eliminating the unwanted terms are discussed in Sections 8.3.3 and 8.3.4. The only modification required in (8.50) is to take account of the finite diameter D'_{zp} of the zone plate by multiplying the infinite series by a circ function. Then we can write

$$g_{zp}(\mathbf{r}') = (\pi i)^{-1} \exp[-i\pi(r'/r'_1)^2] \operatorname{circ}(2r'/D'_{zp}) + \text{dull terms}, \tag{8.64}$$

where r'_1 and D'_{zp} are measured in the $\mathbf{r}'$ plane.

For a point source, $f^{\delta}(\mathbf{r}) = \delta(\mathbf{r} - \mathbf{r}_s)$, the coded image is [cf. (8.11)]

$$\begin{aligned} h^{\delta}(\mathbf{r}'') &= C g_{zp}(a\mathbf{r}'' + b\mathbf{r}_s) \\ &= (C/\pi i)\exp[(-i\pi/r_1'^2)|a\mathbf{r}'' + b\mathbf{r}_s|^2]\,\mathrm{circ}[(2/D'_{zp})|a\mathbf{r}'' + b\mathbf{r}_s|] + \ldots . \end{aligned} \tag{8.65}$$

If a reduced-scale copy of the coded image is made, and the photographic gamma is adjusted properly, the resulting transparency can have an optical amplitude transmittance given by

$$t_{ci}^{\delta}(\mathbf{r}) = K h^{\delta}(\mathbf{r}/m_0), \tag{8.66}$$

where K is a constant, m_0 is the optical magnification in the copying step (typically, $m_0 \approx \frac{1}{20}$), and the subscript ci stands for coded image.

Optical reconstruction consists of illuminating the transparency with a plane wave and observing the diffraction pattern a distance z away. For simplicity, we assume that the plane wave has unit amplitude and is traveling parallel to the z axis and hence perpendicular to $t_{ci}^{\delta}(\mathbf{r})$. It is known from Fresnel diffraction theory that propagation of light through free space is equivalent to a linear filtering operation, with the filter impulse response given by

$$p_{\mathrm{dif}}(\mathbf{r}) = \frac{\exp(2\pi i z/\lambda)}{i\lambda z}\exp\left[\left(\frac{i\pi}{\lambda z}\right)r^2\right], \tag{8.67}$$

where λ is the optical wavelength. The optical amplitude on a screen a distance z from $t_{ci}^{\delta}(\mathbf{r})$ is thus given by

$$\psi_z(\mathbf{r}) = t_{ci}^{\delta}(\mathbf{r}) ** p_{\mathrm{dif}}(\mathbf{r}). \tag{8.68}$$

The close similarity between $p_{\mathrm{dif}}(\mathbf{r})$ and $g_{zp}(\mathbf{r}')$ should not be overlooked. When we illuminate the coded image with coherent light and observe the diffraction pattern on a screen an appropriate distance away, we are basically correlating the coded image with one term in the infinite series for $g_{zp}(\mathbf{r}')$. Loosely speaking, free space is a matched filter for a zone-plate image.

The essential features of (8.68) can be seen most easily by temporarily assuming an infinite zone plate $D'_{zp} \to \infty$ and setting $\mathbf{r}_s = 0$. We then have

$$\psi_z(\mathbf{r}) = \mathrm{const} \cdot \int_{\infty} \exp[(i\pi/\lambda z)r'^2]\exp[(-i\pi a^2/r_1'^2 m_0^2)|\mathbf{r} - \mathbf{r}'|^2]\, d^2r'. \tag{8.69}$$

This is a complicated integral in general, but it simplifies greatly if we place our viewing screen at a distance z given by

$$\pi/\lambda z = \pi a^2/r_1'^2 m_0^2 \tag{8.70}$$

or

$$z = r_1'^2 m_0^2/a^2\lambda. \tag{8.71}$$

But $1/a$ is the usual projection magnification and m_0 is the optical magnification. The quantity $r_1'^2 m_0^2/a^2$ is thus the square of the radius of the first zone of an elemental zone plate in t_{ci}^{δ}. Comparison with (8.52) then shows that (8.71) places the viewing screen one focal length from the coded image. Mathematically, if (8.70) or (8.71) is satisfied, the quadratic phase factors (i.e., the terms proportional to r'^2) in the integrand of (8.69) cancel, and we have, using (B.92) and (A.17),

$$\begin{aligned}\psi_z(\mathbf{r}) &= \text{const}\cdot\exp(-i\pi a^2 r^2/r_1'^2 m_0^2)\int_{\infty}\exp[(-2i\pi a^2/r_1'^2 m_0^2)(\mathbf{r}\cdot\mathbf{r}')]\,d^2r' \\ &= \text{const}\cdot\delta(\mathbf{r}).\end{aligned} \tag{8.72}$$

In other words, the autocorrelation of a quadratic phase factor is a delta function.

Equation (8.72) says that a perfect reconstruction is obtained—a point source of x rays or gamma rays has been transformed back to a perfect point image. Of course, this conclusion should not be taken at all seriously; it is merely a consequence of our assumption that $D'_{zp}\to\infty$. If we retain the circ function from (8.65), the integral in (8.72) runs over a circular region of diameter $D_{zp}m_0/a$, and the integral does not collapse so neatly into a delta function. Instead, the diffraction pattern is characteristic of a circular aperture, and we obtain for the intensity in the focal plane

$$|\psi_z(\mathbf{r})|^2 = \text{const}\cdot\left|\frac{2J_1(\pi r D'_{zp}a/r_1'^2 m_0)}{\pi r D'_{zp}a/r_1'^2 m_0}\right|^2. \tag{8.73}$$

The diameter of the focal spot, defined as usual as the full width at half maximum, is

$$d_{fs} = 1.40 r_1'^2 m_0/aD'_{zp}. \tag{8.74}$$

However d_{fs} should not be equated with the spatial resolution δ_{zp}. The latter is determined by finding how much $\mathbf{r}_s$ must be changed to shift the center of the focal spot by d_{fs}. Some simple algebra (Barrett and Horrigan, 1973) gives

$$\delta_{zp} = 1.40 r_1'^2/bD'_{zp}. \tag{8.75}$$

To put this result in a more useful form, note that the width of the outermost zone in the zone plate is given by

$$\Delta r'_{min} = r'_N - r'_{N-1} \approx r'_1/2\sqrt{N} = r_1'^2/D'_{zp}, \tag{8.76}$$

where r'_N is the radius of the outermost zone,

$$r'_N = \tfrac{1}{2}D'_{zp} = r'_1\sqrt{N}. \tag{8.77}$$

Therefore

$$\delta_{zp} = 1.40\,\Delta r'_{min}/b. \tag{8.78}$$

Comparison of this result with the corresponding result for a pinhole, (4.35), shows that the zone plate aperture gives approximately the same resolution as the pinhole that just fits into the outermost zone.

8.3.3 The Off-Axis Zone Plate in Radiography

Coded-aperture imaging with an on-axis zone plate suffers from the same problem as on-axis Gabor holography. In the reconstruction step, the unwanted terms in t_{zp} produce waves that overlap the desired focal spot and reduce its contrast. The more resolvable point sources there are in the original emissive object, the more overlapping zone plates there are in the coded image and the more the contrast is reduced. In practice, the on-axis zone plate is a useful coded aperture only for very dilute objects such as x-ray stars; it is virtually useless in nuclear medicine. (See, however, Section 8.3.4.)

Just as in optical holography, one way to image large objects with a zone-plate coded aperture is to use an off-axis zone plate. Then, as we discussed in Section 8.3.1, there is a spatial separation of the diffracted orders and one may indeed treat $g_{zp}(\mathbf{r}')$ as being composed of only a single quadratic phase factor. The other terms are of no concern.

However, if the on-axis zone plate aperture is simply replaced by an off-axis one, it is usually found that there is no reconstruction at all. From a physical point of view, it is easiest to appreciate the source of this difficulty by considering what an extended source looks like from positions in the detector plane. If the source is large enough that several opaque zones of the zone plate can be seen across it, moving from point to point in the detector plane will vary the position of these zones relative to the object, but the total radiation collected at each point will vary only little. The result is a very low-contrast coded image that does not contain much information. Stated differently, a large, structureless object casts a large structureless shadow of a fine aperture; the coded image is more or less a uniform gray and cannot diffract much light in the reconstruction step.

From a more mathematical point of view, the difficulty is that there is very little overlap between the scaled Fourier transforms of the object and the aperture transmittance. Equation (4.22) tells us that the transform of the coded image is

$$H(\boldsymbol{\rho}'') = C(a/b)^2 \tilde{F}(\boldsymbol{\rho}'')\tilde{G}_{zp}(\boldsymbol{\rho}''). \tag{8.79}$$

If the object is broad and structureless, $\tilde{F}(\boldsymbol{\rho}'')$ is nonzero only for small values of $\boldsymbol{\rho}''$. The scaled aperture transform $\tilde{G}(\boldsymbol{\rho}'')$, on the other hand, has a bandpass character as shown in Fig. 8.28 (Barrett and Horrigan, 1973). The off-axis zone plate thus acts as a bandpass filter that rejects all spatial frequencies in the object except those within a circular passband in the ξ–η plane. In

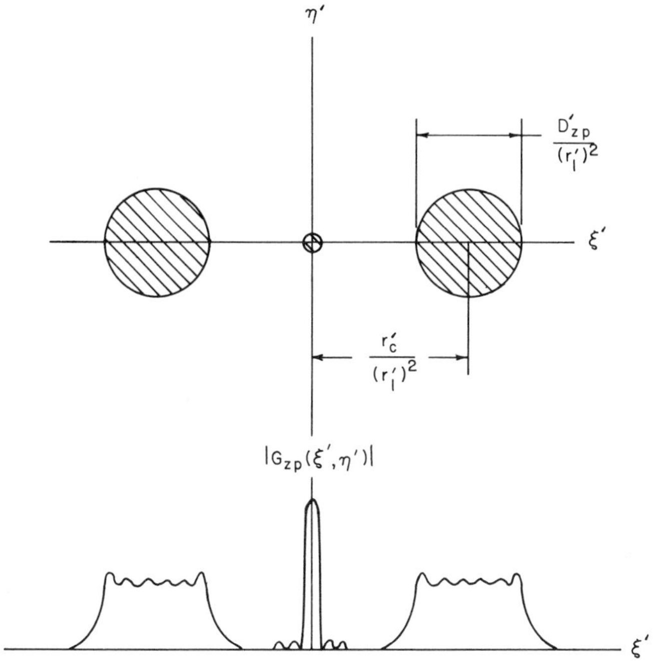

Fig. 8.28 Illustration of the Fourier transform of an off-axis zone plate $G_{zp}(\xi', \eta')$. The upper part of the figure shows an aerial view of the two-dimensional spatial-frequency plane. The function $G_{zp}(\xi', \eta')$ is nonzero over a small region near the origin and in two circular regions displaced an amount $r'_c/r_1'^2$ from the origin, where r'_c is the distance from the center of curvature of the zones to the center of the aperture, and r'_1 is the radius of the first zone (which is not necessarily within the aperture). There are also other circular regions, not shown, which are displaced still further from the origin, and in which $G_{zp}(\xi', \eta')$ is small but nonzero. These regions correspond to higher-order terms in the zone-plate transmission. The lower portion of the figure shows (schematically) the magnitude of the complex quantity $G_{zp}(\xi', \eta')$ along the ξ' axis.

particular, very low frequencies are rejected. If $\tilde{F}(\boldsymbol{\rho}'')$ is nonzero only when $\tilde{G}(\boldsymbol{\rho}'')$ is near zero and vice versa, the coded image $H(\boldsymbol{\rho}'')$ contains essentially no information.

The solution to this dilemma is to artifically introduce into the object high spatial frequencies that can be recorded with good fidelity by the off-axis system. This is accomplished by modulating the object with a periodic pattern of opaque and transparent bars as shown in Fig. 8.29. In optical parlance, the modulating pattern is known as a *Ronchi ruling*, while in the literature on coded apertures it is frequently called a *halftone screen*. This latter appellation, however, is misleading since a halftone screen as used in the printing trade serves to correct for a nonlinear imaging system, not necessarily one that is unresponsive to low frequencies.

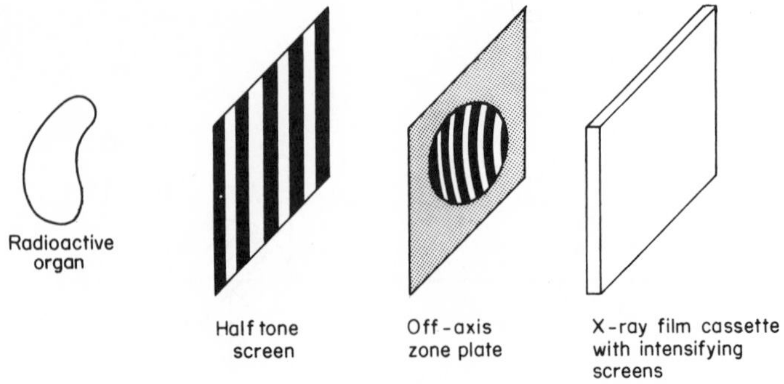

Fig. 8.29 Coded-aperture system using an off-axis zone plate with a modulating grid ("half-tone screen") near the object. The grid serves to spatially heterodyne the object spectrum into the pass band of the zone plate.

The combination of the modulating grid and the original object can be thought of as an effective object that has been artifically divided into parts that are small enough to be imaged by the zone plate. Another viewpoint is that the modulating grid *samples* the object (see Section 2.5). If the grid frequency satisfies the Nyquist condition (2.82), then no information about the object is lost in recording the coded image, and the effects of the grid can be readily removed from the final image by using an appropriate low-pass filter in the reconstruction process.

Still another physical interpretation of the action of the modulating grid is that a moiré fringe pattern is formed on the detector. As shown in Fig. 8.30, there are some places on the detector plane where the transparent bars on the grid appear to line up with the transparent zones in the center of the zone

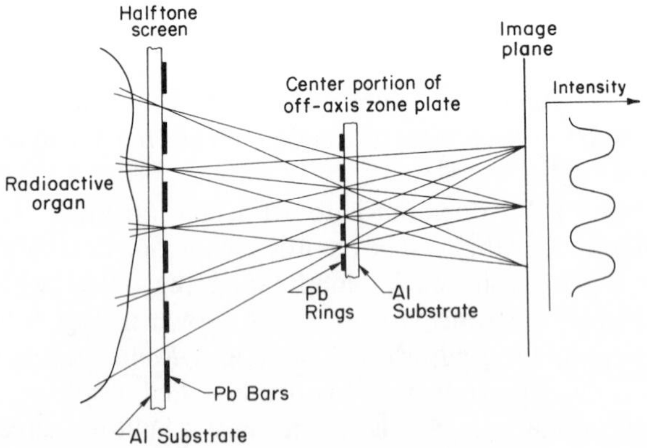

Fig. 8.30 Illustration of the action of the modulating grid. The coded image is a moiré pattern formed by the zone plate and the modulated object.

plate. A relatively large radiation flux is received at these points. Conversely, there are some detector points from which the opaque bars on the grid appear to line up with the transparent center zones, and a relatively smaller flux is received. It is diffraction from these moiré fringes that ultimately forms the reconstruction.

In a more formal way, the use of a modulating grid can be shown to be equivalent to a heterodyne technique for matching the Fourier spectrum of the object to that of the off-axis zone plate. For simplicity, assume that the object is planar and that the modulating grid is in direct contact with it. (Neither of these assumptions is essential.) Let the gamma-ray transmission of the modulating grid be denoted by $g_{mg}(\mathbf{r})$, and let its Fourier transform be $G_{mg}(\boldsymbol{\rho})$. The effective object is then given by

$$f_{eff}(\mathbf{r}) = f(\mathbf{r})g_{mg}(\mathbf{r}), \tag{8.80}$$

or, in the frequency domain

$$F_{eff}(\boldsymbol{\rho}) = F(\boldsymbol{\rho}) ** G_{mg}(\boldsymbol{\rho}). \tag{8.81}$$

The usual equations for image formation are still applicable with $f_{eff}(\mathbf{r})$ appearing in place of $f(\mathbf{r})$. In particular, (8.79) becomes

$$H(\boldsymbol{\rho}'') = C(a/b)^2 \tilde{F}_{eff}(\boldsymbol{\rho}'')\tilde{G}_{zp}(\boldsymbol{\rho}''), \tag{8.82}$$

where [cf. (4.20)]

$$\begin{aligned}\tilde{F}_{eff}(\boldsymbol{\rho}'') &= \mathscr{F}_2\{f(-a\mathbf{r}''/b)g_{mg}(-a\mathbf{r}''/b)\}\\ &= (b/a)^2 F_{eff}(-b\boldsymbol{\rho}''/a)\\ &= (b/a)^2[F(-b\boldsymbol{\rho}''/a) ** G_{mg}(-b\boldsymbol{\rho}''/a)].\end{aligned} \tag{8.83}$$

To avoid carrying along the scale factors, we define

$$\tilde{G}_{mg}(\boldsymbol{\rho}'') = (b/a)^2 G_{mg}(-b\boldsymbol{\rho}''/a). \tag{8.84}$$

Note that the tilde on $\tilde{G}_{mg}$ has a different meaning from the one on $\tilde{G}_{zp}$; since G_{mg} is originally in the same plane as F, it has the same scaling property as F. From (8.84) and (8.83) it is easy to show, by writing out the convolution integral in detail, that

$$\tilde{F}_{eff}(\boldsymbol{\rho}'') = \tilde{F}(\boldsymbol{\rho}'') ** \tilde{G}_{mg}(\boldsymbol{\rho}''), \tag{8.85}$$

and therefore (8.82) becomes

$$H(\boldsymbol{\rho}'') = C(a/b)^2[\tilde{F}(\boldsymbol{\rho}'') ** \tilde{G}_{mg}(\boldsymbol{\rho}'')]\tilde{G}_{zp}(\boldsymbol{\rho}''). \tag{8.86}$$

To interpret this equation, we must use the fact that $g_{mg}(\mathbf{r})$ is a periodic function in one dimension. Therefore $\tilde{g}_{mg}(\mathbf{r}'')$ is also a periodic function and its Fourier transform must be nonzero only for a discrete set of frequencies [see Appendix B, especially (B.87)]. We can then write

$$\tilde{G}_{\text{mg}}(\boldsymbol{\rho}'') = \sum_{n=-\infty}^{\infty} \tilde{G}_n \delta(\boldsymbol{\rho}'' - n\boldsymbol{\rho}_{\text{g}}''), \tag{8.87}$$

where the $\tilde{G}_n$ are constants (Fourier components of the grid) and $\boldsymbol{\rho}_{\text{g}}''$ is the fundamental frequency of $\tilde{G}_{\text{mg}}(\boldsymbol{\rho}'')$. The scaled frequency $\boldsymbol{\rho}_{\text{g}}''$ is related to the fundamental frequency of the grid before scaling by $\boldsymbol{\rho}_{\text{g}}'' = -a\boldsymbol{\rho}_{\text{g}}/b$.

The use of (8.87) allows the convolution in (8.86) to be readily performed since convolution of a function with a delta function just reproduces the original function with a shift. The result is

$$H(\boldsymbol{\rho}'') = C\left(\frac{a}{b}\right)^2 \tilde{G}_{\text{zp}}(\boldsymbol{\rho}'') \sum_{n=-\infty}^{\infty} \tilde{G}_n \tilde{F}(\boldsymbol{\rho}'' - n\boldsymbol{\rho}_{\text{g}}''). \tag{8.88}$$

Equations of this form were also encountered in the discussion of sampling in Chapter 2. Sampling a function in the space domain corresponds to replicating its transform in the frequency domain. For the present purposes, the importance of this result is that $\boldsymbol{\rho}_{\text{g}}''$ can be chosen so that one of the replicas of $\tilde{F}(\boldsymbol{\rho}'')$ falls in the passband of $\tilde{G}_{\text{zp}}(\boldsymbol{\rho}'')$.

Thus, with the modulating grid the problem of spectral overlap between $\tilde{G}_{\text{zp}}$ and $\tilde{F}$ has been solved. The resulting coded image is fully analogous to an off-axis Leith and Upatnieks hologram, and high-quality images of extended objects can be formed. Some examples will be shown in Section 8.3.5.

Further details on the off-axis zone plate, including expressions for its resolution and depth of field, are given by Barrett and Horrigan (1973).

An interesting variation on the basic off-axis zone plate system was proposed by Wilson *et al.* (1973). They replaced the Ronchi modulation grid by a second off-axis zone plate. For $s_1 = s_2$, the scale of the modulation zone plate is chosen to be exactly twice the scale of the imaging aperture. The space-domain counterpart of (8.82) then becomes

$$h(\mathbf{r}'') = C(a/b)^2[\tilde{f}(\mathbf{r}'')\tilde{g}_{\text{zp}}(\mathbf{r}'')] ** \tilde{g}_{\text{zp}}(\mathbf{r}''). \tag{8.89}$$

Since the two zone plates are identical after projection to the detector, they are both described by the *same* function $\tilde{g}_{\text{zp}}(\mathbf{r}'')$. This function is given by

$$\tilde{g}_{\text{zp}}(\mathbf{r}'') = \left(\frac{1}{2} + \frac{1}{\pi i}\exp\left(-\frac{i\pi a^2 r''^2}{r_1'^2}\right) + \frac{1}{\pi i}\exp\left(\frac{i\pi a^2 r''^2}{r_1'^2}\right)\right)$$
$$\cdot \operatorname{circ}\left[\left(\frac{2a}{D_{\text{zp}}'}\right)|a\mathbf{r}'' - \mathbf{r}_c|\right] + \text{higher-order terms}, \tag{8.90}$$

where the vector $\mathbf{r}_c$ defines the location of the center of curvature of the zones. The easiest way to understand the operation of this system is to consider an infinite zone plate ($D_{\text{zp}}' \to \infty$) and concentrate on selected terms from (8.90). In particular, we pick the term $\exp(-i\pi a^2 r''^2/r_1'^2)$ for the first appearance of $\tilde{g}_{zp}(\mathbf{r}'')$ in (8.89) and the term $\exp(+i\pi a^2 r''^2/r_1'^2)$ for the second appearance of $\tilde{g}_{zp}(\mathbf{r}'')$, or vice versa. We then have

$$h(\mathbf{r}'') = -C\left(\frac{a}{\pi b}\right)^2 \int_\infty \tilde{f}(\mathbf{r}_0'')\exp\left(-\frac{i\pi a^2 r_0''^2}{r_1'^2}\right) \cdot \exp\left[\left(\frac{i\pi a^2}{r_1'^2}\right)|\mathbf{r}'' - \mathbf{r}_0''|^2\right] d^2 r_0'' + \text{cc} + \text{other terms}, \tag{8.91}$$

where cc denotes the complex conjugate of the previous term. If we expand out the factor $|\mathbf{r}'' - \mathbf{r}_0''|^2$, we see that the terms proportional to $r_0''^2$ cancel and we are left with

$$h(\mathbf{r}'') = -C(a/\pi b)^2 \exp(i\pi a^2 r''^2/r_1'^2) \cdot \int_\infty \tilde{f}(\mathbf{r}_0'')\exp\left[-2\pi i\left(\frac{a^2}{r_1'^2}\right)\mathbf{r}'' \cdot \mathbf{r}_0''\right] d^2 r_0'' + \text{cc} + \text{other terms}. \tag{8.92}$$

However, this integral is just the Fourier transform of $\tilde{f}(\mathbf{r}'')$ with a frequency variable $\boldsymbol{\rho}'' = a^2\mathbf{r}''/r_1'^2$. Therefore we may write

$$h(\mathbf{r}'') = -C(a/\pi b)^2 \exp(i\pi a^2 r''^2/r_1'^2)\,\tilde{F}(a^2\mathbf{r}''/r_1'^2) + \text{cc} + \text{other terms}. \tag{8.93}$$

This equation shows that the coded image has the same structure as a Fraunhofer diffraction pattern (Goodman, 1968; Gaskill, 1978) and may therefore be regarded as a Fraunhofer hologram. Reconstruction is accomplished with a coherent optical system in which suitable apertures are used to eliminate the unwanted terms (Wilson *et al.*, 1973).

To gain some physical insight into (8.93), consider what the object looks like when viewed from a point in the detector plane. From this point one zone plate is projected onto the other, but with a lateral shift that depends on the location of the viewing point. When two identical zone plates are superimposed with a shift, a set of regularly spaced moiré fringes is produced as shown in Fig. 8.31. The detector therefore receives a flux of radiation proportional to the spatial integral of the product of the object distribution $f(\mathbf{r})$ and the modulating moiré pattern. But this is just a literal interpretation of a two-dimensional Fourier integral; a Fourier sine transform is formed by multiplying a function by a sinusoidal pattern and integrating. To the extent that the fringes are sinusoidal [which means neglecting the higher-order terms in $g_{zp}(\mathbf{r}')$] the flux is thus proportional to one Fourier component of $f(\mathbf{r})$. A different detector point records a different Fourier component since the vector spatial frequency of the moiré fringes is proportional to the vector displacement between the two zone plates, and this displacement depends on the location of the detector point due to parallax. Furthermore, a small displacement of the detector point produces only a small change in the spatial frequency of the fringes, but a substantial change in their phase, causing

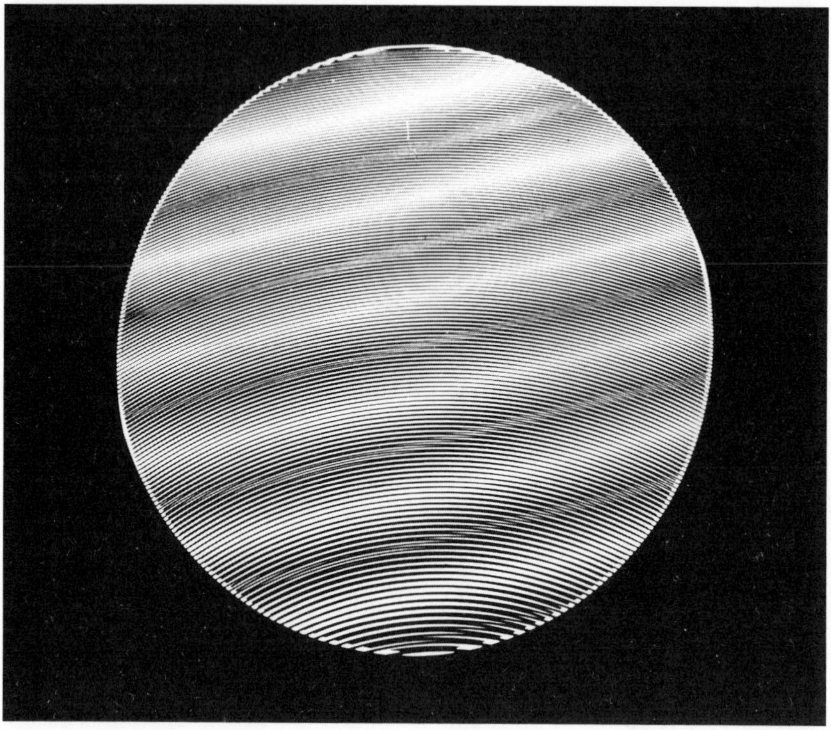

Fig. 8.31 Moiré fringe pattern produced by two off-axis zone plates.

sinusoidal fringes to become cosinusoidal. Thus the complete Fourier transform, sine and cosine terms over a wide range of frequencies, is recorded in the coded image.

8.3.4 Multiple Zone Plates

Although the off-axis zone plate yields high-quality images of large objects, it has one important drawback that has seriously limited its use. For zone plates with the same r_1' and D_{zp}', an off-axis zone plate has substantially finer zones than an on-axis one. Therefore the detector must have a higher spatial resolution in the off-axis case in order to resolve the fine detail in the coded image. Alternatively, for a given detector a coarser off-axis zone plate (larger r_1') must be used and spatial resolution in the decoded image must be sacrificed. Numerically, the resolution will be about a factor of three worse in the off-axis case. Since the resolution of an Anger camera is rather poor to begin with, a further three-fold loss is unacceptable and the off-axis zone plate is not usable with an Anger camera. Since no other detector is widely used in nuclear medicine, the off-axis zone plate has found very little clinical applicability.

One solution to this dilemma is to use on-axis zone plates but find other ways to eliminate the unwanted terms in $g_{zp}(\mathbf{r}')$. This goal can be achieved if more than one coded image is formed from the same object, and information from all coded images is combined in the decoding step. The procedure is reminiscent of the two-annulus algorithm described in Section 8.2.4. Suppose, for example, that we construct four on-axis zone plates with transmissions given by

$$\begin{aligned} g_1(\mathbf{r}') &= \tfrac{1}{2}[1 + \sin(\pi r'^2/r_1'^2)]\,\mathrm{circ}(2r'/D'_{zp}), \\ g_2(\mathbf{r}') &= \tfrac{1}{2}[1 + \cos(\pi r'^2/r_1'^2)]\,\mathrm{circ}(2r'/D'_{zp}), \\ g_3(\mathbf{r}') &= \tfrac{1}{2}[1 - \sin(\pi r'^2/r_1'^2)]\,\mathrm{circ}(2r'/D'_{zp}), \\ g_4(\mathbf{r}') &= \tfrac{1}{2}[1 - cos(\pi r'^2/r_1'^2)]\,\mathrm{circ}(2r'/D'_{zp}). \end{aligned} \tag{8.94}$$

Note that all of these functions are positive definite and less than one everywhere; they thus represent physically realizable gamma-ray transmittances. The corresponding coded images, denoted by $h_i(\mathbf{r}'')$ $(i = 1\text{–}4)$, are given by

$$h_i(\mathbf{r}'') = C(a/b)^2\tilde{f}(\mathbf{r}'') ** \tilde{g}_i(\mathbf{r}''), \qquad i = 1\text{–}4, \tag{8.95}$$

where the tildes imply projection to the image plane as usual.

If all four of the coded images are stored in a computer, we can form an auxiliary complex function $h_c(\mathbf{r}'')$ defined by

$$h_c(\mathbf{r}'') = [h_2(\mathbf{r}'') - h_4(\mathbf{r}'')] - i[h_1(\mathbf{r}'') - h_3(\mathbf{r}'')]. \tag{8.96}$$

Since $h_c(\mathbf{r}'')$ does not represent any physically measurable quantity, but only numbers in a computer, there is nothing to prohibit it from being complex.

Using (8.94) and (8.95), it is easy to show that

$$h_c(\mathbf{r}'') = C(a/b)^2\tilde{f}(\mathbf{r}'') ** \tilde{g}_{czp}(\mathbf{r}''), \tag{8.97}$$

where

$$\tilde{g}_{czp}(\mathbf{r}'') = \exp(-i\pi a^2 r''^2/r_1'^2)\,\mathrm{circ}(2ar''/D'_{zp}). \tag{8.98}$$

Here czp means "complex zone plate". Comparison of (8.98) with (8.64) shows that we have succeeded in isolating the interesting term in $\tilde{g}_{zp}(\mathbf{r}'')$.

Decoding can now be carried out by several means. For example, we can perform a matched filtering operation in the computer by correlating $h_c(\mathbf{r}'')$ with a function proportional to $\tilde{g}_{czp}(\mathbf{r}'')$. Or we can produce an optical transparency for which the complex amplitude transmittance is proportional to $h_c(\mathbf{r}'')$. If this transparency is illuminated with a plane wave, a nearly exact image of $f(\mathbf{r})$ is formed [see (8.67)–(8.69)]. More details on this optical approach are given by Barrett *et al.* (1974).

If, instead of using four zone plates, we had used just two (say g_1 and g_3), there would be no way to eliminate the twin-image term. However, we could eliminate the dc term by simply subtracting the two coded images (Macdonald *et al.*, 1974):

$$h_1(\mathbf{r}'') - h_3(\mathbf{r}'') = C(a/b)^2\tilde{f}(\mathbf{r}'') ** \{[\sin(\pi a^2 r''^2/r_1'^2)]\,\mathrm{circ}(2ar''/D'_{zp})\}. \quad (8.99)$$

In other words, the difference image is equivalent to an image formed with a physically unrealizable bipolar (but real) coded aperture. For objects of modest size, this approach can produce acceptable images. It can be shown that three on-axis zone plates are the least that can be used and still produce a complete separation of terms.

One drawback to the use of multiple zone plates is that the object must not change during the entire sequence of exposures. Therefore this technique is unsuited for rapid dynamic studies.

8.3.5 Practical Results

The earliest example of the successful use of a zone-plate coded aperture was the work of Mertz and Young (1961). Using an off-axis zone plate and film recording, they produced a good reconstruction of a star field. Because the object consisted mainly of a set of discrete points, no modulating grid was necessary.

Initial attempts to use a zone plate with an Anger camera were largely unsuccessful (Barrett, 1972). However, higher-resolution detectors such as an image intensifier camera (Rogers *et al.*, 1972) and x-ray film cassettes (Barrett *et al.*, 1973), which permitted the use of off-axis zone plates and modulating grids, did produce good images. Examples are shown in Figs. 8.32–8.35. Some clinical studies were carried out using film cassettes by Farmelant *et al.* (1975). In this work, the poor quantum efficiency of x-ray film-screen systems at 140 keV led to an exposure time that was usually a factor of 4–6 longer than with an Anger camera and collimator. Even though the images, especially of the thyroid, had high resolution, and the tomographic capability was sometimes useful, the long exposure times prevented wide use.

This same system—an off-axis zone plate, modulating grid, and screen-film detector—was used successfully by Holman *et al.* (1977) to study myocardial infarction in dogs (see Fig. 8.35). These workers were able to quantitatively determine the volume of the infarct to an accuracy of about 15% from the optically reconstructed images. For animal studies, large doses could be used to circumvent the poor quantum efficiency of the screens.

The results of a study performed with an Anger camera and multiple on-axis zone plates are shown in Fig. 8.36. Although the image quality is

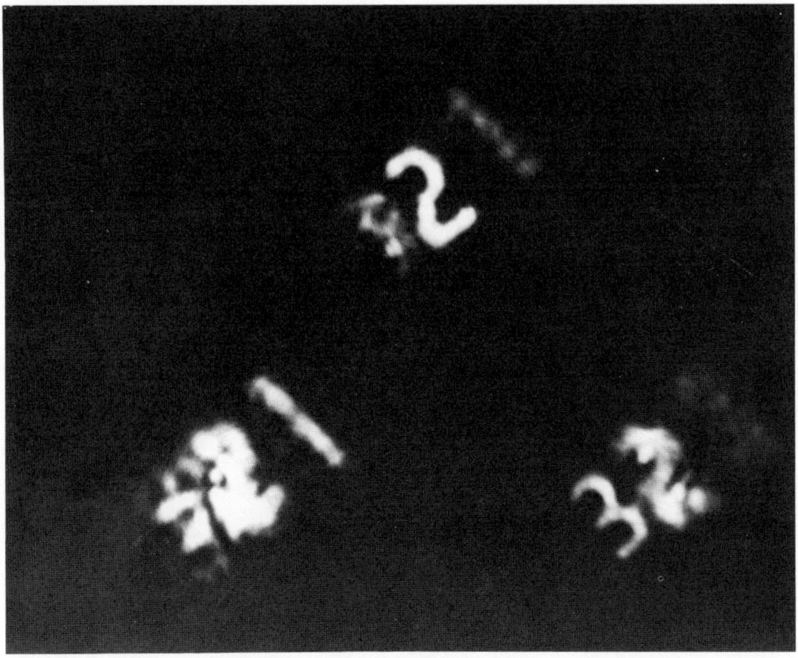

Fig. 8.32 Illustration of the tomographic capability of the off-axis zone plate system. The object consisted of three radioactive numerals in three different planes. Reconstruction was carried out with a coherent optical system. Shown here are three different reconstructed images, focused on each of the numerals. Note the considerable out-of-focus artifacts.

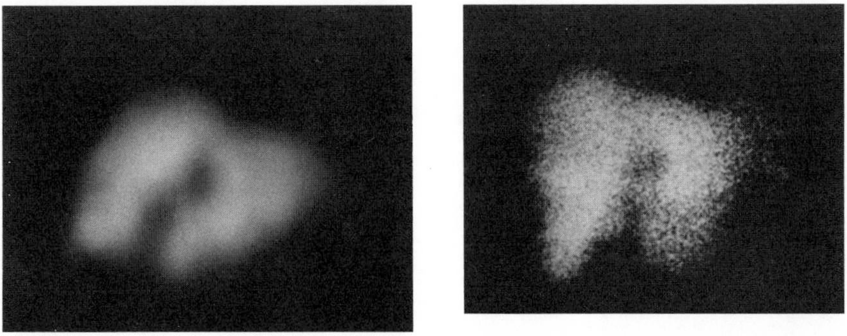

Fig. 8.33 ^{99m}Tc sulfur colloid images of a patient showing considerable hepatomegaly Left: Image from zone plate-film cassette system. Right: Image from Anger Camera and collimator. (From Farmelant *et al.*, 1975.)

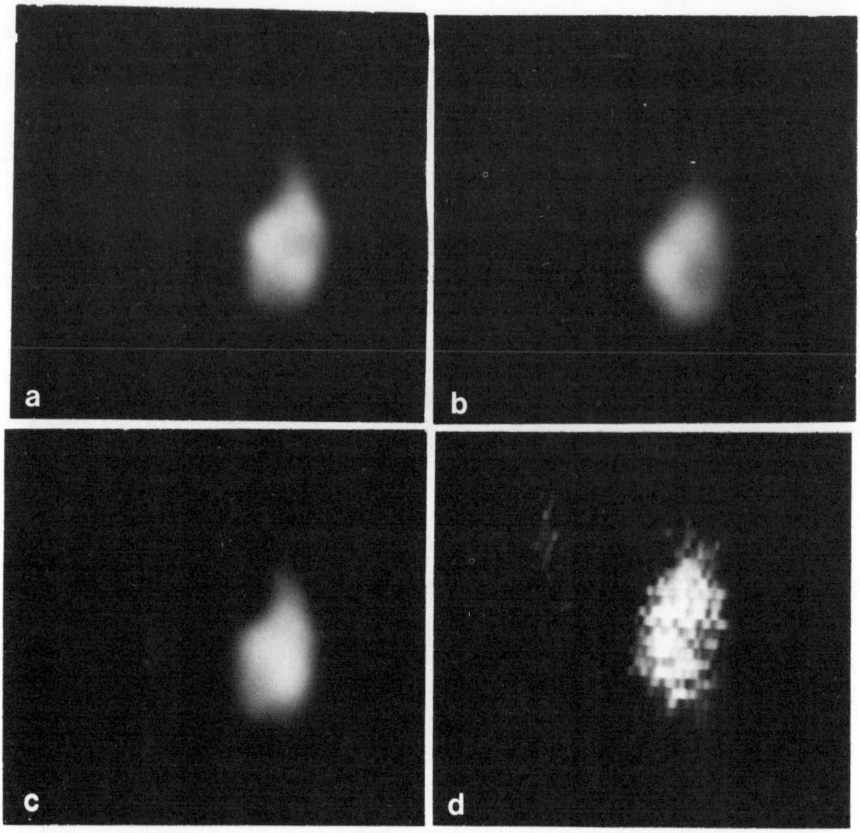

Fig. 8.34 Images of the thyroid gland of a patient who has had a partial thyroidectomy. (a)–(c) are three different planes reconstructed from a coded image obtained with the zone plate-film cassette system. Note the cold nodule in (b) that was confirmed by palpation. (d) is a conventional image obtained with a rectilinear scanner. (From Farmelant *et al.*, 1975.)

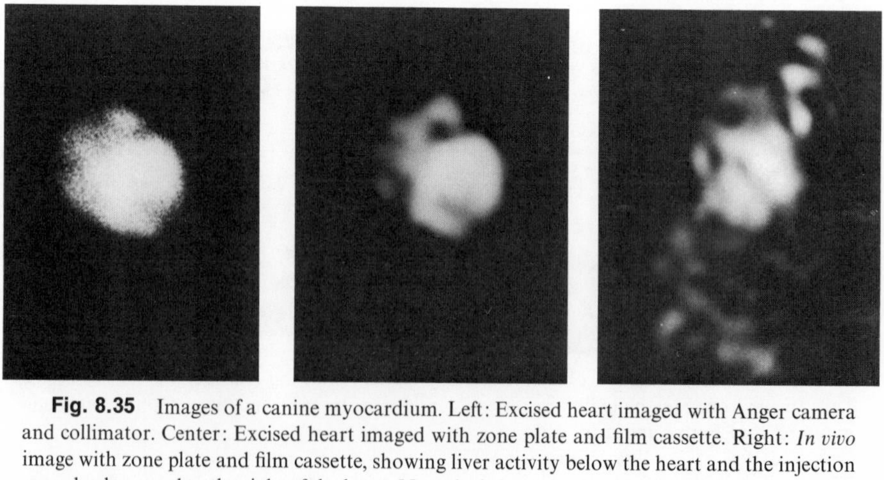

Fig. 8.35 Images of a canine myocardium. Left: Excised heart imaged with Anger camera and collimator. Center: Excised heart imaged with zone plate and film cassette. Right: *In vivo* image with zone plate and film cassette, showing liver activity below the heart and the injection cannula above and to the right of the heart. Note the infarct clearly visualized in both zone-plate images as a cold line extending to the apex of the heart. (From Farmelant *et al.*, 1975.)

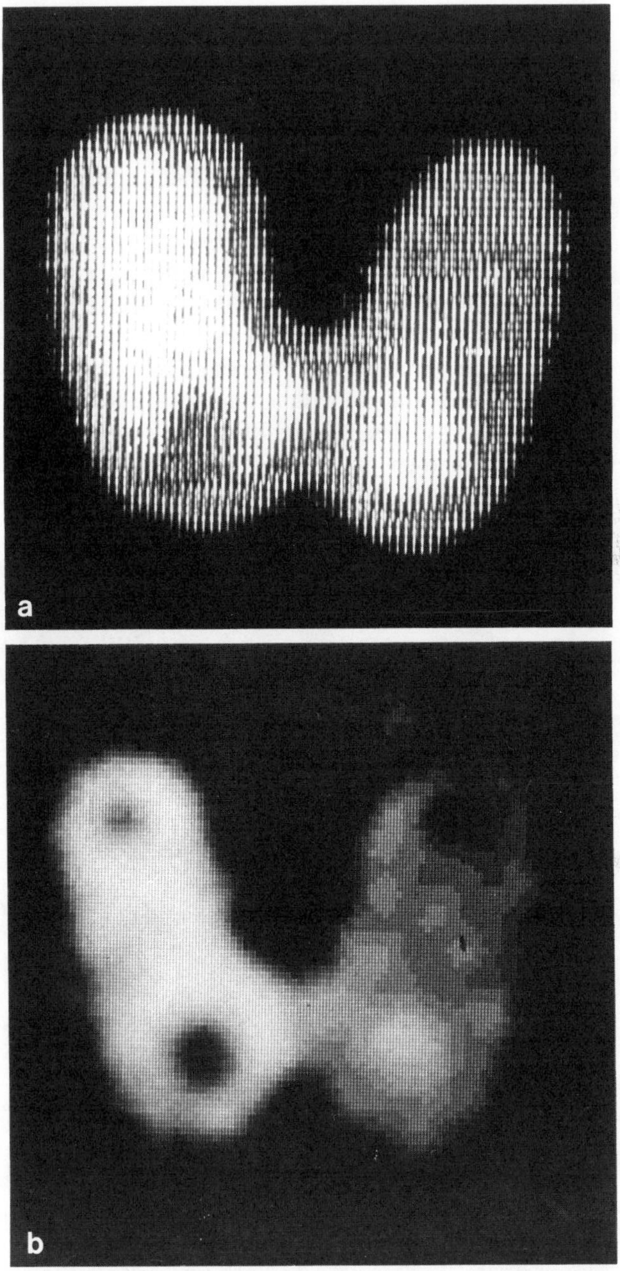

Fig. 8.36 Images of the Picker thyroid phantom with a Picker Dynacamera 4/15. (a) Image with conventional multihole collimator. (b) Image at same total exposure time with three on-axis zone plates. (Unpublished work of E. R. Reinhardt, G. Laub, and W. H. Bloss, University of Stuttgart, and U. Feine and W. Müller-Schauenburg, University of Tübingen.)

good, changing the plates is mechanically cumbersome, and the limited count-rate capability of the Anger camera nullifies part of the advantage of the more efficient aperture.

Further work with the zone plate must await the development of better detectors. For example, a screen-film system with a spatial resolution better than 1 mm and a quantum efficiency in excess of 50% could theoretically be constructed using cesium iodide or bismuth germanate. Such a detector could again make the zone plate into a competitive clinical tool.

In the nonmedical arena, the zone plate has been used to image laser fusion pellets (Ceglio *et al.*, 1977a,b), and fuel pins in a nuclear reactor (Stalker and Kelly, 1980; Kelly *et al.*, 1979). The latter work is particularly interesting because an elaborate detector system based on image intensifiers was constructed specifically for use with a zone plate aperture.

The zone plate has also been used for coded-source imaging, and a reconstructed image is shown in Fig. 8.37. Perhaps the most interesting feature of this image is that the finest bars in the resolution test target, with

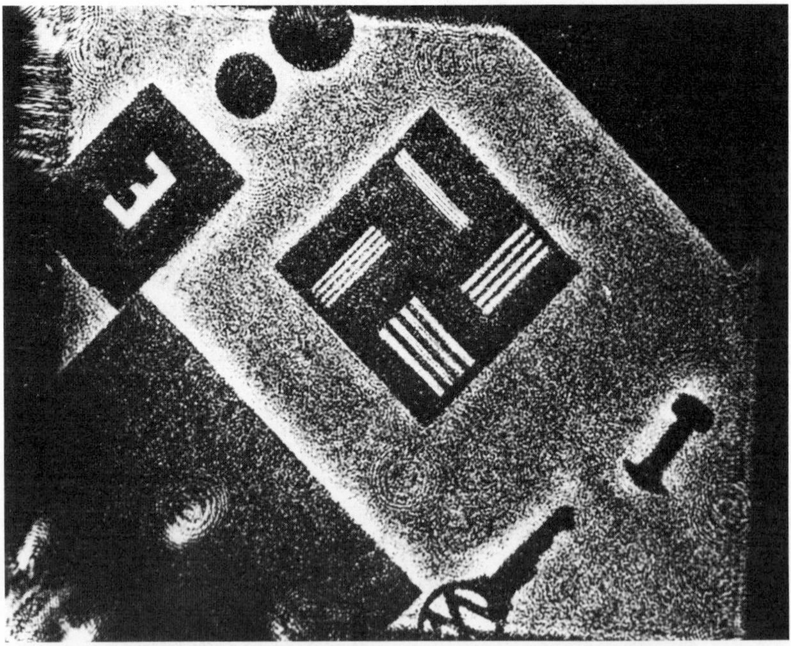

Fig. 8.37 Transmission radiograph obtained with a zone-plate coded-source imaging system. A large disk source of x rays, about 5 cm in diameter, was coded with an off-axis zone plate. The magnification was 2:1 ($s_1 = s_2$), and the object was covered with a modulating grid made of thin tungsten wires. Reconstruction was accomplished with a coherent optical system. (From Stoner *et al.*, 1976.)

a bar width of 0.5 mm, are clearly resolved. Since the overall diameter of the x-ray source was 5 cm and 2:1 magnification was used, the resolution without coding and reconstruction would have been 2.5 cm. Thus the linear resolution in the image was increased a factor of 50 and the number of resolvable spots in the image was increased a factor of 2500.

8.4 PINHOLE ARRAYS

For best signal-to-noise ratio, as we shall see in Chapter 10, a coded image should be decoded by matched filtering. The resulting point spread function, the autocorrelation of the aperture transmission, should be as similar to a delta function as possible for good image fidelity. For this reason considerable effort has been devoted to finding aperture patterns with deltalike autocorrelation functions. In Section 8.2 we saw that the annulus does *not* have a particularly desirable autocorrelation, but requires an inverse filter that degrades the SNR. In the case of the zone plate, any one term in the infinite-series expansion for g_{zp} has a sharply peaked autocorrelation (identically a delta function in the limit $D'_{zp} \to \infty$), but some compromises must be made in order to separate out unwanted terms.

However, there are a number of coded apertures, all arrays of pinholes, that have desirable autocorrelation properties. Three variations on this basic approach are described below.

8.4.1 Random and Pseudorandom Pinhole Arrays

One of the earliest coded apertures was the random pinhole array suggested by Dicke (1968). His prescription for constructing the aperture was to lay out a square grid of points, then either make each point into a pinhole or leave it opaque according to a table of random numbers. A typical array and its autocorrelation function are shown in Fig. 8.38. Dicke suggested a number of specific ways to decode the image obtained with a random pinhole array, but all of them amount to matched filtering. One can, for example, use the incoherent correlator shown in Fig. 8.6. In any event, the PSF is the autocorrelation of the aperture pattern with suitable scale factors.

A deficiency in this aperture is readily apparent from Fig. 8.38. The PSF has a nice central core, but it does not go to zero away from the core. There is a triangular base, characteristic of the overall size of the aperture, and also small fluctuations around this triangle. For an array of N pinholes, the

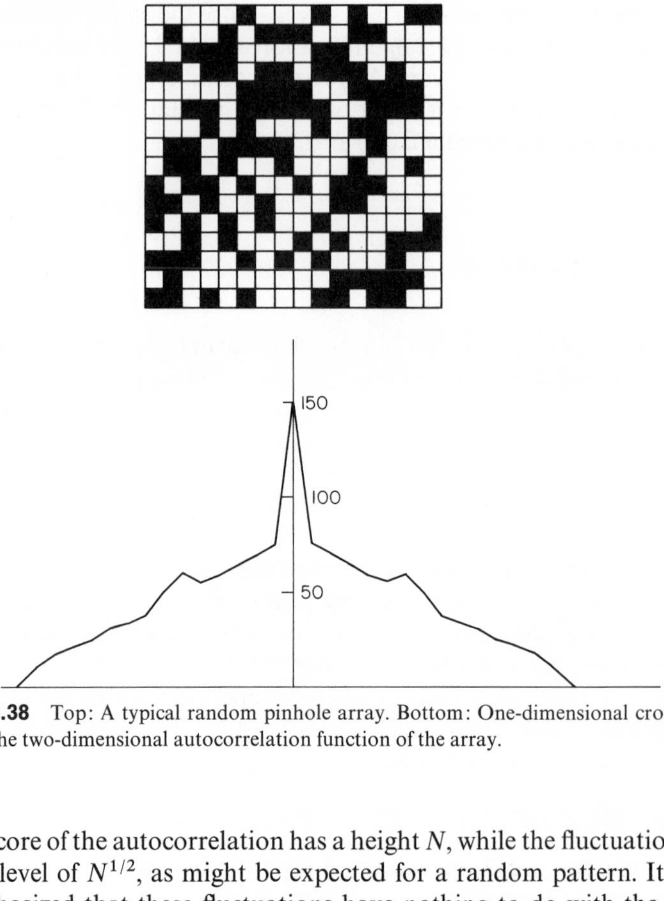

Fig. 8.38 Top: A typical random pinhole array. Bottom: One-dimensional cross section through the two-dimensional autocorrelation function of the array.

central core of the autocorrelation has a height N, while the fluctuations have an rms level of $N^{1/2}$, as might be expected for a random pattern. It should be emphasized that these fluctuations have nothing to do with the photon statistics of the radiation source. They would persist in the limit that an infinite number of photons were detected. These fluctuation are sometimes called *intrinsic noise*, although they are really not noise at all but rather a deterministic feature of the aperture code.

Minor modifications of the aperture and decoding function can improve the PSF. Brown (1972, 1974) suggested that the decoding function be essentially the same random array as the aperture, but take on both positive and negative values. Specifically, if a pinhole occurs at some location in the aperture, the corresponding location in the decoding function is assigned a value $+1$. Conversely, if a location in the aperture has no pinhole, the corresponding location in the decoding function is set to -1. This modification effectively eliminates the triangular base seen in Fig. 8.38. Brown also modified the code function itself to reduce the fluctuations further. One of his suggestions was to form two coded images with two complementary arrays—basically the approach we discussed in Section 8.3.4 with zone plates.

8.4.2 Nonredundant Pinhole Arrays

The next step in the development of pinhole arrays as coded apertures was the use of nonredundant arrays (Chang *et al.*, 1974; Wouters *et al.*, 1973), an example of which is shown in Fig. 8.39. The term nonredundant means that a particular vector displacement between any two pinholes in the array is not repeated. If $\mathbf{r}_i$ and $\mathbf{r}_j$ are the locations of the ith and jth pinholes, the quantity $\mathbf{r}_i - \mathbf{r}_j$ is different for all choices of i and j.

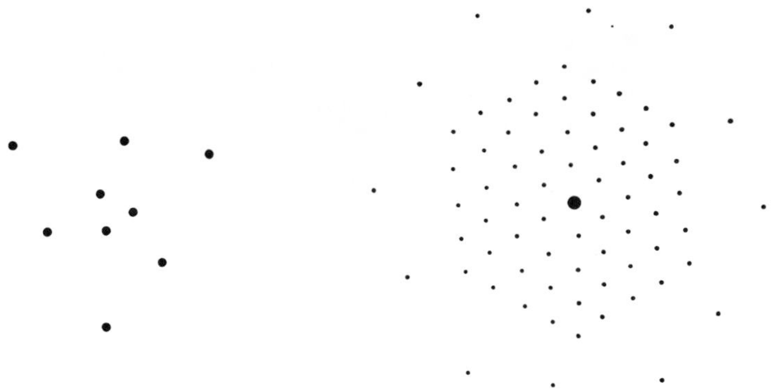

(a) (b)

Fig. 8.39 Nonredundant pinhole array (a) and its autocorrelation (b). The central peak in the autocorrelation has a value of 9, which is the number of pinholes in the array, while all other peaks are of unit height. (Courtesy of J. E. Dowdy.)

The advantage of the nonredundant array is apparent from Fig. 8.39: the side lobes in the PSF have a maximum height of unity, compared to the central core of height N, where N is the number of pinholes. However, in practice N cannot be made very large because the pinholes must have a finite diameter. Therefore even this N:1 peak-to-sidelobe ratio is not really satisfactory.

The nonredundant array can also be used as the source configuration for coded-source imaging. An example of a transmission image obtained in this way is shown in Fig. 8.40.

An ingenious iterative algorithm devised by Tipton *et al.* (1976) can be used to further reduce the sidelobes. Basically, the idea is to use the matched filter output as merely a first estimate of the object, and from this estimate

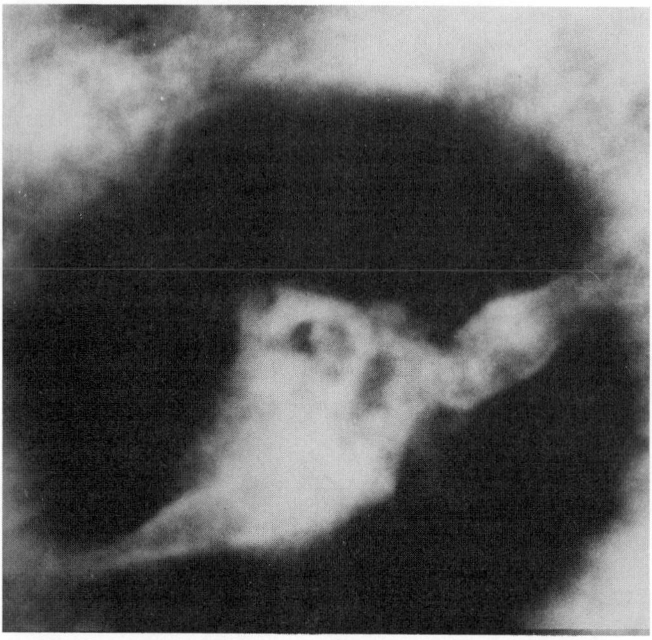

Fig. 8.40 Reconstructed tomorgraphic image of the bones of the inner ear (shown light) of a 3M skull phantom. The exposure was made on a prototype flashing tomosynthesis coded-source system and reconstructed digitally by W. J. Dallas, E. Klotz, R. Linde, W. Mauser, and H. Weiss (unpublished).

to calculate an estimate of the undesired background due to the sidelobes. The background estimate is then subtracted from the object estimate to get an improved object estimate, and the process is repeated iteratively (see Fig. 8.41).*

8.4.3 Uniformly Redundant Arrays

Since the sidelobes in the autocorrelation function are a crucial factor in image quality, considerable effort has been expended on reducing their influence. The nonredundant arrays are important because the magnitude of the sidelobes never exceeds $1/N$ of the peak height. There is another class of codes, called uniformly redundant arrays, in which the sidelobes are large but spatially uniform. The term "uniformly redundant" implies that every vector displacement $\mathbf{r}_i - \mathbf{r}_j$ recurs exactly M times. A one-dimensional example is shown in Fig. 8.42. Notice that the decoding function in Fig. 8.42

* Ohyama *et al.* (1981) have also had good results with a similar algorithm.

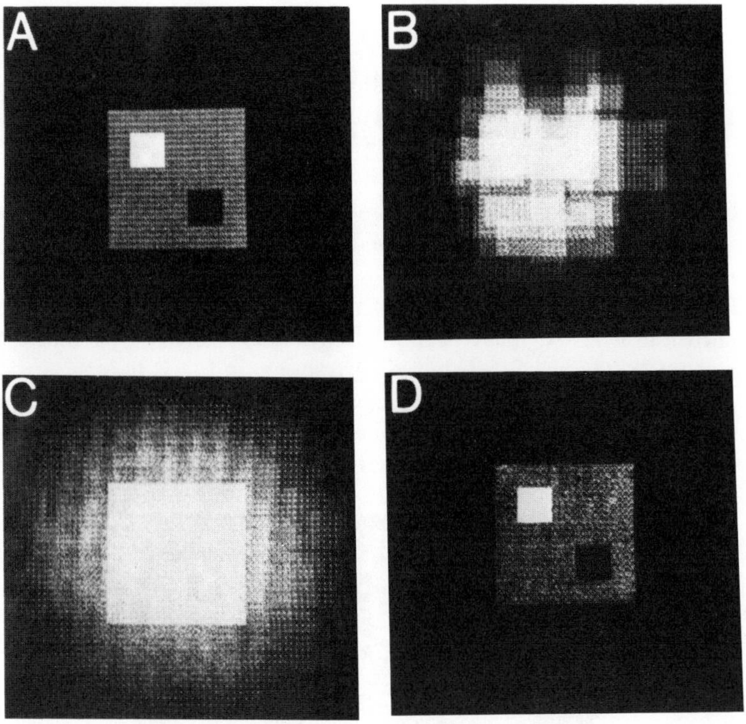

Fig. 8.41 Illustrations of the iterative decoding scheme devised by Tipton. (a) Test object used in computer simulation; (b) coded image formed with a non-redundant pinhole array; (c) Decoded image produced by matched filtering; (d) Decoded image by iterative algorithm. (Courtesy of J. E. Dowdy and M. D. Tipton. See Tipton, 1978.)

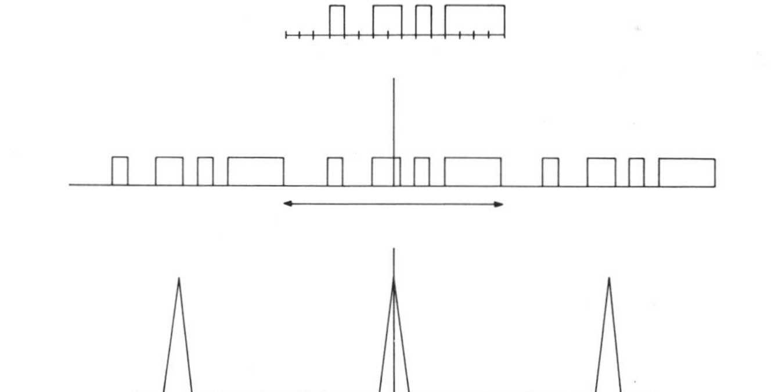

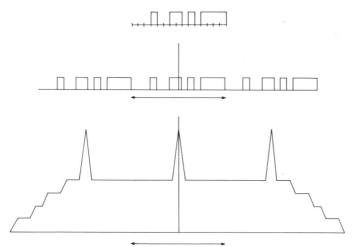

Fig. 8.42 One-dimensional uniformly redundant array and its decoded PSF. Top: The aperture code. Center: The decoding function, which is a cyclically repeated version of the basic code. Bottom: The PSF, which is the convolution of the top and center functions.

is not the aperture code itself, but rather a cyclically repeated version of the aperture. The uniformly redundant codes have the nice property that their correlation with this kind of decoding function produces a sharp central peak surrounded by sidelobes of uniform height over a substantial region. If the object is not too large, the effect of the sidelobes is to produce a uniform background level that can be removed by subtracting a constant bias level from the image.

Two-dimensional versions of the uniformly redundant codes, such as the one shown in Fig. 8.43, have been investigated extensively by Fenimore and Cannon (1978). Some of their images are shown in Fig. 8.44.

We should comment that the nice correlation property of the uniformly redundant codes holds only if the coded image and decoding functions have the same scale. If there is a mismatch in scales, nonuniformities in the

Fig. 8.43 Apertures used in computer simulations by Fenimore and Cannon (1978). Top: Uniformly redundant array. Bottom: Random array.

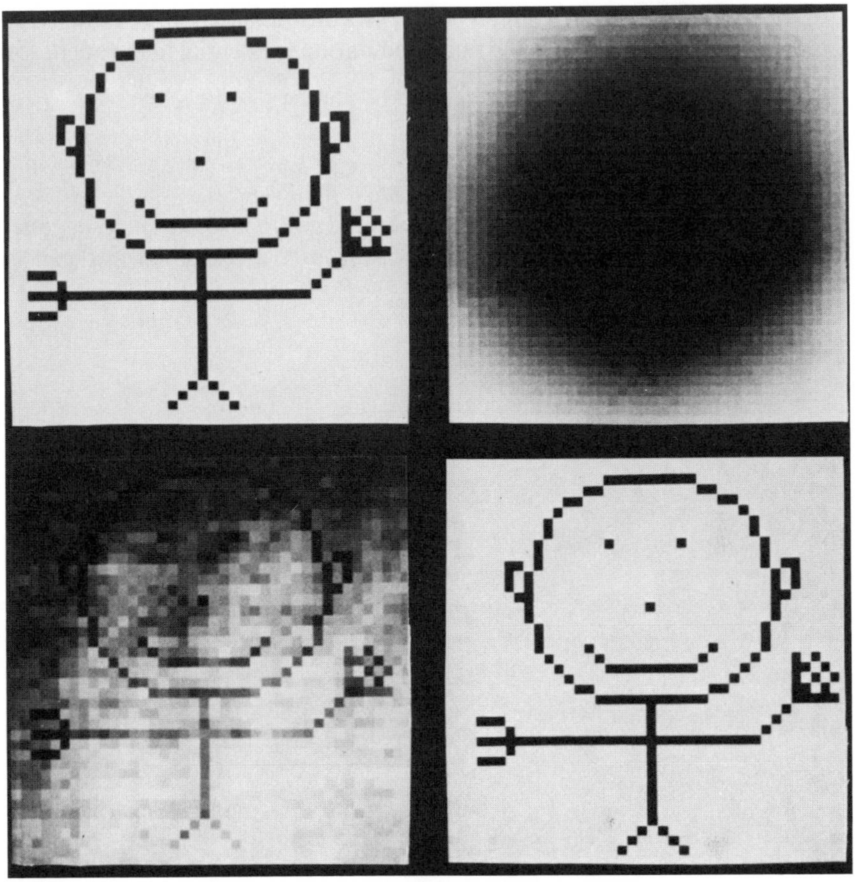

Fig. 8.44 Reconstructed images obtained by Fenimore and Cannon (1978) using arrays of Fig. 8.43. Top left: Original object. Top right: Reconstruction from random array with matched filter decoding. Bottom left: Reconstruction from random array with bipolar decoding functions. Bottom right. Reconstruction from uniformly redundant array.

sidelobes appear. Nevertheless the tomographic properties of these apertures do not appear to be any worse than other coded apertures, and Fenimore and Cannon have obtained excellent images of three-dimensional objects.

8.5 TIME-MODULATED CODED APERTURES

We have encountered several examples of time-modulated coded apertures, such as multiple annuli or zone plates. However, in these cases only a relatively small number (2–4) of individual aperture codes were used.

In this section we discuss three systems in which a large number of discrete codes are used and in which the time modulation is essential to the operation, not merely a way of improving the PSF.

8.5.1 The Rotating Slit

The rotating slit coded aperture, illustrated in Fig. 8.45, was first suggested by Tanaka and Iinuma (1975) and subsequently investigated in detail by Miller (1978).

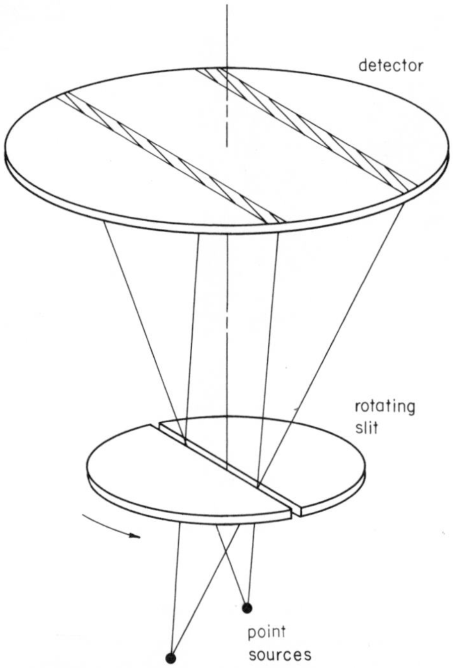

Fig. 8.45 Rotating slit coded aperture.

The aperture function for a slit of width w and length l is (see Fig. 8.46)

$$g_{\mathrm{rs}}^{\phi}(\mathbf{r}') = \mathrm{rect}[l^{-1}(x'\cos\phi + y'\sin\phi)]\,\mathrm{rect}[w^{-1}(y'\cos\phi - x'\sin\phi)], \quad (8.100)$$

where $\mathbf{r}' = (x', y')$, and ϕ is the angle between the long axis of the slit and the x' axis. A useful approximation is that l is very large and w is very small. If the length of the slit image is so large that the ends of the slit do not fall on the detector, the first rect function in (8.100) is always unity. If w is so small that the slit image appears to be an unresolvable line, the second rect function

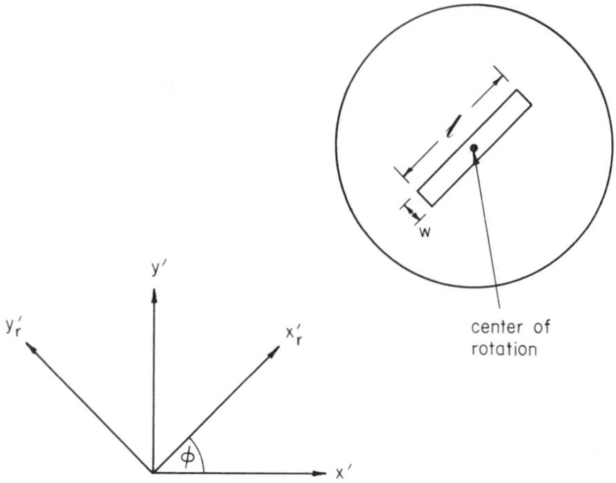

Fig. 8.46 Geometry for the rotating slit.

may be replaced with a delta function. We then have

$$g_{\mathrm{rs}}^{\phi}(\mathbf{r}') \approx w\,\delta(y'\cos\phi - x'\sin\phi). \tag{8.101}$$

Note that this is a one-dimensional delta function describing a line in the x'–y' plane. It is analogous to the ring delta function used to describe the annulus.

To simplify the impending algebra, we define a rotated coordinate system by (see Fig. 8.46)

$$x'_{\mathrm{r}} = x'\cos\phi + y'\sin\phi, \qquad y'_{\mathrm{r}} = y'\cos\phi - x'\sin\phi. \tag{8.102}$$

Similar rotated coordinates may be defined in the $\mathbf{r}$ and $\mathbf{r}''$ planes. In terms of these coordinates,

$$g_{\mathrm{rs}}^{\phi}(\mathbf{r}') \approx w\,\delta(y'_{\mathrm{r}}). \tag{8.103}$$

The coded image for one particular slit orientation is given by

$$\begin{aligned} h^{\phi}(\mathbf{r}'') = h^{\phi}(x''_{\mathrm{r}}, y''_{\mathrm{r}}) &= C\int_{\infty} f(\mathbf{r})g_{\mathrm{rs}}^{\phi}(a\mathbf{r}'' + b\mathbf{r})\,d^2r \\ &= C\int_{\infty} f(x_{\mathrm{r}}, y_{\mathrm{r}})w\,\delta(ay''_{\mathrm{r}} + by_{\mathrm{r}})\,dx_{\mathrm{r}}\,dy_{\mathrm{r}} \\ &= C\left(\frac{w}{b}\right)\int_{-\infty}^{\infty} f(x_{\mathrm{r}}, -ay''_{\mathrm{r}}/b)\,dx_{\mathrm{r}}, \end{aligned} \tag{8.104}$$

where $f(x_{\mathrm{r}}, y_{\mathrm{r}})$ is the source distribution $f(\mathbf{r})$ expressed in the rotated coordinates, and similarly for $h^{\phi}(x''_{\mathrm{r}}, y''_{\mathrm{r}})$.

The structure of (8.104) is familiar from the discussion of transaxial tomography in Chapter 7. The coded image $h^{\phi}(x_r'', y_r'')$ exists as a two-dimensional distribution on the detector, but it contains no information in one direction. If we simply ignore the unimportant x_r'' dependence of $h^{\phi}(x_r'', y_r'')$ and regard the image as a one-dimensional function of y_r'', it is formally identical to a one-dimensional projection at angle ϕ of the planar object distribution $f(\mathbf{r})$. Then any of the algorithms of transaxial tomography can be used to reconstruct $f(\mathbf{r})$. We can, for example, sum the back projections and then apply a two-dimensional ρ filter as described in Section 7.2.5. It might seem that $h^{\phi}(x_r'', y_r'')$ is already a back projection and all we have to do is sum the individual coded images to obtain the unfiltered summation image. Deterministically this procedure is correct, but it is less than optimum when noise is considered. Although the image information in $h^{\phi}(x_r'', y_r'')$ is one dimensional, the noise is two dimensional. That is, the Wiener spectrum of the noise extends to high frequency in all directions in the ξ''–η'' plane. Therefore a considerable noise reduction can be effected by filtering the coded image with a filter for which the bandwidth is very narrow in the direction parallel to the slit. Stated differently, the coded image can be averaged along the x_r'' direction to reduce the noise without loss of image information.

After such prefiltering, the summation image is formed by adding the individual coded images. Let us calculate the summation image for a point source at the origin, $f(\mathbf{r}) = \delta(\mathbf{r})$. For simplicity, we assume that the discrete sum over slit angles can be replaced by a continuous integral. By analogy to (7.24), (8.104) now becomes

$$\begin{aligned} h^{\delta}(\mathbf{r}'') &= \left(\frac{\pi}{M}\right) \int_0^{\pi} h^{\phi}(\mathbf{r}'')\, d\phi \\ &= C\left(\frac{\pi}{M}\right) \int_0^{\pi} d\phi \int_{\infty} \delta(\mathbf{r}) g_{\mathrm{rs}}^{\phi}(a\mathbf{r}'' + b\mathbf{r})\, d^2r \\ &\approx Cw\left(\frac{\pi}{M}\right) \int_0^{\pi} d\phi\, \delta(ay_r'') \\ &= Cw\left(\frac{\pi}{M}\right) \int_0^{\pi} d\phi\, \delta(ay'' \cos\phi - ax'' \sin\phi) \\ &= Cw(\pi/M)(1/ar''), \end{aligned} \tag{8.105}$$

where the last step follows by the same arguments that led to (7.26).

The point spread function, obtained by rescaling $h^{\delta}(\mathbf{r}'')$ back to the object plane, is [cf. (4.36)]

$$p_{\mathrm{rs}}(\mathbf{r}) = (b/a)^2 h^{\delta}(-b\mathbf{r}/a) = \mathrm{const} \cdot 1/r, \tag{8.106}$$

which, not unexpectedly, is just the PSF obtained in transaxial tomography by summation of unfiltered back projections. Thus a suitably apodized two-dimensional ρ filter will suffice to produce a quite acceptable image. An example is shown in Fig. 8.47.

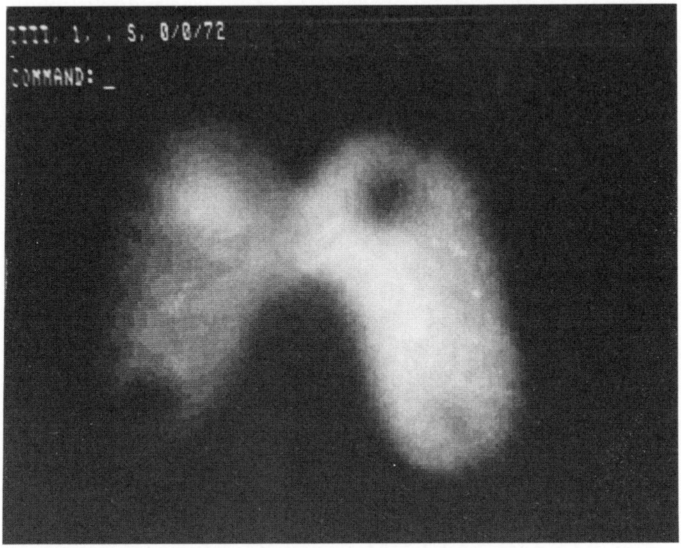

Fig. 8.47 Image of the Picker thyroid phantom obtained with a rotating slit coded aperture and an Anger camera. Reconstruction utilized an algorithm from transaxial tomography. (Unpublished work of G. Gindi, C. L. Giles, and H. H. Barrett.)

It must be emphasized that the analogy between the rotating slit and transaxial tomography is just a formal mathematical one. Both systems involve a $1/r$ PSF, but the physical nature of the images is quite different. Transaxial tomography gives an image of one isolated section of a three-dimensional object. Rotating slit images, on the other hand, are completely *non*tomographic. The development above was for a planar object, but a three-dimensional object may be thought of as a stack of planes. Then *each* plane in the object gives a $1/r$ PSF and there is no way of separating the planes during reconstruction. All planes are collapsed into one, just as in pinhole or collimator imaging, and there is no preferential plane of focus. The rotating slit is unique in this respect—it is the *only* nontomographic coded aperture.

The basic reason for the lack of tomography is that $1/r$ is a function without a characteristic scale. If $p(\mathbf{r}) = K/r$, then $p(\alpha\mathbf{r}) = K/\alpha r = (1/\alpha) \cdot p(\mathbf{r})$. Scaling the dimensions of the function is indistinguishable from changing its magnitude. Only power-law functions r^β have this property. If there should be any reason to synthesize other power-law functions ($\beta \neq -1$), this can be accomplished by changing the profile of the slit in the y_r'' direction. However it can be argued that $\beta = -1$ is optimum (Miller, 1978).

Two variations on the rotating slit theme should be mentioned. If tomographic information should be desired, all that is necessary is to displace the slit from the rotation axis. The coded images now "view" the object from different directions and can be processed so that one plane is in sharp focus and all others are blurred (Kujoory *et al.*, 1980).

The other variation is the slat collimator shown in Fig. 8.48 (Keyes, 1975). This collimator gives the same point image as a slit—each point is encoded as a stripe on the detector—but offers the same improvement in geometric efficiency and freedom from obliquity problems as a conventional collimator offers in comparison to a pinhole (see Section 4.5.5).

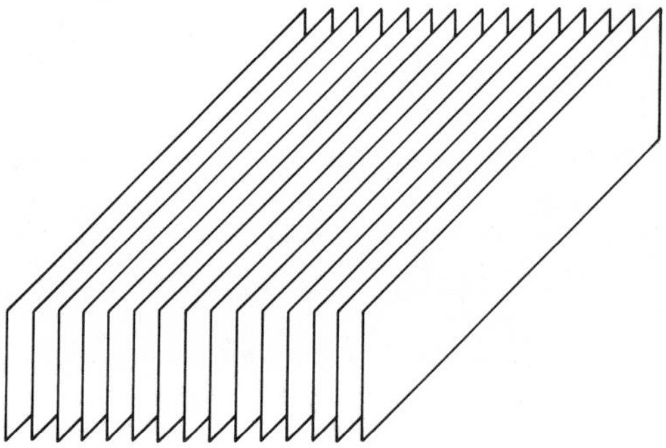

Fig. 8.48 A slat collimator which gives the same PSF as an on-axis rotating slit, but better geometric efficiency.

8.5.2 The Stochastic Aperture

Workers at the University of Michigan (May *et al.*, 1974; Akcasu *et al.*, 1974; Koral *et al.*, 1975) have developed a time-modulated coded aperture that they call the stochastic aperture. One way of looking at this aperture is that it is a uniformly redundant array in the time domain rather than the space domain. Consider the geometry shown in Fig. 8.49 and suppose first that only one point source is present. As the aperture is moved in its plane, the signal from any one detector has a temporal dependence that is identical to the spatial dependence of the one-dimensional aperture code. Information about the location of the point source is encoded as the phase or starting time of the temporal signal. Correlation of the signal with a suitable decoding function is a way of determining the phase and hence the location of the point.

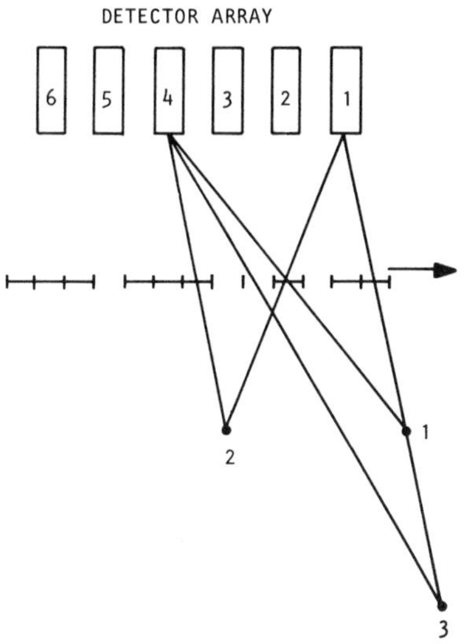

Fig. 8.49 Geometry for a one-dimensional time-modulated coded-aperture system. The aperture plate is stepped through a sequence of positions and the output of each detector for each position of the aperture is recorded. (From Simpson, 1980.)

Note that an imaging detector is not essential in this system—an image could be formed from the signal from a single detector. If, however, an array of detectors is used as shown in Fig. 8.49, then tomographic information can be obtained. Points 1 and 3 in this figure, for example, give identical signals in detector No. 1 and could not be distinguished from this signal alone. Only a single correlation peak is observed during decoding for these two points. However, detector No. 4 views points 1 and 3 from a different angle and gives two resolvable correlation peaks during decoding. Thus, with an array of detectors there is parallax and hence the potential for tomography. The algorithms devised at the University of Michigan for realizing this potential will be discussed further in Section 9.5.2.

We have mentioned that the aperture code in the stochastic aperture is basically a uniformly redundant array. In our previous discussion of such arrays, it was shown that the best decoding function was not the aperture code itself, but rather a cyclically repeated replica of it. In the stochastic aperture, the cyclic property is built into the aperture rather than the decoding function. As illustrated in one dimension in Fig. 8.50, a cyclic aperture can be moved behind a stationary window so that one basic period of the code is always in use.

An interesting feature of this arrangement is that the field of view can be quite large. Point 3 in Fig. 8.50 is so far to the right that only detector 6 receives any radiation at all from it. Nevertheless, the signal from detector 6 is quite sufficient to reconstruct point 3 with as much lateral resolution as any other point. Of course. there is no tomographic information about point 3 since, as far as it is concerned, there is only one detector in the array.

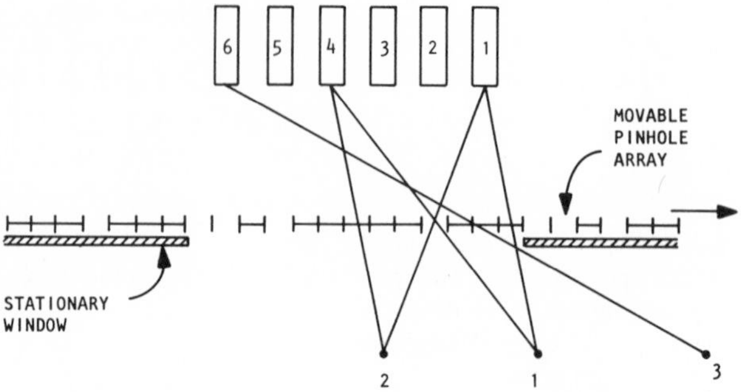

Fig. 8.50 Illustrations of how the stochastic aperture can be implemented by moving a cyclic aperture behind a stationary window. (From Simpson, 1980.)

8.5.3 The Fourier Aperture

The last time-modulated aperture we shall discuss is called the Fourier aperture (Mertz, 1974; Chou and Barrett, 1978). Its most interesting feature is that each individual aperture pattern in the sequence is used to measure one Fourier component in the object.

The operation of this aperture is most easily understood by considering a planar gamma-ray emitter described by a source distribution $f(x, y)$. Suppose it is desired to measure the Fourier cosine component of $f(x, y)$ for a particular spatial frequency having Cartesian components ξ_1 and η_1. This Fourier component is defined by

$$F_c(\xi_1, \eta_1) = \int_{-\infty}^{\infty} dx \int_{-\infty}^{\infty} dy\, f(x, y) \cos[2\pi(\xi_1 x + \eta_1 y)]. \qquad (8.107)$$

To measure $F_c(\xi_1, \eta_1)$, we can use a coded aperture with a transmission specified by

$$g_c(x, y; \xi_1, \eta_1) = \tfrac{1}{2}\{1 + \cos[2\pi(\xi_1 x + \eta_1 y)]\}. \qquad (8.108)$$

This aperture is placed in direct contact with the gamma-ray source. The source is then observed through the aperture by a *nonimaging* detector such as a scintillator–photomultiplier combination. If the detector subtends a solid angle Ω_d and has unity quantum efficiency, the mean number of recorded counts after an exposure time τ is

$$\begin{aligned} N_c(\xi_1, \eta_1) &= \frac{\Omega_d \tau}{4\pi} \int_{-\infty}^{\infty} dx \int_{-\infty}^{\infty} dy\, f(x, y) g_c(x, y; \xi_1, \eta_1) \\ &= \frac{\Omega_d \tau}{8\pi} [F_c(\xi_1, \eta_1) + F_c(0, 0)]. \end{aligned} \qquad (8.109)$$

The quantity $F_c(0,0)$ is merely the integral of $f(x, y)$ over the x–y plane; it can easily be determined, for example by removing the aperture and counting for a suitable period. Thus $N_c(\xi_1, \eta_1)$ is a direct measure of $F_c(\xi_1, \eta_1)$.

This process can, in principle, now be repeated many times with a whole family of apertures, each having a different spatial frequency (ξ_i, η_i). Furthermore, the Fourier sine components $F_s(\xi_i, \eta_i)$ can be obtained by using sinusoidal rather than cosinusoidal apertures. In this way we can conceive of sampling $F_c(\xi, \eta)$ and $F_s(\xi, \eta)$ at a sufficient number of points to permit reconstruction of $f(x, y)$ by a discrete inverse Fourier transform.

One problem with the scheme just described is that it is mechanically cumbersome. Even though all spatial-frequency vectors with the same magnitude $[\rho = (\xi^2 + \eta^2)^{1/2}]$ can be obtained by rotating a single aperture, and the sinusoidal and cosinusoidal apertures differ by only a lateral shift, the number of required apertures is still large. A more practical approach is to obtain *all* of the necessary patterns by superposing two identical periodic grids (e.g., Ronchi rulings) as illustrated in Fig. 8.51. The composite transmission function for the two grids is just the product of the individual transmissions:

$$g_{\mathrm{Fa}}(\mathbf{r}) = g_1(\mathbf{r}) g_2(\mathbf{r}), \tag{8.110}$$

where Fa stands for Fourier aperture. For simplicity we assume that the individual grids are cosinusoidal, so that

$$g_i(\mathbf{r}) = \tfrac{1}{2}[1 + \cos(2\pi \boldsymbol{\rho}_i \cdot \mathbf{r})], \qquad i = 1, 2, \tag{8.111}$$

where the two frequencies $\boldsymbol{\rho}_1$ and $\boldsymbol{\rho}_2$ have the same magnitude but not necessarily the same orientation. Substituting (8.111) into (8.110) and using some familiar trigonometric identities yields

$$\begin{aligned} g_{\mathrm{Fa}}(\mathbf{r}) = \tfrac{1}{4} + \tfrac{1}{8}\cos[2\pi(\boldsymbol{\rho}_1 - \boldsymbol{\rho}_2) \cdot \mathbf{r}] + \tfrac{1}{8}\cos[2\pi(\boldsymbol{\rho}_1 + \boldsymbol{\rho}_2) \cdot \mathbf{r}] \\ + \tfrac{1}{4}\cos(2\pi \boldsymbol{\rho}_1 \cdot \mathbf{r}) + \tfrac{1}{4}\cos(2\pi \boldsymbol{\rho}_2 \cdot \mathbf{r}). \end{aligned} \tag{8.112}$$

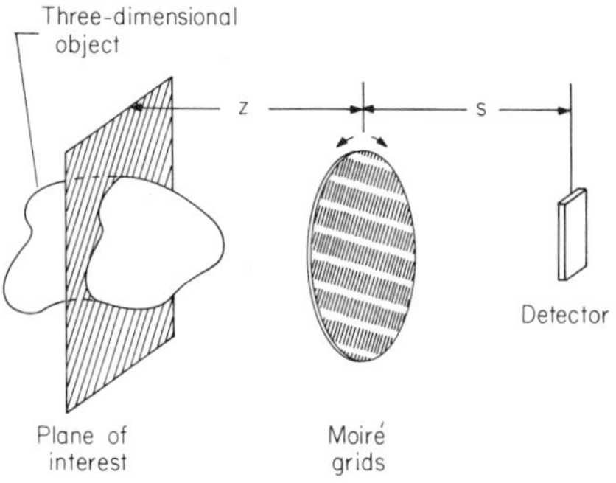

Fig. 8.51 Basic geometry for the Fourier aperture. (From Chou and Barrett, 1978.)

The composite transmission thus contains a moiré or difference-frequency term similar in form to (8.107). Present also are terms having the frequencies of the individual apertures, a sum-frequency term, and a constant term. If we had used Ronchi rulings with a square-wave profile instead of cosinusoidal grids, there would also be higher harmonics. If all of these unwanted terms can be neglected, a point we shall return to shortly, then the difference-frequency term provides the desired aperture function. The difference frequency can be scanned over the ξ–η plane by changing the orientation of the two grids, and the moiré pattern can be changed from sinusoidal to cosinusoidal simply by shifting *either* grid by a quarter period. Thus sufficient data can be obtained to reconstruct $f(x, y)$.

The discussion to this point has been unrealistic in one important respect. We seldom deal with planar objects, let alone ones so accessible that we can place the aperture in direct contact with them. A better model is to consider a general, three-dimensional object as divided into a set of planes parallel to the aperture. If self-absorption of the radiation in the object is negligible (an assumption we have been making throughout this chapter), we can calculate the detector response for each plane independently and sum the results. To do this, two modifications of the previous discussion must be made. First, we must allow for the emitting plane being some distance from the aperture plane. Second, we must now take proper account of the finite detector size. The analysis proceeds exactly as in earlier sections of this chapter and only the result will be given here. Again assuming an aperture transmission in the form of (8.108), we find that the number of recorded counts from the plane at distance z from the aperture is given by

$$N_{\mathrm{c}}(\xi_1, \eta_1) = \frac{L_x L_y}{8\pi(s+z)^2}\left[F_{\mathrm{c}}\left(\frac{s\xi_1}{s+z}, \frac{s\eta_1}{s+z}\right)\operatorname{sinc}\left(\frac{z\xi_1 L_x}{s+z}\right)\right.$$
$$\left.\times \operatorname{sinc}\left(\frac{z\eta_1 L_y}{s+z}\right) + F_{\mathrm{c}}(0,0)\right]. \tag{8.113}$$

Here the detector is assumed to be a rectangle, centered on the origin, with sides of length L_x and L_y oriented parallel to the x and y axes, and s is the distance from the detector to the aperture plane.

Note that if $z = 0$, both sinc functions equal unity, $L_x L_y/s^2 = \Omega_{\mathrm{d}}$, and (8.109) is recovered. If, however, $z \neq 0$, the size of the detector controls the frequency response of the system. Furthermore, different planes are imaged at different scales because of the scale factor $s/(s+z)$ in the argument of F_{c}.

We are now in a position to discuss the undesired frequency components in the composite transmission of the two grids. Regarded as vectors in the ξ–η plane, the sum-frequency term and the difference-frequency term are orthogonal. Furthermore, if the fundamental grid frequency is large so that the maximum desired difference frequency can be obtained with a small angle between the grids, then the fundamental-frequency vectors are also nearly orthogonal to the difference frequency. Therefore, if the detector is a long, slender rectangle with its long axis parallel to the moiré fringes, one of the sinc functions in (8.113) will serve to suppress the unwanted terms. (Of course, the detector orientation must be changed as the orientation of the fringes is changed, but this motion is not difficult mechanically.) This approach fails if z is small, but in most practical situations a judicious choice of detector dimensions should permit adequate suppression of the fundamental and sum-frequency terms. Harmonics of the difference frequency cannot be suppressed in this way since they are parallel to the difference frequency, but they can be eliminated by using sinusoidal (and hence harmonic-free) grids in the first place, or by using the method devised by Coltman (1954) for determining sine-wave response from a series of measurements using square-wave inputs.

Further discussion of the Fourier aperture, especially its three-dimensional properties, will be found in Chapter 9.

9

Three-Dimensional Imaging

9.1 INTRODUCTION

In the preceding three chapters we considered various aspects of the tomographic imaging of three-dimensional objects. The classical tomography systems of Chapter 6 and the multiplex tomography systems of Chapter 8 usually produce a very imperfect kind of tomographic image in which a selected plane is in focus and all other planes are more or less blurred. Multiplex tomography is multiplanar, since many object planes can be reconstructed from a single coded image. In this sense it is a three-dimensional imaging technique, but the presence of the blurred out-of-focus planes is a serious flaw. Computed tomography, as discussed in Chapter 7, yields an uncorrupted image of a single plane. It is a three-dimensional technique since a three-dimensional (3D) volume can be built up as a stack of two-dimensional (2D) planes.

The methods to be discussed in this chapter are *inherently* three dimensional. They produce 3D images directly, not as stacks of 2D images. In these methods, the entire data set must be collected and processed to get any reconstruction at all of the 3D object. It is not possible to take some subset of the data and process it to reconstruct a 2D plane as in computed tomography.

The imaging performance of a 3D system can be described by a 3D PSF, just as a 2D PSF is used to describe a 2D image. In classical tomography or multiplex tomography, the 3D PSF is usually shaped somewhat like an hourglass, as shown schematically in Fig. 9.1. There is a focal plane, plane A in Fig. 9.1, passing through the thin neck of the hourglass. A cross section

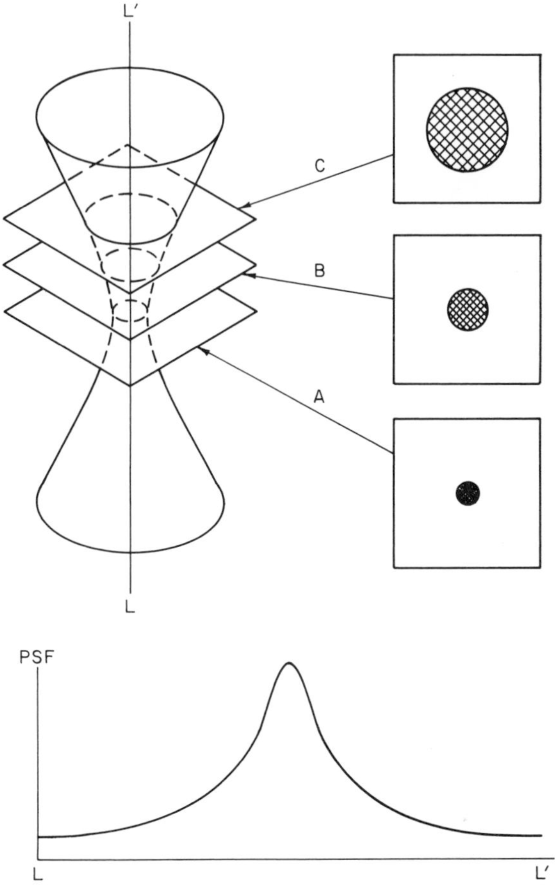

Fig. 9.1 Illustration of a 3D PSF of the kind that might apply to a classical tomography or multiplex tomography system. Although plane *A* is in sharp focus, there is considerable out-of-focus contribution from other planes such as *B* and *C*.

of the PSF in this plane is very compact, approximating a delta function. In other planes, however, the PSF is broad and has appreciable amplitude. A vertical section through the PSF, like the line LL' in Fig. 9.1, shows considerable "spillover" from the focal plane to adjacent planes. This PSF is quite far from the ideal 3D PSF which is a compact ball or 3D delta function. True 3D imaging systems, to perform well, must produce a PSF that is compact in all directions.

The 3D systems described in this chapter use various kinds of projection data as the starting point for a 3D reconstruction. We must distinguish between 2D projections, formed by integrating the 3D object along a set of lines, and 1D projections, formed by integrating over a set of parallel planes. Note that the term 1D or 2D refers to the dimensionality of the data set after projection. A 1D projection requires a 2D (planar) integral, while a 2D projection requires a 1D (line) integral.

9.2 MATHEMATICAL PRELIMINARIES

9.2.1 Notation

The 3D position vector will be denoted by $\mathfrak{r}$, while $\mathbf{r}$ will be reserved for 2D vectors. In cases where an axis of symmetry exists, that axis will always be the z axis. Hence

$$\mathfrak{r} = (\mathbf{r}, z) = (x, y, z). \tag{9.1}$$

Similarly, a 3D spatial-frequency vector will be denoted by $\boldsymbol{\sigma}$ with components (ξ, η, ζ), while $\boldsymbol{\rho}$ is the usual 2D frequency vector:

$$\boldsymbol{\sigma} = (\boldsymbol{\rho}, \zeta) = (\xi, \eta, \zeta). \tag{9.2}$$

The 3D Fourier transform and its inverse are given by

$$F(\boldsymbol{\sigma}) = \mathscr{F}_3\{f(\mathfrak{r})\} = \int_\infty d^3r \exp(-2\pi i \boldsymbol{\sigma} \cdot \mathfrak{r}) f(\mathfrak{r}), \tag{9.3}$$

$$f(\mathfrak{r}) = \mathscr{F}_3^{-1}\{F(\boldsymbol{\sigma})\} = \int_\infty d^3\sigma \exp(+2\pi i \boldsymbol{\sigma} \cdot \mathfrak{r}) F(\boldsymbol{\sigma}). \tag{9.4}$$

We shall also continue the convention of using $\delta(\ )$ as a delta function in any number of dimensions, as distinguished by the dimensionality of the argument. For example, $\delta(\mathfrak{r})$ is a 3D delta function, $\delta(\mathbf{r})$ is 2D, but $\delta(\mathfrak{r}_1 \cdot \mathfrak{r}_2)$ and $\delta(\mathbf{r}_1 \cdot \mathbf{r}_2)$ are both 1D.

The 3D object will be denoted by $f(\mathfrak{r})$. If emission imaging is under discussion, $f(\mathfrak{r})$ is defined such that $Tf(\mathfrak{r})\, d^3\mathfrak{r}$ is the mean number of photons emitted from the volume element $d^3\mathfrak{r}$ in time T. For transmission problems, $f(\mathfrak{r})$ is simply the linear attenuation coefficient $\mu(\mathfrak{r})$. Self-absorption of the radiation in emission imaging is neglected throughout this chapter.

9.2.2 Central Slice Theorem for Line Integrals

If the 3D object $f(\mathfrak{r})$ or $f(x, y, z)$ is projected along a set of rays parallel to the z axis, the result is a 2D projection on the x–y plane given by

$$\lambda(x, y) = \int_{-\infty}^{\infty} f(x, y, z)\, dz. \tag{9.5}$$

The symbol $\lambda(\ )$ is used for projections, just as in Chapter 7; the distinction between 1D and 2D projections is made through the argument of λ.

The Fourier transform of $\lambda(x, y)$ is

$$\Lambda(\xi,\eta) = \int_{-\infty}^{\infty} dx \int_{-\infty}^{\infty} dy \int_{-\infty}^{\infty} dz\, f(x,y,z) \exp[-2\pi i(\xi x + \eta y)]$$
$$= \mathscr{F}_3\{f\}|_{\zeta=0} = F(\xi,\eta,0). \tag{9.6}$$

This is the counterpart of (7.18) for 3D objects. *The 2D transform of a 2D projection yields one plane through the 3D transform of the original object.* In this case the relevant plane is $\zeta = 0$.

If the projection direction is not the z axis, it is a simple matter to find a rotated coordinate frame (x_r, y_r, z_r) such that the projection is along z_r. Then the projection is denoted $\lambda_{\theta_r\phi_r}(x_r, y_r)$, where θ_r and ϕ_r are the polar and azimuthal angles of the z_r axis. The central slice theorem (9.6) becomes

$$\mathscr{F}_2\{\lambda_{\theta_r\phi_r}(x_r, y_r)\} = \Lambda_{\theta_r\phi_r}(\xi_r,\eta_r) = F_r(\xi_r,\eta_r,0), \tag{9.7}$$

where F_r is the same distribution as F but expressed in rotated frequency-space coordinates. Again, a plane in 3D frequency space is obtained, this time the plane $\zeta_r = 0$. *In all cases the plane passes through the origin,* just as in the case of 1D projections of a 2D object, where we showed in Section 7.2.2 that each projection yields information on a *line* through the origin of a 2D frequency space.

9.2.3 Central Slice Theorem for Planar Integrals

If the 3D object $f(\mathbf{r})$ is imaged with a system that integrates over a series of planes normal to the x axis, the resulting image is a 1D projection given by

$$\lambda(x) = \int_{-\infty}^{\infty} dy \int_{-\infty}^{\infty} dz\, f(x,y,z). \tag{9.8}$$

For example, $\lambda(x)$ is a good approximation to the image obtained with the slat collimator shown in Fig. 8.48. Planar integrals arise also in imaging with nuclear magnetic resonance. [See Shepp (1980).]

The 1D Fourier transform of $\lambda(x)$ is

$$\mathscr{F}_1\{\lambda(x)\} = \Lambda(\xi) = \int_{-\infty}^{\infty} dx \int_{-\infty}^{\infty} dy \int_{-\infty}^{\infty} dz\, f(x,y,z)\exp(-2\pi i \xi x)$$
$$= \mathscr{F}_3\{f\}|_{\eta=0,\zeta=0} = F(\xi,0,0). \tag{9.9}$$

If the planes of integration are not normal to the x axis, a rotated coordinate system (x_r, y_r, z_r) must again be used. The 1D projection can then be written in any of the following equivalent forms:

$$\lambda_{\hat{\mathbf{n}}}(x_r) = \int_{-\infty}^{\infty} dy_r \int_{-\infty}^{\infty} dz_r\, f_r(x_r, y_r, z_r)$$
$$= \int_{-\infty}^{\infty} dx_r' \int_{-\infty}^{\infty} dy_r' \int_{-\infty}^{\infty} dz_r'\, f_r(x_r', y_r', z_r')\,\delta(x_r - x_r')$$
$$= \int_{\infty} d^3r'\, f(\mathbf{r}')\,\delta(x_r - \hat{\mathbf{n}}\cdot\mathbf{r}'), \tag{9.10}$$

where $\hat{\mathbf{n}}$ is a 3D unit vector in the x_r direction, i.e., normal to the planes of integration. In the last form of (9.10), note that the 1D delta function reduces the 3D volume integral to a 2D integral over the plane $\hat{\mathbf{n}} \cdot \mathbf{r}' = x_r$, which is normal to $\hat{\mathbf{n}}$ and a distance x_r from the origin.

The counterpart of the central slice theorem for this situation is

$$\Lambda_{\hat{\mathbf{n}}}(\xi_r) = F_r(\xi_r, 0, 0). \tag{9.11}$$

Thus, *the 1D transform of a 1D projection gives information about the object along a line through the origin in 3D space.* The line is, of course, the ξ_r axis.

9.3 RECONSTRUCTION BY BACK-PROJECTION AND SUMMATION

9.3.1 Unfiltered Back-Projection of One-Dimensional Projections

Since 1D projections are obtained by integrating over planes, back projection means smearing the data back uniformly over the original planes. The 3D back-projected image associated with the 1D data set $\lambda_{\hat{\mathbf{n}}}(x_r)$ is given by [cf. (7.19)]

$$g_{\hat{\mathbf{n}}}[x_r, y_r, z_r] = \lambda_{\hat{\mathbf{n}}}(x_r). \tag{9.12}$$

Of course, $g_{\hat{\mathbf{n}}}(x_r, y_r, z_r)$ is actually independent of y_r and z_r. In terms of the unrotated coordinates,

$$g_{\hat{\mathbf{n}}}(\mathbf{r}) = \lambda_{\hat{\mathbf{n}}}(\mathbf{r} \cdot \hat{\mathbf{n}}), \tag{9.13}$$

since $x_r = \mathbf{r} \cdot \hat{\mathbf{n}}$ defines the original plane of integration.

The summation image $b(\mathbf{r})$ is formed by summing $g_{\hat{\mathbf{n}}}(\mathbf{r})$ over all orientations $\hat{\mathbf{n}}$. For a discrete set of orientations,

$$b(\mathbf{r}) = \sum_i g_{\hat{\mathbf{n}}_i}(\mathbf{r}). \tag{9.14}$$

The discrete sum can be replaced with an integral if a dense set or continuum of projection directions is available.

We shall now calculate the PSF in the unfiltered summation image (Chiu, 1980). For a point object at the origin, $f^\delta(\mathbf{r}) = \delta(\mathbf{r})$, each projection is given by

$$\lambda^\delta_{\hat{\mathbf{n}}}(x_r) = \delta(x_r). \tag{9.15}$$

Since each projection gives information on only one frequency line, the orientation vector $\hat{\mathbf{n}}$ must cover all possible directions in a hemisphere (or 2π solid angle) to completely sample the 3D frequency space. The PSF is thus given by

$$p_u(\mathbf{r}) = \frac{1}{2\pi} \int_{2\pi} d\Omega_n \, \delta(\mathbf{r} \cdot \hat{\mathbf{n}}), \tag{9.16}$$

where the subscript u denotes "unfiltered," and $d\Omega_n = \sin\theta_n \, d\theta_n \, d\phi_n$, with θ_n and ϕ_n being the polar and azimuthal angles of $\hat{\mathbf{n}}$. We denote the polar coordinates of $\mathbf{r}$ by $(\mathrm{r}, \theta, \phi)$. Since $p_u(\mathbf{r})$ is spherically symmetric, there is no loss of generality if we set $\theta = \phi = 0$. Then (9.16) becomes

$$p_u(\mathbf{r}) = \frac{1}{2\pi} \int_0^{\pi/2} \sin\theta_n \, d\theta_n \int_0^{2\pi} d\phi_n \, \delta(\mathrm{r}\cos\theta_n)$$

$$= \int_0^1 \delta(\mathrm{r}\cos\theta_n) \, d(\cos\theta_n) = \frac{1}{2\mathrm{r}}, \tag{9.17}$$

the factor of $\frac{1}{2}$ coming because the argument of the delta function vanishes exactly at the lower limit of integration.

Equation (9.17) shows that the PSF for the unfiltered summation image is proportional to $1/\mathrm{r}$, just as in the case of 2D reconstruction from 1D line-integral projections. [cf. (7.26)]. However, it must be kept in mind that r is the magnitude of a 3D vector. It is *not* correct to infer from (9.17) that the MTF in the summation image is $1/\sigma$, where σ is the magnitude of the 3D spatial frequency vector. To find the transfer function, we must take the 3D Fourier transform of $1/(2\mathrm{r})$:

$$P_u(\boldsymbol{\sigma}) = \mathscr{F}_3\left\{\frac{1}{2\mathrm{r}}\right\} = \int_\infty d^3\mathrm{r}\left(\frac{1}{2\mathrm{r}}\right)\exp(-2\pi i \boldsymbol{\sigma} \cdot \mathbf{r}). \tag{9.18}$$

If we orient the coordinate system so that $\boldsymbol{\sigma}$ is parallel to the z axis, $\boldsymbol{\sigma} \cdot \mathbf{r} = \sigma \mathrm{r} \cos\theta$, and

$$P_u(\boldsymbol{\sigma}) = \int_0^{2\pi} d\phi \int_{-1}^{1} d(\cos\theta) \int_0^\infty \mathrm{r}^2 \, d\mathrm{r}\left(\frac{1}{2\mathrm{r}}\right)\exp(-2\pi i \sigma \mathrm{r}\cos\theta)$$

$$= 4\pi \int_0^\infty \frac{1}{2\mathrm{r}} \operatorname{sinc}(2\sigma \mathrm{r}) \mathrm{r}^2 \, d\mathrm{r} = \frac{1}{\sigma}\int_0^\infty \sin(2\pi\sigma \mathrm{r}) \, d\mathrm{r}. \tag{9.19}$$

This last integral is not well behaved, since the integrand oscillates indefinitely with constant amplitude. However, if we interpret it as

$$\lim_{\alpha \to 0} \int_0^\infty e^{-\alpha \mathrm{r}} \sin(2\pi\sigma \mathrm{r}) \, d\mathrm{r} = \frac{1}{2\pi\sigma}, \tag{9.20}$$

then the transfer function becomes

$$P_u(\boldsymbol{\sigma}) = 1/(2\pi\sigma^2). \tag{9.21}$$

The falloff at high frequencies is now even more severe than for 2D reconstruction: $1/(\text{frequency})^2$ rather than just $1/(\text{frequency})$. Clearly a correction filter is required, and it will be introduced in Sections 9.3.3 and 9.3.5.

There is a simple geometrical interpretation of (9.21). The set of projections for all $\hat{\mathbf{n}}$ recreates the object Fourier transform on a set of lines radiating out in all directions from the origin in frequency space. For a point object, all of these lines have equal weight. The density of lines is proportional to $1/\sigma^2$ since the total number of lines crossing a spherical surface of radius σ is constant. The construction is analogous to the lines of electric force emanating from a static point charge, where the electric field obeys an inverse-square law like (9.21).

9.3.2 Unfiltered Back-Projection of Two-Dimensional Projections

We have seen that a 2D line-integral projection gives information on a plane in 3D Fourier space. This plane, defined by $\zeta_r = 0$, has a normal vector $\hat{\mathbf{n}}_r$ that is oriented with respect to the unrotated (ξ, η, ζ) axes by the same polar and azimuthal angles θ_r and ϕ_r that specify the orientation of the projection axis z_r in the unrotated space-domain frame (x, y, z). There are many ways in which all or part of the volume in 3D Fourier space can be mapped out by varying θ_r and ϕ_r. It is definitely *not* necessary for the vector $\hat{\mathbf{n}}_r$ to explore all possible directions. Ordinary computed tomography, for example, corresponds to fixing θ_r at $\pi/2$ and varying ϕ_r from 0 to π. As shown in Fig. 9.2, the plane normal to $\hat{\mathbf{n}}_r$ then sweeps out the full volume in Fourier space, and no further information can be gained by varying θ_r. More generally, a complete data set is generated whenever $\hat{\mathbf{n}}_r$ traces out one-half of a great circle; the full hemisphere is not required (Orlov, 1975a,b).

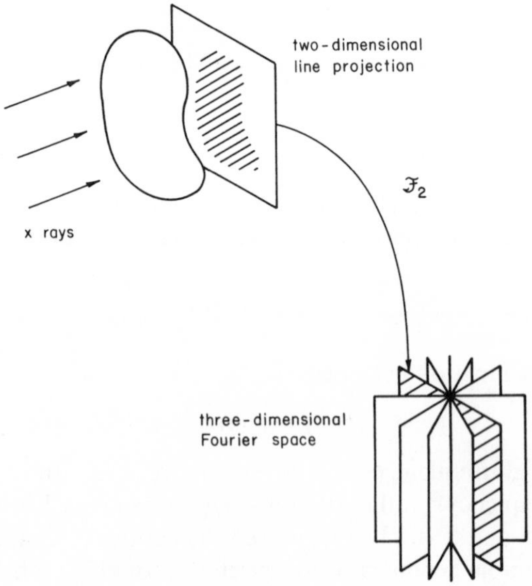

Fig. 9.2 Illustration showing that the full 3D Fourier space is sampled by 2D projections whenever the projection direction $\mathbf{n}_r$ sweeps out half of a great circle.

There is, however, some theoretical interest in systems where $\hat{\mathbf{n}}_r$ covers a hemisphere (Tanaka, 1979; Levitan, 1979; Nalcioglu and Cho, 1978).* We emphasize that these hypothetical systems collect much more information than is required for an unambiguous reconstruction, but they may offer some advantage in terms of noise and photon utilization (Nalcioglu and Cho, 1978). To the authors' knowledge, no practical systems using such redundant data have been constructed. Nevertheless, for completeness, we briefly consider this case here. Our derivation follows Chiu (1980).

For a point object at the origin, every 2D projection is given by

$$\lambda^{\delta}_{\theta_r \phi_r}(x_r, y_r) = \delta(x_r)\,\delta(y_r). \tag{9.22}$$

The summation image is

$$p_u(\mathbf{r}) = b^{\delta}_u(\mathbf{r}) = \frac{1}{2\pi}\int_{2\pi} d\Omega_r\, \delta(x_r)\,\delta(y_r), \tag{9.23}$$

where $d\Omega_r = \sin\theta_r\, d\theta_r\, d\phi_r$. Since $p_u(\mathbf{r})$ is spherically symmetric, we again take $\theta = \phi = 0$, where $\mathbf{r} = (\mathrm{r}, \theta, \phi)$, so that

$$x_r = \mathrm{r}\sin\theta_r\cos\phi_r, \tag{9.24a}$$

$$y_r = \mathrm{r}\sin\theta_r\sin\phi_r, \tag{9.24b}$$

$$p_u(\mathbf{r}) = \frac{1}{2\pi}\int_0^{2\pi} d\phi_r \int_0^{\pi/2} \sin\theta_r\, d\theta_r\, \delta(\mathrm{r}\sin\theta_r\cos\phi_r)\,\delta(\mathrm{r}\sin\theta_r\sin\phi_r). \tag{9.25}$$

The delta function $\delta(\mathrm{r}\sin\theta_r\cos\phi_r)$ has singularities at $\phi_r = \pi/2$ and $3\pi/2$. By (A.24) we can write

$$\delta(\mathrm{r}\sin\theta_r\cos\phi_r) = \frac{\delta[\phi_r - \pi/2] + \delta[\phi_r - 3\pi/2]}{|\mathrm{r}\sin\theta_r|}. \tag{9.26}$$

The other delta function in (9.25) is equal to $\delta(\mathrm{r}\sin\theta_r)$ at both of the singularities. Hence

$$p_u(\mathbf{r}) = \frac{1}{\pi}\int_0^{\pi/2} \sin\theta_r \frac{\delta(\mathrm{r}\sin\theta_r)}{|\mathrm{r}\sin\theta_r|}\, d\theta_r = \frac{1}{2\pi \mathrm{r}^2}. \tag{9.27}$$

Thus the PSF varies as $1/\mathrm{r}^2$ in this case, a result that also follows from the geometric picture given at the end of Section 9.3.1. The main difference is that Section 9.3.1 dealt with a superposition of radial lines in *frequency* space, so the *transfer function* had an inverse square behavior. Here the lines are in real space, so the *PSF* is the quantity that obeys an inverse-square law.

* The intermediate case where $\hat{\mathbf{n}}_r$ covers more than a great circle but less than a full hemisphere has also been treated by Ra and Cho (1981).

Here the transfer function is given by [cf. (9.19)]

$$P_u(\boldsymbol{\sigma}) = \mathscr{F}_3\left\{\frac{1}{2\pi r^2}\right\} = 4\pi \int_0^\infty \frac{1}{2\pi r^2}\,\mathrm{sinc}(2\sigma r) r^2\, dr$$

$$= 2\int_0^\infty \mathrm{sinc}(2\sigma r)\, dr = \frac{1}{2\sigma}, \tag{9.28}$$

where the last step follows from the central ordinate theorem (B.15) and (B.25).

9.3.3 Three-Dimensional Filter Functions

In Sections 9.3.1 and 9.3.2, we have seen that the 3D image formed by unfiltered back projection and summation of either 1D or 2D projections falls off rapidly at high frequencies. A compensating filter is required.

Consider first the case of 1D projections. Equation (9.21) shows that the appropriate filter function to apply to the summation image has the form

$$Q_3^{(1)}(\boldsymbol{\sigma}) = 2\pi\sigma^2 A(\sigma), \tag{9.29}$$

where $A(\sigma)$ is a 3D apodizing function. The subscript on $Q_3^{(1)}$ indicates that the filter operates in 3D frequency space, while the superscript is a reminder that we started with 1D projections or planar integrals. After application of this filter, the final 3D MTF is just $A(\sigma)$.

It is also possible in principle to do a direct space-domain convolutional filtering on the 3D summation image. In this case, the required filter function is the inverse 3D Fourier transform of $Q_3^{(1)}(\boldsymbol{\sigma})$, which has been calculated by Chiu (1980). By analogy to (9.19)

$$q_3^{(1)}(\mathbf{r}) = \mathscr{F}_3^{-1}\{Q_3^{(1)}(\boldsymbol{\sigma})\} = 4\pi\int_0^\infty 2\pi\sigma^2 A(\sigma)\,\mathrm{sinc}(2\sigma r)\sigma^2\, d\sigma. \tag{9.30}$$

If we take $A(\sigma) = 1$ so that the MTF will be perfect at all frequencies, then

$$q_3^{(1)}(\mathbf{r}) = 4\pi\int_0^\infty 2\pi\sigma^2 \frac{\sin(2\pi\sigma r)}{2\pi\sigma r}\sigma^2\, d\sigma = \frac{4\pi}{r}\int_0^\infty \sigma^3 \sin(2\pi\sigma r)\, d\sigma. \tag{9.31}$$

This integral, even though wildly divergent, can be expressed as a derivative of a delta function as defined by (A.26). If $\delta'''(x)$ denotes the third derivative of the 1D delta function $\delta(x)$, its 1D Fourier transform is, by use of (A.26),

$$\mathscr{F}_1\{\delta'''(x)\} = \int_{-\infty}^{\infty} \delta'''(x)\exp(-2\pi i\xi x)\, dx$$

$$= -\left(\frac{d^3}{dx^3}\exp(-2\pi i\xi x)\right)_{x=0} = (2\pi i\xi)^3. \tag{9.32}$$

Hence the inverse transform is

$$\begin{aligned}\delta'''(x) &= \mathscr{F}_1^{-1}\{(2\pi i\xi)^3\} = \int_{-\infty}^{\infty} (2\pi i\xi)^3 \exp(2\pi i\xi x)\, d\xi \\ &= (2\pi)^3 \int_{-\infty}^{\infty} \xi^3 \sin(2\pi\xi x)\, d\xi \\ &= 16\pi^3 \int_0^{\infty} \xi^3 \sin(2\pi\xi x)\, d\xi. \end{aligned} \tag{9.33}$$

Using (9.33), we can rewrite (9.31)

$$q_3^{(1)}(\mathbf{r}) = (1/4\pi^2 \mathrm{r})\, \delta'''(\mathrm{r}). \tag{9.34}$$

Note that $\delta'''(\mathrm{r})$ is still the third derivative of a 1D delta function. It can be used to perform only one of the three integrals in the 3D convolution of the summation image with $q_3^{(1)}(\mathbf{r})$.

Next we turn to the case treated in Section 9.3.2 where the 3D summation image is formed from 2D projections. From (9.28) the required filter in the 3D frequency domain is

$$Q_3^{(2)}(\boldsymbol{\sigma}) = 2\sigma A(\sigma). \tag{9.35}$$

We shall not dwell on this case because it is of little practical importance. Tanaka (1979) has shown that, for $A(\sigma) = 1$, the space-domain filter $q_3^{(2)}$ is a generalized function that behaves as $-1/\mathrm{r}^4$ for $\mathrm{r} \neq 0$, with a strong positive singularity at $\mathrm{r} = 0$.

9.3.4 Two-Dimensional Filter Functions

In Chapter 7, we showed that the functional form of the frequency-domain filter function was the same whether it was a 1D filter applied to the projection data or a 2D filter applied to the summation image. The same conclusion holds for 3D imaging (Levitan, 1979). Therefore, if we have the 2D data set of Section 9.3.2 where $\hat{\mathbf{n}}_r$ covers a full hemisphere, we can perform a 2D filtering operation on it before back-projection. The appropriate filter to use has the same form as (9.35) but with the 2D frequency $\boldsymbol{\rho}$ appearing in place of $\boldsymbol{\sigma}$:

$$Q_2^{(2)}(\boldsymbol{\rho}) = 2\rho A(\rho), \tag{9.36}$$

where $\boldsymbol{\rho}$ has components (ξ_r, η_r) in the rotated frame in which the data are recorded.

This filter was also considered by Tanaka (1979) who showed that its space-domain counterpart is a generalized function which behaves as $-1/r^3$ for $r \neq 0$, with $r = (x_r^2 + y_r^2)^{1/2}$.

9.3.5 One-Dimensional Filter Functions

A rather interesting situation arises if we contemplate filtering a 1D data set before back-projection. By the same argument as in Section 9.3.4, the appropriate filter in the 1D frequency domain is [cf. (9.29)]

$$Q_1^{(1)}(\xi_r) = 2\pi\xi_r^2 A(\xi_r). \tag{9.37}$$

An argument similar to the one leading to (9.34) (Chiu, 1980) shows that, if $A(\xi_r) = 1$,

$$q_1^{(1)}(x_r) = -\delta''(x_r)/(2\pi). \tag{9.38}$$

Since convolution of a function with the second derivative of a delta function is equivalent to taking the second derivative of the function, the filtered 1D projection is

$$\lambda_{\hat{\mathbf{n}}}^{\dagger}(x_r) = \lambda_{\hat{\mathbf{n}}}(x_r) * q_1^{(1)}(x_r) = -\frac{1}{2\pi}\frac{\partial^2}{\partial x_r^2}\lambda_{\hat{\mathbf{n}}}(x_r). \tag{9.39}$$

Note that this is a purely *local* operation. A discrete approximation to the second derivative involves the values of $\lambda_{\hat{\mathbf{n}}}(x_r)$ at just three consecutive values of x_r. By contrast, in the usual CT case of reconstructing a 2D object from 1D projections, the filter function extends to $\pm\infty$ (falling off as $-1/x_r^2$), so that the whole data set for each projection angle is required in order to calculate the filtered projection at one point.

The reconstructed object $f(\mathbf{r})$ is obtained by back-projecting and summing $\lambda_{\hat{\mathbf{n}}}^{\dagger}(x_r)$. As discussed in Section 9.3.1, back-projection is equivalent to the substitution of $\mathbf{r} \cdot \hat{\mathbf{n}}$ for x_r, yielding

$$\begin{aligned} f(\mathbf{r}) &= -\frac{1}{4\pi^2}\int_{2\pi} d\Omega_n \left.\frac{\partial^2 \lambda_{\hat{\mathbf{n}}}(x_r)}{\partial x_r^2}\right|_{x_r = \mathbf{r}\cdot\hat{\mathbf{n}}} \\ &= -\frac{1}{4\pi^2}\int_{2\pi} d\Omega_n \lambda''_{\hat{\mathbf{n}}}(\mathbf{r}\cdot\hat{\mathbf{n}}). \end{aligned} \tag{9.40}$$

This equation is one form of the 3*D inverse Radon transform.* It is worth noting that Radon's original work involved determination of an N-dimensional object from its integrals over $(N-1)$-dimensional hyperplanes. For $N = 3$, this means that the basic input data for an inverse Radon transform are integrals over 2D planes, i.e., 1D projections.

An equivalent form of the 3D inverse Radon transform is

$$f(\mathbf{r}) = -\frac{1}{4\pi^2}\nabla^2 \int_{2\pi} d\Omega_n \lambda_{\hat{\mathbf{n}}}(\mathbf{r}\cdot\hat{\mathbf{n}}). \tag{9.41}$$

One way to prove that (9.41) is equivalent to (9.40) is to take the operator ∇^2 under the integral. Straightforward evaluation of the Laplacian in spherical coordinates with $\hat{\mathbf{n}}$ along the polar axis shows that

$$\nabla^2 \lambda(\mathrm{r}\cos\theta) = \left.\frac{\partial^2 \lambda(x_\mathrm{r})}{\partial x_\mathrm{r}^2}\right|_{x_\mathrm{r} = \mathrm{r}\cos\theta} \tag{9.42}$$

and (9.40) follows at once. A more revealing way to show the equivalence is to use the result from Section 9.3.1 that the PSF for the unfiltered summation image is just $1/(2\mathrm{r})$. If we denote the image obtained by unfiltered back-projection and summation as $b(\mathbf{r})$, we can write

$$\begin{aligned} b(\mathbf{r}) &= \frac{1}{2\pi}\int_{2\pi} d\Omega_n\, \lambda_{\hat{\mathbf{n}}}(\mathbf{r}\cdot\hat{\mathbf{n}}) = f(\mathbf{r}) *** \left(\frac{1}{2\mathrm{r}}\right) \\ &= \frac{1}{2}\int_\infty d^3\mathrm{r}'\, f(\mathbf{r}')\frac{1}{|\mathbf{r}-\mathbf{r}'|}. \end{aligned} \tag{9.43}$$

The Laplacian of $b(\mathbf{r})$ is

$$\nabla^2 b(\mathbf{r}) = \frac{1}{2}\int_\infty d^3\mathrm{r}' f(\mathbf{r}')\nabla^2 \frac{1}{|\mathbf{r}-\mathbf{r}'|}. \tag{9.44}$$

But it is well known from electrostatics (Jackson, 1975) that

$$\nabla^2 \frac{1}{|\mathbf{r}-\mathbf{r}'|} = -4\pi\,\delta(\mathbf{r}-\mathbf{r}'). \tag{9.45}$$

Equation (9.45) is simply Poisson's equation for the potential of a point charge.

Combining (9.43)–(9.45) gives

$$\frac{1}{2\pi}\nabla^2 \int_{2\pi} d\Omega_n\, \lambda_n(\mathbf{r}\cdot\hat{\mathbf{n}}) = -2\pi\int_\infty d^3\mathrm{r}'\, f(\mathbf{r}')\,\delta(\mathbf{r}-\mathbf{r}') = -2\pi f(\mathbf{r}), \tag{9.46}$$

in agreement with (9.41).

Thus a local Laplacian operation on the 3D summation image yields an accurate reconstruction. Equation (9.46) is mathematically equivalent to the filtering operation described by (9.34) (Chiu, 1980; Chiu *et al.*, 1980).

9.3.6 Spherically Symmetric Objects

An interesting application of the results of Section 9.3.5 is to spherically symmetric objects $f(\mathrm{r})$ (Vest and Steel, 1978; Chiu, 1980). Each projection is given by the same function $\lambda(x)$, and the subscripts $\hat{\mathbf{n}}$ and r are unnecessary. The filtered projection is $(-1/2\pi)\lambda''(x)$, where the double prime denotes second derivative. The reconstructed 3D object is

$$f(\mathrm{r}) = \frac{-1}{4\pi^2}\int_{2\pi} d\Omega_n\, \lambda''(\mathbf{r}\cdot\hat{\mathbf{n}}). \tag{9.47}$$

Since the object is symmetric, we can take $\theta = \phi = 0$, so that $\mathbf{r} \cdot \hat{\mathbf{n}} = \mathrm{r} \cos \theta_n$. Then

$$f(\mathrm{r}) = -\frac{1}{4\pi^2} \int_0^{2\pi} d\phi_n \int_0^{\pi/2} \sin \theta_n \, d\theta_n \, \lambda''(\mathrm{r} \cos \theta_n) = \frac{-1}{2\pi} \int_0^1 du \, \lambda''(\mathrm{r}u)$$

$$= \frac{-1}{2\pi \mathrm{r}} \int_0^{\mathrm{r}} dv \, \lambda''(v) \tag{9.48}$$

where $u = \cos \theta_n$ and $v = \mathrm{r}u$. The integrand in (9.48) is now a perfect differential $d(\lambda')$. Furthermore, since $\lambda(x)$ is an even function, $\lambda'(0) = 0$, and we have

$$f(\mathrm{r}) = -\frac{1}{2\pi \mathrm{r}} \lambda'(\mathrm{r}) = -\frac{1}{2\pi \mathrm{r}} \left. \frac{d\lambda(x)}{dx} \right|_{x=\mathrm{r}}. \tag{9.49}$$

This remarkable result, first obtained by Vest and Steel, shows that a simple derivative suffices to reconstruct a spherically symmetric 3D object from its 1D projection. *Back-projection is not required.*

9.4 COORDINATE TRANSFORMATIONS

In most radiographic systems, the recorded image is a projection of the object, but the lines (or planes) of integration are not parallel. For example, a pinhole image is a set of line integrals along converging lines passing through the pinhole. A transmission radiograph obtained with a point source is a set of line integrals along lines diverging from the source. A rotating-slit image is a set of planar integrals along planes passing through the slit. In this section we show that such systems can be analyzed by Fourier methods, especially the central slice theorem, if we use a distorted object space (Chiu *et al.*, 1979; Chiu, 1980). Basically, the function of the distortion is to convert divergent-ray projections into parallel-ray projections.

9.4.1 Pinhole Imaging

Consider the pinhole camera shown in Fig. 9.3. This geometry differs from the one used in Chapter 4 in two minor respects: the plane $z = 0$ has been displaced a distance s_1 so that the origin of coordinates lies within the object, and the pinhole is displaced away from the z axis by a 2D vector $\mathbf{r}_0'$. The 3D object is specified by $f(\mathbf{r})$ or $f(\mathbf{r}, z)$. With these changes, (4.210) for the 2D image distribution $h(\mathbf{r}'')$ becomes

$$h(\mathbf{r}'') = \frac{T}{4\pi} \int_\infty d^2 r \int_{-\infty}^{\infty} dz \, \frac{f(\mathbf{r}, z) g(a\mathbf{r}'' + b\mathbf{r})}{(s_1 + s_2 + z)^2}, \tag{9.50}$$

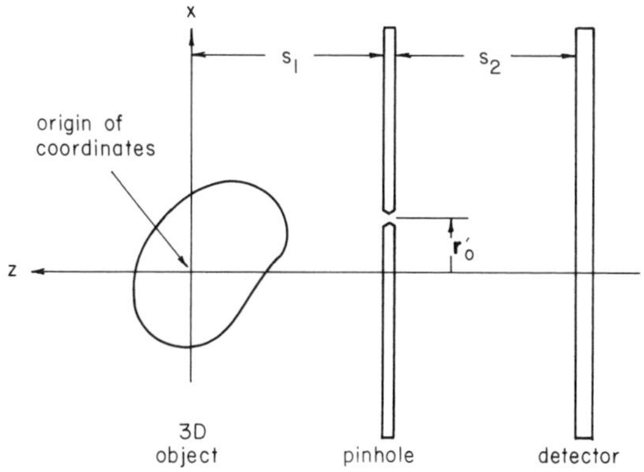

Fig. 9.3 Geometry of a pinhole imaging system.

where now

$$a = (s_1 + z)/(s_1 + s_2 + z), \tag{9.51}$$

$$b = s_2/(s_1 + s_2 + z). \tag{9.52}$$

For a small pinhole of area $\mathscr{A}_{ph}$, the aperture transmission function $g(\mathbf{r}')$ may be approximated as

$$g(\mathbf{r}') = \mathscr{A}_{ph}\,\delta(\mathbf{r}' - \mathbf{r}'_0). \tag{9.53}$$

We define a new set of coordinates $(\tilde{r}, \tilde{z})$ or $(\tilde{x}, \tilde{y}, \tilde{z})$ by (Chiu *et al.*, 1979)

$$\tilde{z} = \frac{s_1}{s_1 + z}\, z, \qquad \tilde{\mathbf{r}} = \frac{s_1}{s_1 + z}\,\mathbf{r}. \tag{9.54}$$

The inverse transformation is

$$z = \frac{s_1}{s_1 - \tilde{z}}\,\tilde{z}, \qquad \mathbf{r} = \frac{s_1}{s_1 - \tilde{z}}\,\tilde{\mathbf{r}}. \tag{9.55}$$

Note that the origins of the two coordinate systems coincide, but that there is a highly nonlinear distortion of the z axis. The plane $z = \infty$ maps to $\tilde{z} = s_1$, while the aperture plane $z = -s_1$ maps to $\tilde{z} = -\infty$.

To understand the effect of this transformation, consider a family of rays that pass through the pinhole (see Fig. 9.4). The jth ray, characterized by the 2D vector slope parameter $\mathbf{m}_j$, satisfies the equation

$$\mathbf{r} - \mathbf{r}'_0 = \mathbf{m}_j(z + s_1). \tag{9.56}$$

Note that the lateral coordinate of all rays is $\mathbf{r} = \mathbf{r}'_0$ when $z = -s_1$, i.e., when the rays pass through the aperture plane.

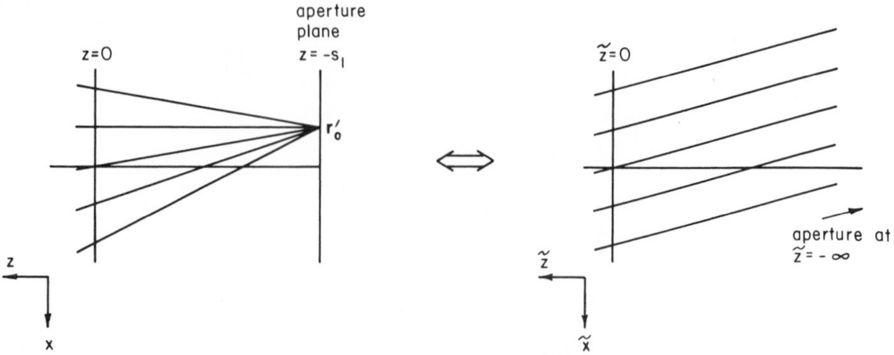

Fig. 9.4 Illustration of the coordinate transformation specified by (9.54) and (9.55). The family of divergent rays through the point $\mathbf{r}_0'$ at left is mapped into a family of parallel rays in the distorted space as shown at right.

In the distorted frame, (9.56) becomes

$$\tilde{\mathbf{r}} - \mathbf{r}_0' = \mathbf{m}_j s_1 - \mathbf{r}_0' \tilde{z}/s_1 \tag{9.57}$$

This is now the equation for a family of *parallel* lines as illustrated in Fig. 9.4. The slope of each line is $-\mathbf{r}_0'/s_1$, independent of j. The intercepts of the lines with the plane $\tilde{z} = 0$ are the same as with the plane $z = 0$, but the transformation has effectively moved the pinhole to $\tilde{z} = -\infty$ while preserving the slope of the central ray that passes through the origin of coordinates.

To incorporate this new coordinate system into (9.50), we define a distorted object function $\tilde{f}(\tilde{\mathbf{r}}, \tilde{z})$. We could obtain this new function by merely using (9.55) to reexpress $f(\mathbf{r}, z)$ in the new system, forming $\tilde{f}(\tilde{\mathbf{r}}, \tilde{z}) = f[\mathbf{r}\,(\tilde{\mathbf{r}}, \tilde{z}), z(\tilde{z})]$, but it is more convenient to also scale the magnitude of the function, defining it by

$$\tilde{f}(\tilde{\mathbf{r}}, \tilde{z}) d^2\tilde{r}\, d\tilde{z} = [s_1/(s_1 + z)]^2 f(\mathbf{r}, z)\, d^2 r\, dz, \tag{9.58}$$

where $\mathbf{r}$ and z on the right-hand side are to be expressed by (9.55). With this definition, the Jacobian of the transformation is built into the new function $\tilde{f}$ and is not needed in the integrals. It should also be noted that the tilde on $\tilde{f}$ implies a different sort of scaling here than in Chapter 4 [cf. (4.15)].

Substituting (9.53) and (9.58) into (9.50) gives

$$\begin{aligned} h(\mathbf{r}'') &= \frac{T\mathscr{A}_{\text{ph}}}{4\pi} \int_\infty d^2\tilde{r} \int_{-\infty}^{\infty} d\tilde{z} \left(\frac{s_1 + z}{s_1}\right)^2 \tilde{f}(\tilde{\mathbf{r}}, \tilde{z}) \frac{\delta(a\mathbf{r}'' + b\mathbf{r} - \mathbf{r}_0')}{(s_1 + s_2 + z)^2} \\ &= \frac{T\mathscr{A}_{\text{ph}}}{4\pi s_1^2} \int_\infty d^2\tilde{r} \int_{-\infty}^{\infty} d\tilde{z}\, \tilde{f}(\tilde{\mathbf{r}}, \tilde{z})\, \delta\!\left(\mathbf{r}'' + \frac{b}{a}\mathbf{r} - \frac{1}{a}\mathbf{r}_0'\right) \end{aligned} \tag{9.59}$$

The 2D Fourier transform of the image is

$$H(\boldsymbol{\rho}'') = \frac{T\mathscr{A}_{\mathrm{ph}}}{4\pi s_1^2} \int_{\infty} d^2\mathbf{r}'' \int_{\infty} d^2\tilde{r} \int_{-\infty}^{\infty} d\tilde{z} \exp(-2\pi i \boldsymbol{\rho}'' \cdot \mathbf{r}'')$$

$$\times \tilde{f}(\tilde{\mathbf{r}}, \tilde{z})\, \delta\left(\mathbf{r}'' + \frac{b}{a}\mathbf{r} - \frac{1}{a}\mathbf{r}'_0\right)$$

$$= \frac{T\mathscr{A}_{\mathrm{ph}}}{4\pi s_1^2} \int_{\infty} d^2\tilde{r} \int_{-\infty}^{\infty} d\tilde{z}\, \tilde{f}(\tilde{\mathbf{r}}, \tilde{z}) \exp\left[-2\pi i \boldsymbol{\rho}'' \cdot \left(-\frac{b}{a}\mathbf{r} + \frac{1}{a}\mathbf{r}'_0\right)\right]. \quad (9.60)$$

We now express a, b, and $\mathbf{r}$ in the exponent in terms of $\tilde{\mathbf{r}}$ and $\tilde{z}$ via (9.51), (9.52), and (9.55). After considerable algebra (Chiu *et al.*, 1979), we find that $H(\boldsymbol{\rho}'')$ has the structure of a 3D Fourier transform of the distorted function $\tilde{f}$. Specifically,

$$H(\boldsymbol{\rho}'') = \frac{T\mathscr{A}_{\mathrm{ph}}}{4\pi s_1^2} \exp\left[-2\pi i\left(1 + \frac{s_2}{s_1}\right)\boldsymbol{\rho}'' \cdot \mathbf{r}'_0\right] \tilde{F}\left(-\frac{s_2}{s_1}\boldsymbol{\rho}'', -\frac{s_2}{s_1^2}\boldsymbol{\rho}'' \cdot \mathbf{r}'_0\right), \quad (9.61)$$

where $\tilde{F}(\tilde{\boldsymbol{\rho}}, \tilde{\zeta})$ is the 3D transform of $\tilde{f}(\tilde{\mathbf{r}}, \tilde{z})$. The form of $\tilde{F}(\tilde{\boldsymbol{\rho}}, \tilde{\zeta})$ that appears in (9.61) is not completely general because $\tilde{\boldsymbol{\rho}}$ and $\tilde{\zeta}$ are not independent. Instead, we see that $\tilde{\boldsymbol{\rho}} = -(s_2/s_1)\boldsymbol{\rho}''$ and $\tilde{\zeta} = -(s_2/s_1^2)\boldsymbol{\rho}'' \cdot \mathbf{r}'_0$, so that

$$\tilde{\zeta} = \tilde{\boldsymbol{\rho}} \cdot (\mathbf{r}'_0/s_1), \quad (9.62)$$

which defines a plane through the origin in the distorted 3D frequency space. The orientation of this plane is determined by the location of the pinhole. If the pinhole lies on the z axis so that $\mathbf{r}'_0 = 0$, then $H(\boldsymbol{\rho}'')$ gives information about $\tilde{F}(\tilde{\boldsymbol{\rho}}, \tilde{\zeta})$ on the plane $\tilde{\zeta} = 0$. As the pinhole moves farther from the z axis, the normal to the relevant plane in distorted frequency space tips farther away from the $\tilde{\zeta}$ axis. Since the frequency space is oriented so that its axes are parallel to the corresponding axes in real space ($\tilde{\zeta}$ parallel to x, etc.), the plane in frequency space is normal to the central ray (from origin to pinhole) in real space. To prove this point, we write the pinhole location as a 3D vector $\mathfrak{r}_0$, which has components $(\mathbf{r}'_0, -s_1)$ since the aperture plane is at $z = -s_1$. This vector $\mathfrak{r}_0$ is also the direction of the central ray. Any vector $\tilde{\boldsymbol{\sigma}}$ in the plane in frequency space, according to (9.62), has components $(\tilde{\boldsymbol{\rho}}, \tilde{\boldsymbol{\rho}} \cdot \mathbf{r}'_0/s_1)$. But

$$\mathfrak{r}_0 \cdot \tilde{\boldsymbol{\sigma}} = \mathbf{r}'_0 \cdot \tilde{\boldsymbol{\rho}} - s_1(\tilde{\boldsymbol{\rho}} \cdot \mathbf{r}'_0/s_1) = 0. \quad (9.63)$$

Therefore, as expected, any $\tilde{\boldsymbol{\sigma}}$ in the plane defined by (9.62) is normal to $\mathfrak{r}_0$.

To summarize, (9.61) shows that pinhole images are similar to 2D parallel-ray projections of 3D objects. The difference is that the 2D Fourier transform of a parallel-ray projection yields information on a plane in an ordinary 3D frequency space, while the 2D transform of a pinhole image yields information on a plane in a *distorted* frequency space. Different planes can be mapped by moving the pinhole to different locations. So long as the pinhole remains in a plane, the same coordinate transformation remains appropriate; it is not necessary to use a different transformation for each pinhole position.

9.4.2 Other Applications of Coordinate Transformation

An approach similar to the one described in Section 9.4.1 can be applied to a wide variety of radiographic systems. One particularly interesting case is the Fourier aperture. In Section 8.5.3 we described the operation of the Fourier aperture with a single detector and a planar object. We saw that, for a single moiré grid frequency, the detector reading gives directly one point in the 2D transform of the object [cf. (8.109)]. For more general 3D objects, each detector reading gives one point in the 3D transform in distorted frequency space (Chiu *et al.*, 1979). A physical interpretation of this result is shown in Fig. 9.5. In the undistorted space domain, rays that reach one detector point are modulated by the moiré grid, forming a set of diverging, sinusoidally modulated fringes in object space. Photons emitted from the "dark" regions of this 3D modulation pattern are blocked by the moiré grid and do not reach the detector, while photons emitted in the "light" region are efficiently detected. The coordinate transformation removes the divergence of the modulation pattern. The detector signal is then the volume integral of the 3D object as modulated by a pattern varying as $\cos(2\pi\boldsymbol{\sigma}_g \cdot \mathbf{r})$ or $\sin(2\pi\boldsymbol{\sigma}_g \cdot \mathbf{r})$. In other words, it is simply one 3D Fourier component of the object. The full set of Fourier components for one detector position and all possible moiré frequencies maps out one plane in the distorted frequency space. Changing the detector location changes the orientation of the plane, just as in the pinhole case. One can, in fact, think of the whole set of moiré frequencies as synthesizing a pinhole.

An interesting conclusion emerges from the coordinate transformation viewpoint when it is applied to a general coded-aperture system. It turns out that the 2D Fourier transform of a single coded image yields information over some volume in 3D distorted frequency space, but that the information is in an ambiguous multiplexed form. If $h(\mathbf{r}'')$ is the coded image, then $H(\boldsymbol{\rho}'')$ for a single $\boldsymbol{\rho}''$ is given by a weighted integral of $\tilde{F}(\tilde{\boldsymbol{\rho}}, \tilde{\zeta})$ along a line in $\tilde{\boldsymbol{\rho}}$–$\tilde{\zeta}$ space. Several coded images must be used if there is to be any hope of demultiplexing these data and obtaining unambiguous information regarding a single object frequency.

Other systems to which coordinate transformations have been applied are transmission radiography, motion tomography, the rotating slit, and multiple coded-aperture systems (Chiu *et al.*, 1979; Chiu, 1980).

One place in which coordinate transformation, as we have described it, is *not* applicable, is in fan-beam projection in ordinary 2D computed

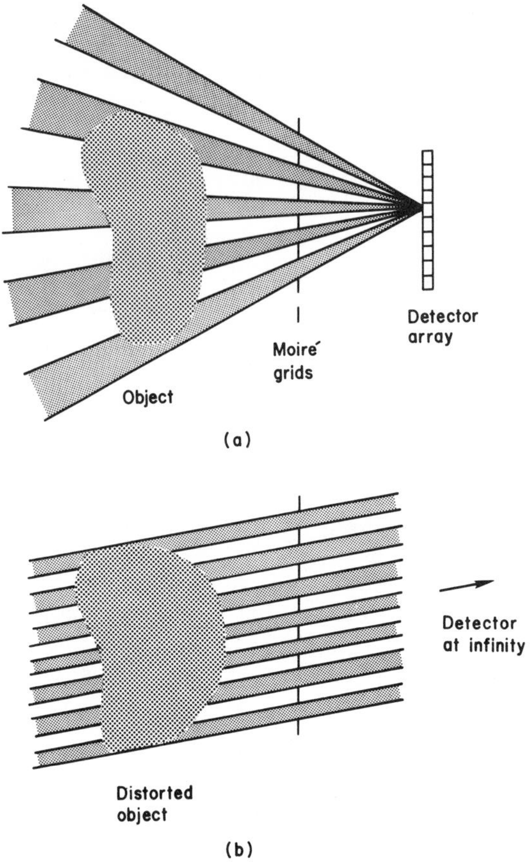

Fig. 9.5 Diagram from Chiu *et al.* (1979) showing how a 3D object is imaged by the Fourier aperture (see text).

tomography. The difficulty in that case is that the projection point is not confined to a plane, so the same transformation is not applicable to all projection directions.

9.5 MULTIPLE-APERTURE SYSTEMS

9.5.1 Three-Dimensional Reconstruction by Matrix Inversion

Chang, Macdonald, and Perez-Mendez (Chang *et al.*, 1974; Chang, 1976) have devised an emission imaging system based on a multiple pinhole array (see Fig. 9.6). The pinholes are opened one at a time, so there is no image

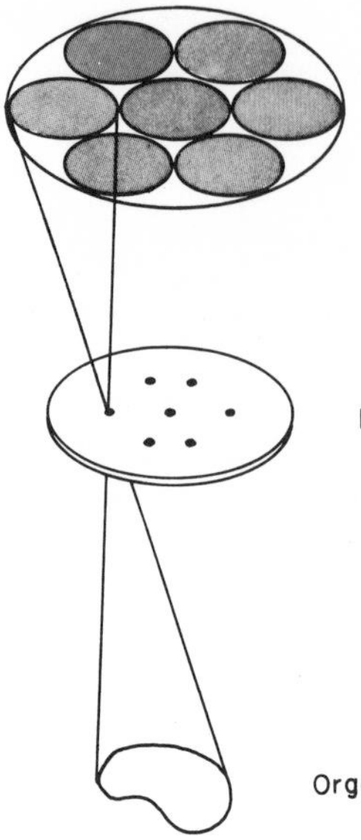

Fig. 9.6 Multiple pinhole system used by Chang *et al.* The pinholes are opened one at a time so there is no image multiplexing.

multiplexing and it is not a coded-aperture system. The interesting feature of this system is the reconstruction method.

Let the kth pinhole in the array be located at point $\mathbf{r}'_k$ in the aperture plane. If the pinhole area $\mathscr{A}_{\text{ph}}$ is small, then the pinhole transmittance can be approximated by a delta function and written, in the notation of Chapter 4, as

$$g_k(\mathbf{r}') = \mathscr{A}_{\text{ph}}\,\delta(\mathbf{r}' - \mathbf{r}'_k). \tag{9.64}$$

We consider the 3D object to be made up of a stack of 2D planes. Each plane is described by a 2D emission density function $f_l(\mathbf{r})$, measured in emitted photons per second per unit area.

We denote the density of detected photons due to the source in the lth plane as viewed with the kth pinhole by $h_{kl}(\mathbf{r}'')$. From (4.13), it is given by

$$h_{kl}(\mathbf{r}'') = C_l \int_\infty g_k(a_l\mathbf{r}'' + b_l\mathbf{r}) f_l(\mathbf{r})\, d^2r, \tag{9.65}$$

$$C_l = \frac{T}{4\pi(s_{1l} + s_2)^2}, \tag{9.66}$$

$$a_l = \frac{s_{1l}}{s_{1l} + s_2}, \tag{9.67}$$

$$b_l = \frac{s_2}{s_{1l} + s_2}, \tag{9.68}$$

where T is the exposure time and s_{1l} is the distance from the aperture plane to the lth object plane. Of course, the aperture-to-detector distance s_2 is the same for all object planes and does not require the subscript l.

Since all object planes are present at once, the composite image through the kth pinhole is

$$h_k(\mathbf{r}'') = \sum_{l=1}^{N_O} h_{kl}(\mathbf{r}''), \tag{9.69}$$

where N_O is the number of object planes. The set of images $h_k(\mathbf{r}'')$, where k ranges from 1 to the number of pinholes N_p, is the basic raw data for reconstruction.

For a point source at the origin of the lth plane, the emission density function is

$$f_l^\delta(\mathbf{r}) = K\,\delta(\mathbf{r}), \tag{9.70}$$

where K is the total number of photons per second emitted by the source. When (9.64) and (9.70) are inserted into (9.65), the kth pinhole image of a point at the origin of the lth plane is found to be

$$\begin{aligned} h_{kl}^\delta(\mathbf{r}'') &= K\mathscr{A}_{\text{ph}} C_l \int_\infty \delta(a_l\mathbf{r}'' + b_l\mathbf{r} - \mathbf{r}_k')\,\delta(\mathbf{r})\,d^2r \\ &= K\mathscr{A}_{\text{ph}} C_l\,\delta(a_l\mathbf{r}'' - \mathbf{r}_k'). \end{aligned} \tag{9.71}$$

The first step in the reconstruction process is to form *tomograms* of each plane. A tomogram is really a 3D summation image evaluated on a discrete set of planes. The contribution of the kth pinhole image $h_k(\mathbf{r}'')$ to the tomogram of the mth plane, $t_m(\mathbf{r})$, is found by back-projecting $h_k(\mathbf{r}'')$ through the pinhole onto the plane. The back-projection process is such that a point at the origin of the mth plane is returned to the origin, and all objects in the plane are rendered with the correct magnification (see Fig. 9.7). Thus, back-projection is essentially a shifting and scaling operation. The image of objects in the mth plane through the kth pinhole is shifted by an amount $\mathbf{r}_k'/a_m$ in the $\mathbf{r}''$ plane. We can shift it back by substituting $\mathbf{r}'' - (-\mathbf{r}_k'/a_m)$ for $\mathbf{r}''$ in $h_k(\mathbf{r}'')$. This shifted image is then corrected for the magnification appropriate to the mth plane by the further substitution $\mathbf{r}'' = -b_m\mathbf{r}/a_m$ [cf. (4.36)]. The process is repeated for each pinhole and the results are added, producing a tomogram or summation image given by

$$\begin{aligned} t_m(\mathbf{r}) &= \sum_{k=1}^{N_P} \left(\frac{b_m}{a_m}\right)^2 h_k\left(\mathbf{r}'' + \frac{\mathbf{r}_k'}{a_m}\right)\Bigg|_{\mathbf{r}''=-b_m\mathbf{r}/a_m} \\ &= \sum_{k=1}^{N_P} \left(\frac{b_m}{a_m}\right)^2 h_k\left(\frac{-b_m\mathbf{r}}{a_m} + \frac{\mathbf{r}_k'}{a_m}\right). \end{aligned} \tag{9.72}$$

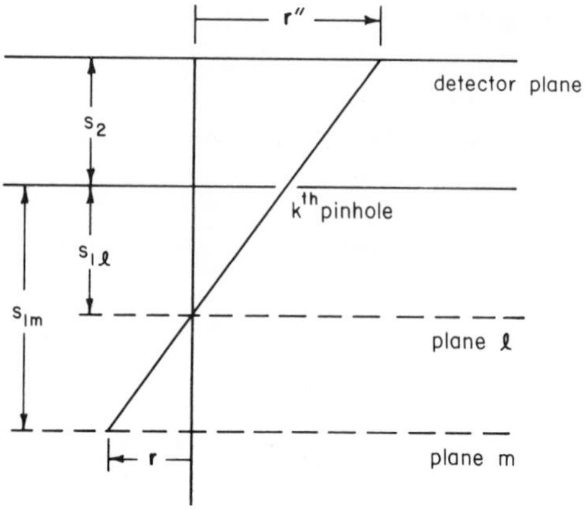

Fig. 9.7 Geometry for forming tomograms. A point actually at the origin in plane l produces an image through the kth pinhole at the point $\mathbf{r}''$ shown. When this image is back-projected to plane m, it is displaced from the origin by $\mathbf{r}$.

The significance of this equation can be better appreciated by considering the special case where the object is a point at the origin of the lth plane, so that $h_k(\mathbf{r}'') = h_{kl}^{\delta}(\mathbf{r}'')$. We shall call the tomogram in this case $p_{ml}(\mathbf{r})$, meaning the tomogram or cross-plane PSF for the mth plane when the object is a point in the lth plane. It is given, from (9.71) and (9.72), by

$$p_{ml}(\mathbf{r}) = \mathscr{A}_{\text{ph}} K \sum_k \left(\frac{b_m}{a_m}\right)^2 C_l \, \delta\left[a_l\left(\frac{-b_m \mathbf{r}}{a_m} + \frac{\mathbf{r}_k'}{a_m}\right) - \mathbf{r}_k'\right]. \tag{9.73}$$

The argument of the delta function vanishes when

$$\frac{a_l b_m}{a_m} \mathbf{r} = \left(\frac{a_l}{a_m} - 1\right) \mathbf{r}_k' \tag{9.74}$$

or

$$\mathbf{r} = \mathbf{r}_k' \frac{s_{1l} - s_{1m}}{s_{1l}}. \tag{9.75}$$

Equation (9.75) also follows from the similar triangles in Fig. 9.7. The delta function in (9.73) therefore represents the intersection with the mth plane of the ray through the kth pinhole and the origin of the lth plane.

In terms of this cross-plane PSF $p_{ml}(\mathbf{r})$, the tomogram of a general multiplanar object is given by

$$t_m(\mathbf{r}) = \sum_{l=1}^{N_O} p_{ml}(\mathbf{r}) ** f_l(\mathbf{r}). \tag{9.76}$$

The frequency-domain version of (9.76) is

$$T_m(\boldsymbol{\rho}) = \sum_{l=1}^{N_0} P_{ml}(\boldsymbol{\rho}) F_l(\boldsymbol{\rho}). \tag{9.77}$$

This is a set of N_0 linear equations in N_0 unknown *functions* $F_l(\boldsymbol{\rho})$. Therefore it can be solved at each frequency $\boldsymbol{\rho}$ by Cramer's rule or any other method of matrix inversion. The requirement for the existence of a solution is that the determinant of $P_{ml}(\boldsymbol{\rho})$ not vanish. Chang (1976) has found that this condition is satisfied for nonredundant pinhole arrays for all frequencies except $\boldsymbol{\rho} = 0$. This exception is no great surprise since a zero-frequency source component (a uniform flood source) looks the same from all pinholes. There is no way to tell how far it is from the aperture plane.

An example of a reconstruction by this method is shown in Fig. 9.8.

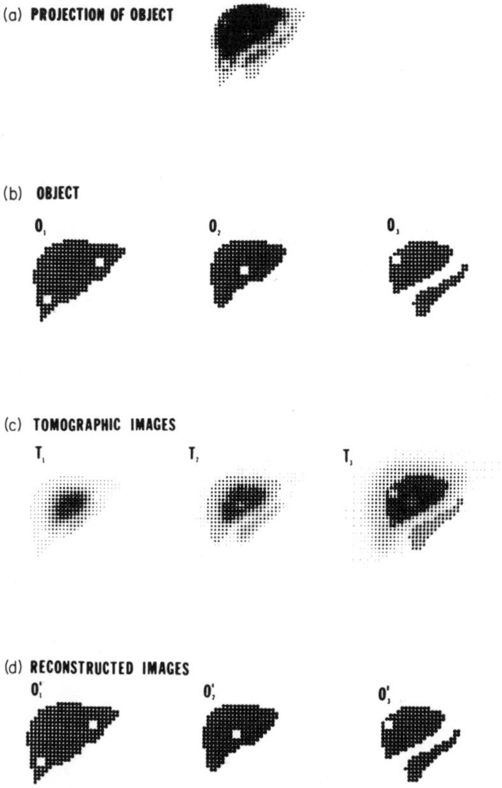

Fig. 9.8 Computer-simulated images obtained by Chang, Macdonald, and Perez-Mendez. The reconstructions in (d) were performed using their matrix inversion algorithm.

9.5.2 Iterative Reconstruction Based on Three-Dimensional Back-Projection

Kirch and co-workers (Vogel *et al.*, 1978) have used a multiple pinhole array similar to the one described in Section 9.5.1. By using just seven pinholes and using a large-field Anger camera as the detector, they were able to produce all of the pinhole images simultaneously without image overlap. Their basic data are still individual unmultiplexed pinhole images just as in the work of Chang (1976).

Kirch has devised an interesting variation of 3D back-projection which he refers to as *impedance estimation.* Rather than back-projecting $h_k(\mathbf{r}'')$ through the kth pinhole, he forms the reciprocal image $[h_k(\mathbf{r}'')]^{-1}$, back-projects and sums, and then takes the reciprocal of the summation image. His basic tomogram is thus [cf. (9.72)]

$$t_m(\mathbf{r}) = \left\{ \sum_{k=1}^{N_P} \left(\frac{a_m}{b_m} \right)^2 \left[h_k\left(\frac{-b_m \mathbf{r}}{a_m} + \frac{\mathbf{r}'_k}{a_m} \right) \right]^{-1} \right\}^{-1}. \tag{9.78}$$

This addition rule—the reciprocal of the sum of the reciprocals—is the same as the rule for adding impedances in parallel, hence the designation impedance estimator. The advantage of this rule in the present problem is that it emphasizes "cold" regions where $h_k(\mathbf{r}'')$ is small. In many applications, the cold regions are medically the most significant.

Kirch uses the tomograms of (9.78) as just the first estimate of the object. He then calculates what the kth pinhole image would be if this estimate were correct and compares it with the actual measured $h_k(\mathbf{r}'')$. A correction is then made to the tomograms in a manner similar to the SIRT algorithm (Section 7.3.5) and the object estimate is updated and the process repeated. In practice, one or two iterations often suffices to yield an excellent image. An example is shown in Fig. 9.9.

Closely related to this work is the approach used at the University of Michigan for 3D reconstruction from stochastic-aperture images (see Section 8.5.2). After the temporal correlation operation, the data from one detector element produce one pinholelike projection of the object. The only difference is that the projection point where all rays converge is the detector element rather than an actual pinhole in the aperture plane. A 3D back-projection operation again produces a first estimate of the object, which can be improved upon by various iterative procedures such as ART (Koral and Rogers, 1979). The main advantage of this approach over Kirch's system is that many more projections are available in the data set, giving a denser sampling in 3D Fourier space. The disadvantage is the time required to accumulate these data.

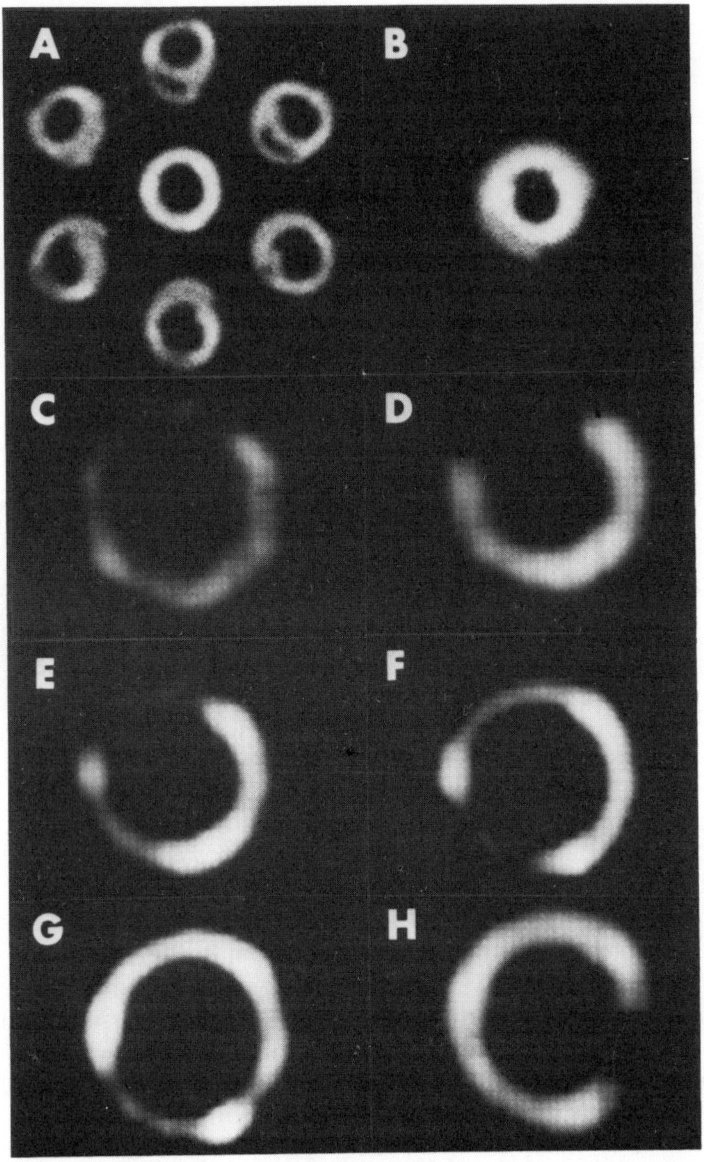

Fig. 9.9 Myocardial phantom images obtained by Kirch and co-workers (Vogel *et al.*, 1978). A: Composite pinhole image; B: Image with a parallel-hole collimator; C–H: Reconstructed sectional images.

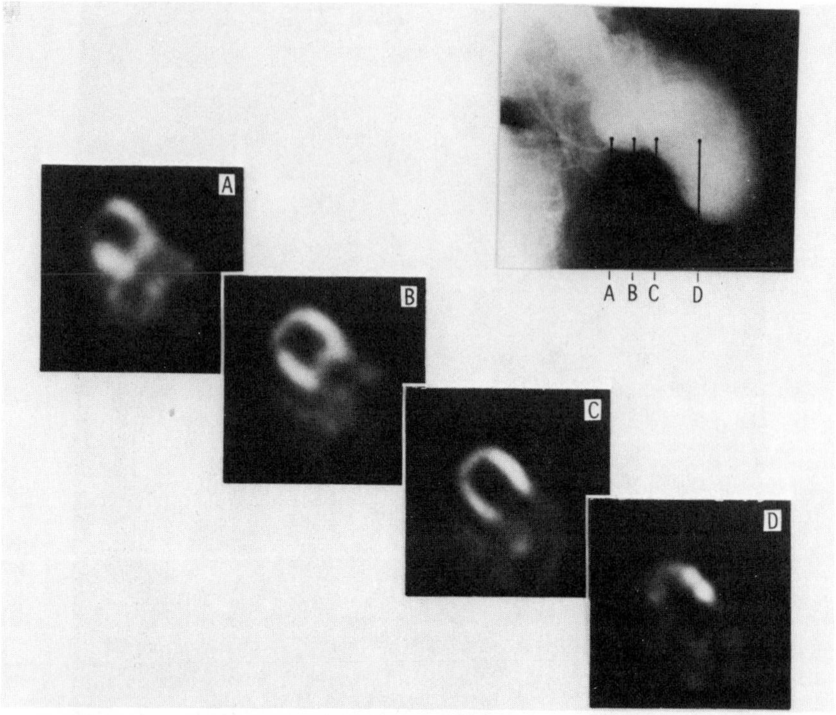

Fig. 9.10 Reconstructed myocardial images obtained by Rogers *et al.* (1980). Radiograph at upper right shows location of reconstructed sections.

Some examples of stochastic aperture reconstructions are shown in Figs. 9.10 and 9.11. It is also possible to use similar iterative reconstruction algorithms with multiplexed multiple-pinhole data sets (Ohyama *et al.*, 1981).

9.5.3 Multiple Coded Apertures Derived from Bessel Functions

Joy and co-workers (Renaud *et al.*, 1979) at the University of Toronto have used a multicoding system with interesting 3D properties. Rather than beginning with the actual apertures used by these workers, we consider instead a set of apertures with transmittance given by

$$g_k(\mathbf{r}') = \tfrac{1}{2}[1 + J_0(2\pi\alpha_k r')] \qquad (k = 1, 2, \ldots, N_a), \tag{9.79}$$

where $J_0(\ )$ is the usual zero-order Bessel function. These are physically realizable apertures since $0 < g_k(\mathbf{r}') \leqslant 1$, but they would be difficult to construct since they are not binary apertures. Furthermore, we are not yet considering any limitation to the overall size of the aperture or detector.

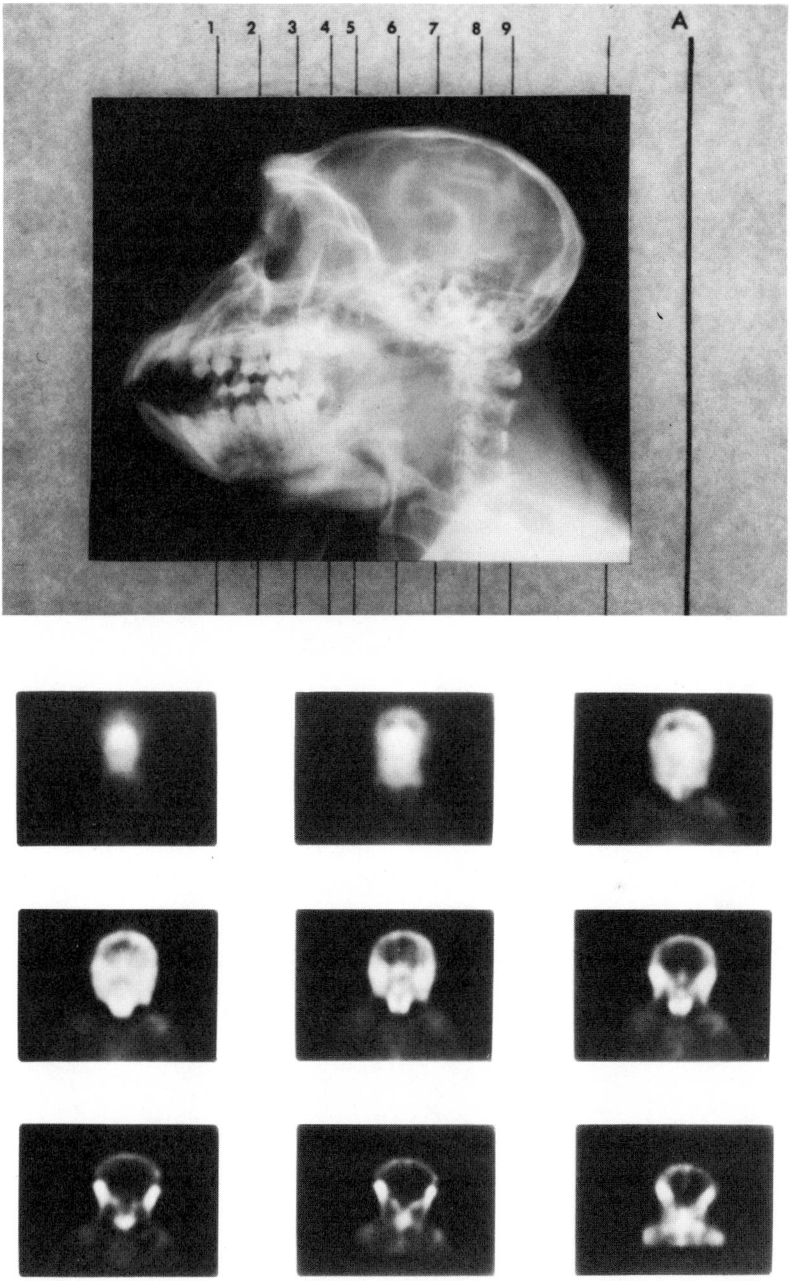

Fig. 9.11 Top: Radiograph of a monkey's head. Bottom: Successive reconstructed sections obtained with a stochastic aperture and an iterative reconstruction algorithm. The nine images from upper left to lower right correspond to sections 1–9 labeled on the radiograph. (Unpublished work of W. L. Rogers and K. F. Koral.)

From (B.106), the 2D Fourier transform of $g_k(\mathbf{r}')$ is

$$G_k(\boldsymbol{\rho}') = \tfrac{1}{2}[\delta(\boldsymbol{\rho}') + (1/2\pi\alpha_k)\,\delta(\rho' - \alpha_k)]. \tag{9.80}$$

Note that $\delta(\boldsymbol{\rho}')$ is a 2D delta function but $\delta(\rho' - \alpha_k)$ is a 1D ring delta function.

Again we consider a multiplanar object where $f_l(\mathbf{r})$ is the 2D emission function for the lth plane . From (4.22) and (9.66)–(9.68), the kth coded image in the frequency domain is

$$H_k(\boldsymbol{\rho}'') = \sum_l \left(\frac{C_l}{a_l^2}\right) F_l\left(\frac{-b_l\boldsymbol{\rho}''}{a_l}\right) G_k\left(\frac{\boldsymbol{\rho}''}{a_l}\right). \tag{9.81}$$

The important point here is that the ring delta function in $G_k(\boldsymbol{\rho}'')$ is a filter that passes only the frequencies $\boldsymbol{\rho}''$ whose magnitude satisfies

$$\rho'' = a_l \alpha_k. \tag{9.82}$$

An object frequency $\boldsymbol{\rho}$ associated with plane l can contribute to $H_k(\boldsymbol{\rho}'')$ only if its magnitude satisfies

$$\rho = b_l \rho''/a_l = b_l \alpha_k, \tag{9.83}$$

which is different for every plane l. Thus annular regions in $H_k(\boldsymbol{\rho}'')$ can be identified with specific object planes. Each coded image can be filtered into contributions from individual planes. Consider, for example, the filter given by

$$Q_{kl}(\boldsymbol{\rho}'') = \mathrm{circ}\left(\frac{\rho''}{a_l\alpha_k + \Delta/2}\right) - \mathrm{circ}\left(\frac{\rho''}{a_l\alpha_k - \Delta/2}\right), \tag{9.84}$$

which describes an annular region of width Δ and mean radius $a_l\alpha_k$ in the 2D frequency plane. When this filter is applied to $H_k(\boldsymbol{\rho}'')$, the result is

$$\begin{aligned} H_k(\boldsymbol{\rho}'')Q_{kl}(\boldsymbol{\rho}'') &= Q_{kl}(\boldsymbol{\rho}'') \sum_{l'} \frac{C_{l'}}{4\pi\alpha_k a_{l'}^2} F_{l'}\left(\frac{-b_{l'}\boldsymbol{\rho}''}{a_{l'}}\right) \delta\left[\frac{\rho''}{a_{l'}} - \alpha_k\right] \\ &= \frac{C_l}{4\pi\alpha_k a_l^2} F_l\left(\frac{-b_l\boldsymbol{\rho}''}{a_l}\right) \delta\left(\frac{\rho''}{a_l} - \alpha_k\right), \end{aligned} \tag{9.85}$$

where the last step follows because only the term with $l' = l$ falls within the passband of the filter if Δ is sufficiently small. Even the zero-frequency term $\delta(\boldsymbol{\rho}')$ in (9.80) is blocked by the filter. The filtered coded image (9.85) gives information about $F_l(\boldsymbol{\rho})$ along a ring in the frequency plane and *has no contribution from any other plane*. A different filter Q_{kl} with a different value of a_l will select a different plane. The whole set of coded images $H_k(\boldsymbol{\rho}'')$ with different values of α_k then gives information about *each* $F_l(\boldsymbol{\rho})$ on a set of

N_a concentric rings; $F_l(\boldsymbol{\rho})$ is sampled in the radial direction. If the sampling is dense enough, a 2D inverse Fourier transform serves to recover $f_l(\mathbf{r})$ for all l.

The apertures actually used by Joy *et al.* were not the ones described by (9.79), but rather had transmittances of

$$g_k(\mathbf{r}') = \tfrac{1}{2}\{1 \pm \operatorname{sgn}[J_0(2\pi\alpha_k r')]\} \operatorname{circ}(r'/R), \tag{9.86}$$

$$\operatorname{sgn} x = \begin{cases} 1 & \text{if } x > 0 \\ -1 & \text{if } x < 0. \end{cases} \tag{9.87}$$

Equation (9.86) describes a binary function, $g_k = 0$ or 1, of limited radius R. It therefore does not have exactly the desirable transform property (9.80), but seems to be an acceptable approximation if R is large enough.

9.5.4 Restricted View Angle

The systems described in Sections 9.5.1–9.5.3 share one common limitation: they do not fully span the 3D Fourier space because each object point is viewed from a restricted set of angles. Consider, for example, a multiple pinhole system in which all pinholes are contained within a circle of radius R'_m in the aperture plane. As demonstrated in Section 9.4.1, each pinhole image yields information about the object on a plane in a distorted 3D frequency space. The orientation of this plane is determined by the pinhole location. But no matter where the pinhole is within the circle of radius R'_m, there is a region in frequency space defined by two cones of semiangle $\tan^{-1}(R'_m/s_1)$ that is never sampled by any pinhole image (see Fig. 9.12). Object frequencies within these cones are lost and an exact 3D reconstruction is not possible. Similar considerations apply to many other radiographic systems, including any emission imaging system in which the aperture is confined to a single plane, and any transmission imaging system in which the source is confined to a plane. In all of these cases, there are two "missing cones" of data in 3D Fourier space (Chiu *et al.*, 1979).

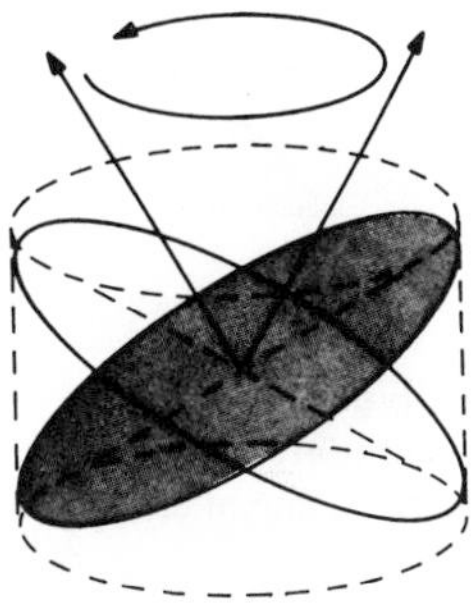

Fig. 9.12 Sampled region in 3D Fourier space for a multiple pinhole system. Each pinhole projection gives information on one plane in a distorted Fourier space. If the pinholes are contained within a finite area, there are two "missing cones" of data.

One manifestation of the missing cones is that uniform flood sources parallel to the aperture plane cannot be imaged properly. Such sources have a 3D Fourier transform that lies entirely along the axis of the cones.

Another description of the problem is the 3D PSF, which cannot be compact in all directions if the cones of information are missing. Suppose our imaging system perfectly determines all Fourier components *outside* the cones. If we simply set the unknown components inside the cones to zero and transform to the space domain, we obtain the PSF shown in Fig. 9.13 (Chiu *et al.*, 1979). In this picture, the direction labeled r can be any direction in the x–y plane, while z is the direction normal to the aperture and detector planes. The significant feature of this PSF is the long low-amplitude tail radiating out from the central core as a conical shell. The size of these tails can be reduced somewhat by proper apodization but they cannot be eliminated by any linear filtering method so long as there are missing cones of data in the other domain.

There is, however, the possibility that nonlinear reconstruction methods can significantly improve the image. There is a great variety of such methods

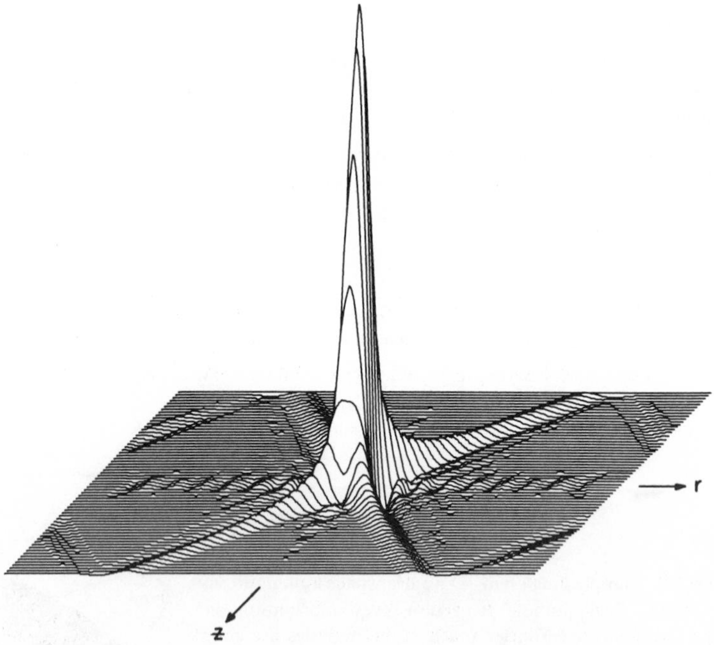

Fig. 9.13 3D PSF obtained in the missing-cone problem. All unmeasured Fourier components are simply set to zero. The three coordinates of this isometric plot are the depth dimension z, a lateral dimension labeled r, which is in the x-y plane, and the PSF. (From Chiu *et al.*, 1979.)

in use in 2D image processing (for a review, see Frieden, 1975), and many of them could be carried over to the 3D problem. Particularly promising is an algorithm proposed independently by Papoulis (1975) and Gerchberg (1974) and applied to radiographic imaging by Tam *et al.* (1979). As a general rule, nonlinear methods succeed where linear methods fail if they effectively incorporate a priori information about the object. In the present problem, we can use the knowledge that the object is positive definite and limited in spatial extent.

10

Noise in Radiographic Images

10.1 INTRODUCTION

In any physical measurement, there are always errors and uncertainties. We may distinguish between *systematic* and *random* errors. Systematic errors remain the same in every repetition of the measurement. They are more or less under the control of the experimenter or instrument designer, and can, in principle, be reduced to negligible levels if one is willing to accept a costly, complex instrument. Random errors, on the other hand, vary uncontrollably from one repetition of the same basic measurement to the next.

In the context of radiographic imaging, examples of systematic errors include geometric distortion, miscalibration or nonlinearity of the detector, errors due to sampling a continuous image into a discrete set of pixels or quantizing an analog signal into a limited number of digital levels, computation errors when an image is reconstructed from indirect data as in computed tomography, and even uninteresting features of the object itself. Examples of random errors include film grain noise, photon noise, electronic noise, and noise due to scattered radiation.

This chapter will deal exclusively with random noise, and will concentrate heavily on photon noise in x-ray and gamma-ray images. As already noted in Chapter 3, photon noise is usually the predominant source of noise in these images because the allowable dose of radiation to the patient severely limits the number of photons that can be used to form an image.

Before launching into an analysis of noise in radiographic images, we must agree on how to characterize the noise and on how to quantify the degree of noisiness in an image. Ultimately, the only meaningful characterization is in terms of how well the image fulfills its intended purpose and leads to a correct diagnosis. Certainly when comparing two different imaging systems intended for the same diagnostic task, the only proper measure of performance is the correctness of the diagnosis, perhaps measured by true positive, true negative, false positive, and false negative rates.

Nevertheless, an objective physical characterization of image noise is quite useful. For one thing, detailed clinical trials or psychophysical studies of observer performance with different images are difficult to carry out convincingly. For another thing, clinical and psychophysical evaluations tend to be binary comparisons with a restricted applicability, e.g., collimator A is better than collimator B for detecting liver metastases, or x-ray screen X is better than screen Y for imaging 1-cm-diam nodules with 5% contrast. Finally, and perhaps most important, a physical description of the noise can be used to identify potential trade-offs by which the designer or user of the imaging instrument can optimize it for specific tasks.

Even if we agree that a physical characterization of the noise is useful, there is still a bewildering variety of possible things that one can calculate. Broadly speaking, the various measures of noise may be classified as *global* or *local*. Global measures involve the entire image, usually reducing a complex noise pattern to a single number. An example of a global measure is the root-mean-square deviation between the image and the actual object or between the image and its ensemble average. A local measure, on the other hand, varies from point to point in the image. An example would be some sort of local signal-to-noise ratio (SNR). Global measures can be derived from local ones, but the converse is not true except in very special cases. Because of this greater generality, we shall concentrate on local measures in this chapter.

Even if we set out to determine a local SNR, there is still considerable freedom as to what we call signal and what we call noise—one man's signal is another man's noise. Somewhat arbitrarily, we shall regard the signal as the image that would be obtained in the absence of noise, if such a condition were possible. Computationally, the signal may be determined by taking an ensemble average of noisy images. For photon noise, this is equivalent to passing to the limit of an infinite number of detected photons.

With this definition of the signal, a natural choice for the noise is the root-mean-square deviation of the noisy images from the mean or signal image. In general, the noise will vary strongly with position in the image.

10.2 SUMMARY OF BASIC PRINCIPLES

Photon noise in radiographic images may be modeled in terms of the Poisson impulses introduced in Chapter 3. In (3.128) the random process $\mathbf{u}(\mathbf{r})$ was defined as

$$\mathbf{u}(\mathbf{r}) = \sum_{j=1}^{\mathbf{K}} \delta(\mathbf{r} - \mathbf{r}_j), \tag{10.1}$$

where $\mathbf{K}$ and all of the $\mathbf{r}_j$ are random variables. In Chapter 4, we learned how to calculate $h(\mathbf{r}'')$, the mean density of detected photons, for various radiographic systems. From the discussion in Section 3.3, $h(\mathbf{r}'')$ may, with suitable normalization, also be interpreted as the probability density function for $\mathbf{r}_j$. In particular, (3.149) gives

$$\mathrm{pr}_r(\mathbf{r}_j'') = h(\mathbf{r}_j'') \Big/ \int_\infty h(\mathbf{r}'')\, d^2r''. \tag{10.2}$$

From this result, it was shown in (3.150) that

$$\langle \mathbf{u}(\mathbf{r}) \rangle = h(\mathbf{r}). \tag{10.3}$$

The associated nonstationary autocorrelation function is given by (3.151):

$$R_u(\mathbf{r}, \mathbf{r} + \mathbf{L}) = h(\mathbf{r})\,\delta(\mathbf{L}) + h(\mathbf{r})h(\mathbf{r} + \mathbf{L}). \tag{10.4}$$

Thus, knowledge of the average image $h(\mathbf{r})$ *also provides an essentially complete statistical description of the image.*

It will be important to know how $\mathbf{u}(\mathbf{r})$ is affected by a linear filter. In general, when a nonstationary random process $\mathbf{w}_{\text{in}}(\mathbf{r})$ is passed through a linear, shift-invariant filter of impulse response $p_f(\mathbf{r})$, the output autocorrelation function is given by [cf. (3.210)]

$$R_{\text{out}}(\mathbf{r}, \mathbf{r} + \mathbf{L}) = p_f(\mathbf{r}) ** p_f(\mathbf{r} + \mathbf{L}) ** R_{\text{in}}(\mathbf{r}, \mathbf{r} + \mathbf{L}). \tag{10.5}$$

Specifically, if we let

$$\mathbf{w}_{\text{in}}(\mathbf{r}) = \mathbf{u}(\mathbf{r}) \tag{10.6}$$

and

$$\mathbf{w}_{\text{out}}(\mathbf{r}) = \mathbf{u}^\dagger(\mathbf{r}) \equiv \mathbf{u}(\mathbf{r}) ** p_f(\mathbf{r}), \tag{10.7}$$

where the dagger means "filtered," we have [cf. (3.214), where $a(t)$ corresponds to $h(\mathbf{r})$]

$$R_{u\dagger}(\mathbf{r}, \mathbf{r} + \mathbf{L}) = \int_\infty d^2r'\, p_f(\mathbf{r}')p_f(\mathbf{r}' + \mathbf{L})h(\mathbf{r} - \mathbf{r}') + [p_f(\mathbf{r}) ** h(\mathbf{r})][p_f(\mathbf{r} + \mathbf{L}) ** h(\mathbf{r} + \mathbf{L})] \tag{10.8}$$

or, for the zero-mean process $\Delta \mathbf{u}^\dagger(\mathbf{r})$ $(\equiv \mathbf{u}^\dagger(\mathbf{r}) - \langle \mathbf{u}^\dagger(\mathbf{r})\rangle)$,

$$R_{\Delta u^\dagger}(\mathbf{r}, \mathbf{r}+\mathbf{L}) = \int_\infty d^2r'\, p_f(\mathbf{r}')p_f(\mathbf{r}'+\mathbf{L})h(\mathbf{r}-\mathbf{r}'). \tag{10.9}$$

The variance of $\mathbf{u}^\dagger(\mathbf{r})$ is [cf. (3.217)]

$$\sigma^2_{u^\dagger}(\mathbf{r}) = R_{\Delta u^\dagger}(\mathbf{r},\mathbf{r}) = \int_\infty d^2r'\, [p_f(\mathbf{r}')]^2 h(\mathbf{r}-\mathbf{r}')$$
$$= [p_f(\mathbf{r})]^2 ** h(\mathbf{r}). \tag{10.10}$$

Of course, the mean of $\mathbf{u}^\dagger(\mathbf{r})$ is [cf. (3.216)]

$$\langle \mathbf{u}^\dagger(\mathbf{r})\rangle = p_f(\mathbf{r}) ** \langle \mathbf{u}(\mathbf{r})\rangle = p_f(\mathbf{r}) ** h(\mathbf{r}) \equiv h^\dagger(\mathbf{r}). \tag{10.11}$$

We may therefore define a local signal-to-noise ratio as

$$\mathrm{SNR}(\mathbf{r}) \equiv \frac{\langle \mathbf{u}^\dagger(\mathbf{r})\rangle}{\sigma_{u^\dagger}(\mathbf{r})} = \frac{p_f(\mathbf{r}) ** h(\mathbf{r})}{\{[p_f(\mathbf{r})]^2 ** h(\mathbf{r})\}^{1/2}}. \tag{10.12}$$

Notice that $\mathrm{SNR}(\mathbf{r})$ is dimensionless, regardless of the dimensions of $p_f(\mathbf{r})$, since the dimensions of $h(\mathbf{r})$ are 1/area, canceling the dimensions of the area element in the convolution integrals.

Equation (10.12) is the prescription for calculating the local SNR. To apply it to any radiographic system consisting of a source, various attenuating elements, a detector, and any number of filters, we need only identify the last point in the system for which (10.1) is a good description of the image, and calculate the mean image $h(\mathbf{r})$ at that point (see Fig. 10.1). All system elements after that point are then lumped into $p_f(\mathbf{r})$ and the integrals in (10.12) are carried out.

It must be emphasized that the description of the image at the input to the filter as a sum of delta functions is crucial since the uncorrelated nature of $\Delta \mathbf{u}(\mathbf{r})$ was assumed in the derivation of (10.10) [or, equivalently, (3.127)]. Two examples will serve to illustrate this point. Consider first an Anger camera and collimator with an image displayed on a cathode-ray

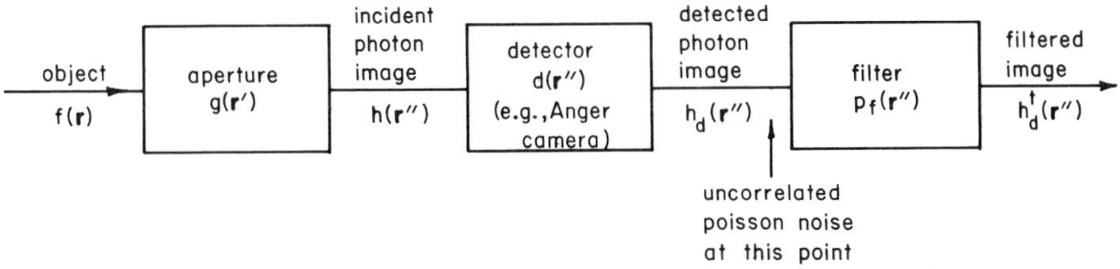

Fig. 10.1 Block diagram of a general radiographic imaging system. For the noise calculation, it is important to identify the last point in the system for which the image consists of a sum of impulses (uncorrelated Poisson noise).

tube (see Fig. 10.2). Each individual gamma ray produces one very small spot of light on the CRT. Thus the light distribution is well characterized by (10.1). Subsequent system elements such as the oscilloscope camera and the observer's eye can be lumped into $p_f(\mathbf{r})$. The intrinsic response of the Anger camera, on the other hand, should *not* be considered in $p_f(\mathbf{r})$. The Anger camera has as its input an array of delta functions, but it does not convolve this input with some impulse response. Rather, each input delta function $\delta(\mathbf{r} - \mathbf{r}_j)$ produces an output delta function $\delta[\mathbf{r} - \mathbf{r}_{jo}]$, where $\mathbf{r}_{jo} - \mathbf{r}_j$ is a random uncertainty in position imparted by the detector. From the results above, we need not concern ourselves with the statistics of $\mathbf{r}_{jo} - \mathbf{r}_j$. All we have to do is calculate the mean image $h(\mathbf{r})$ at the detector output, a task that was accomplished in Chapter 4, and feed the result into (10.12).

As a second example, consider an x-ray screen–film detector. The input to the detector is again a set of Poisson impulses of the form (10.1), but now the action of the detector is rather different. As discussed in Chapter 5,

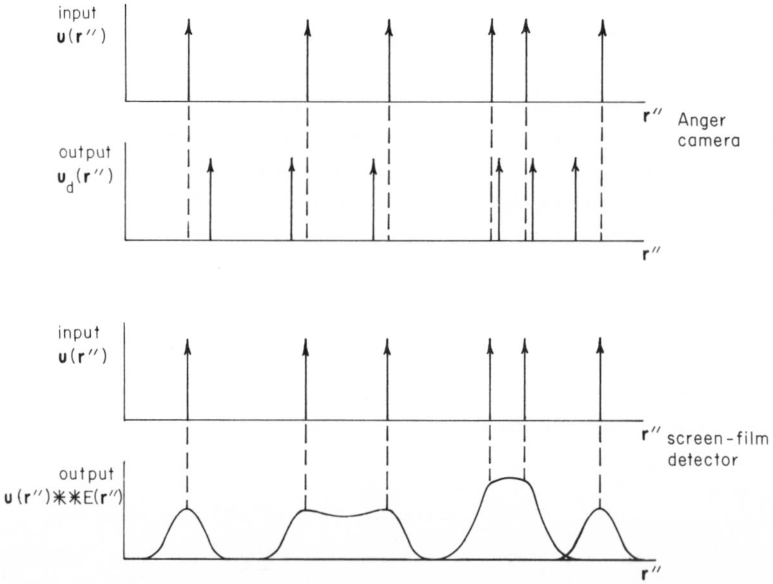

Fig. 10.2 Illustration of a fundamental difference between the noise behavior of an Anger camera and of a screen–film detector. The Anger camera (top) mislocates each scintillation event by some random amount, but always renders it as a sharp impulse. The fluorescent screen (bottom), on the other hand, produces a blurred exposure pattern on the film for each scintillation event. (For purposes of this figure, we have assumed that all x-ray photons produce the same exposure pattern. In reality, the pattern depends also on the depth within the screen at which the photon is absorbed.) Note that $h(\mathbf{r}'')$ is the mean value of the random process $\mathbf{u}(\mathbf{r}'')$ and $h_d(\mathbf{r}'')$ is the mean value of $\mathbf{u}_d(\mathbf{r}'')$.

each absorbed x-ray photon generates a large number of optical photons that diffuse through the screen and expose the film. If the number of optical photons is large enough, it is a good approximation to ignore their statistics and assume that each x-ray photon $\delta(\mathbf{r} - \mathbf{r}_j)$ produces an exposure that is described by the *deterministic* function $E(\mathbf{r} - \mathbf{r}_j)$. In other words, the detector output is *not* of the form (10.1), but rather $\sum_j E(\mathbf{r} - \mathbf{r}_j)$ (see Fig. 10.2). Thus the x-ray screen has to be considered part of the filter $p_f(\mathbf{r})$, and $h(\mathbf{r})$ must be calculated at the detector input [i.e., $h(\mathbf{r})$ represents the mean x-ray fluence incident on the screen].

10.3 NUCLEAR MEDICINE

10.3.1 The Pinhole Camera

An expression for the mean image $h(\mathbf{r}'')$ for a pinhole camera was derived in Chapter 4. Equation (4.18) reads

$$h(\mathbf{r}'') = (a/b)^2 C\tilde{f}(\mathbf{r}'') ** \tilde{g}(\mathbf{r}''), \qquad (10.13)$$

where $\tilde{g}(\mathbf{r}'')$ is the magnified pinhole shadow, given by (4.29) as

$$\tilde{g}(\mathbf{r}'') = \mathrm{circ}(2r''/d''_{\mathrm{ph}}), \qquad (10.14)$$

with $d''_{\mathrm{ph}} \equiv d'_{\mathrm{ph}}/a$. The constants a, b, and C are defined in (4.8), (4.9), and (4.12). For now, we shall assume an ideal detector with unit quantum efficiency and perfect spatial resolution.

To be concrete, we first consider a specific object, a uniform disk source of diameter d_{obj}, for which

$$f(\mathbf{r}) = f_o \,\mathrm{circ}(2r/d_{\mathrm{obj}}). \qquad (10.15)$$

Therefore, by (4.15),

$$\tilde{f}(\mathbf{r}'') = f_o \,\mathrm{circ}(2r''/d''_{\mathrm{obj}}), \qquad (10.16)$$

where $d''_{\mathrm{obj}} = d_{\mathrm{obj}}b/a = d_{\mathrm{obj}}s_2/s_1$. We shall assume that $d''_{\mathrm{obj}} \gg d''_{\mathrm{ph}}$.

To apply (10.12), we must now decide on the filter response $p_f(\mathbf{r}'')$. Motivated by the discussion of matched filters in Chapters 3 and 8, let us take $p_f(\mathbf{r}'')$ in the same form as the aperture shadow:

$$p_f(\mathbf{r}'') = A \,\mathrm{circ}(2r''/d''_f), \qquad (10.17)$$

where A and d''_f are free parameters.

The mean signal, the numerator of (10.12), is given by

$$h(\mathbf{r}'') ** p_f(\mathbf{r}'') = A \int_\infty d^2r''_0 \, h(\mathbf{r}''_0) \,\mathrm{circ}(2|\mathbf{r}'' - \mathbf{r}''_0|/d''_f). \qquad (10.18)$$

For the particular object chosen, $h(\mathbf{r}'')$ is approximately a uniform disk of diameter d''_{obj}. The edge of this disk is blurred by the convolution with $\tilde{g}(\mathbf{r}'')$, but if $d''_{obj} \gg d''_{ph}$, $h(\mathbf{r}'')$ is nearly constant for all points $\mathbf{r}''$ except those within one resolution element of the edge of the disk. Therefore we may write

$$h(\mathbf{r}'') = \begin{cases} h_o & \text{if } r'' < \frac{1}{2}(d''_{obj} - d''_{ph}) \approx \frac{1}{2}d''_{obj} \\ 0 & \text{if } r'' > \frac{1}{2}(d''_{obj} + d''_{ph}) \approx \frac{1}{2}d''_{obj}. \end{cases} \tag{10.19}$$

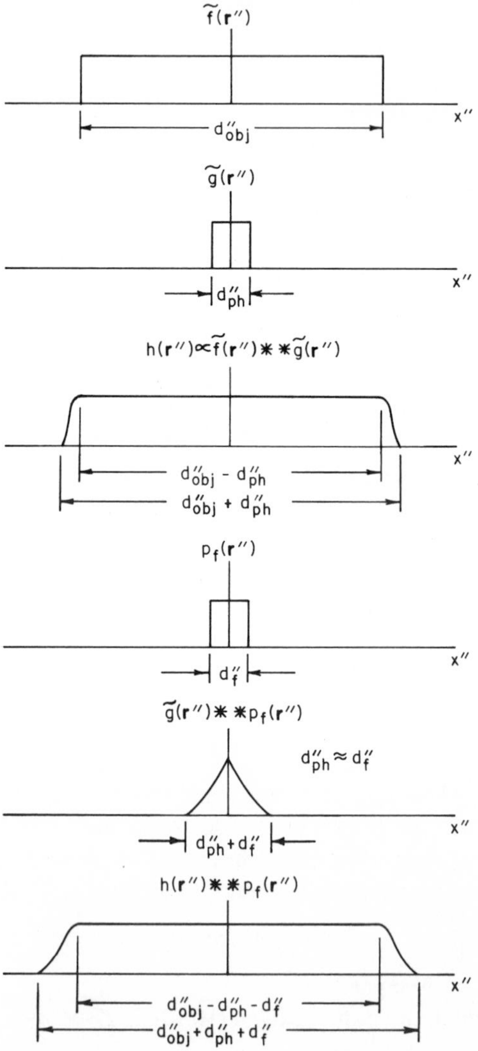

Fig. 10.3 Illustration of various functions that enter into the calculation of the SNR of a pinhole camera viewing a large, uniform disk object. The lower figure represents either the mean image $h(\mathbf{r}'') ** p_f(\mathbf{r}'')$, or the variance pattern $h(\mathbf{r}'') ** [p_f(\mathbf{r}'')]^2$ [see (10.24)].

Note that (10.19) leaves the value of $h(\mathbf{r}'')$ undefined for points $\mathbf{r}''$ within $\pm\frac{1}{2}d''_{\text{ph}}$ of the edge of the disk (see Fig. 10.3). If these points are of interest, a more involved calculation is required.

The constant h_o in (10.19) is the number of detected photons per unit area in the image. From (10.13)–(10.16), it is given by

$$\begin{aligned} h_\text{o} = h(\mathbf{r}'' = 0) &= \left(\frac{a}{b}\right)^2 C[\tilde{f}(\mathbf{r}'') ** \acute{g}(\mathbf{r}'')]_{\mathbf{r}''=0} \\ &= \left(\frac{a}{b}\right)^2 C f_\text{o} \int_\infty d^2r'' \operatorname{circ}\left(\frac{2r''}{d''_{\text{obj}}}\right) \operatorname{circ}\left(\frac{2r''}{d''_{\text{ph}}}\right) \\ &= \left(\frac{a}{b}\right)^2 C f_\text{o}\left(\frac{\pi(d''_{\text{ph}})^2}{4}\right), \end{aligned} \tag{10.20}$$

independent of d''_{obj} so long as $d''_{\text{obj}} > d''_{\text{ph}}$. For a more physical interpretation of (10.20), note that use of (4.12) and (4.35) gives

$$h_\text{o}\, d^2r'' = [T f_\text{o} \pi\, \delta^2_{\text{ph}}/4][d^2r''/4\pi(s_1 + s_2)^2]. \tag{10.21}$$

The quantity in the first set of brackets is the total number of photons emitted from one resolution element of the source in time T, while the quantity in the second set of brackets is the fractional solid angle subtended by the area element d^2r''.

Combining (10.18)–(10.20) and assuming that d''_f is also small compared to d''_{obj}, we have

$$h(\mathbf{r}'') ** p_\text{f}(\mathbf{r}'') = \begin{cases} A h_\text{o}\pi(d''_\text{f})^2/4 & \text{if } \ r'' < \frac{1}{2}(d''_{\text{obj}} - d''_{\text{ph}} - d''_\text{f}) \\ 0 & \text{if } \ r'' > \frac{1}{2}(d''_{\text{obj}} + d''_{\text{ph}} + d''_\text{f}). \end{cases} \tag{10.22}$$

Again, this result does not apply in the blur region at the edge of the filtered disk image, a region of width $(d''_{\text{ph}} + d''_\text{f})$ (see Fig. 10.3).

The denominator in (10.12) is now easy to calculate. Since a circ function takes on only the values zero and one,

$$[p_\text{f}(\mathbf{r}'')]^2 = A^2 \operatorname{circ}(2r''/d''_\text{f}) = A p_\text{f}(\mathbf{r}''). \tag{10.23}$$

Hence,

$$h(\mathbf{r}'') ** [p_\text{f}(\mathbf{r}'')]^2 = A h(\mathbf{r}'') ** p_\text{f}(\mathbf{r}''), \tag{10.24}$$

and (10.22) provides both numerator and denominator of (10.12). The final result for SNR is

$$\text{SNR}(\mathbf{r}'') = \begin{cases} [h_\text{o}\pi(d''_\text{f})^2/4]^{1/2} & \text{if } \ r'' < \frac{1}{2}(d''_{\text{obj}} - d''_{\text{ph}} - d''_\text{f}) \\ 0 & \text{if } \ r'' > \frac{1}{2}(d''_{\text{obj}} + d''_{\text{ph}} + d''_\text{f}). \end{cases} \tag{10.25}$$

The SNR is simply the square root of the number of counts within an area $\pi(d''_\text{f})^2/4$ defined *solely by the width of the filter*. The multiplicative constant A in $p_\text{f}(\mathbf{r}'')$ has dropped out, and the only filter parameter that remains is

d_f''. Of course, h_o is determined by the pinhole diameter, source strength, exposure time, etc., but once the image is recorded, the degree of filtering is crucial.

Note that if there is no filtering at all (i.e., $d_f'' \to 0$), the SNR is zero since at any point in $h(\mathbf{r}'')$ there can be only zero or one detected photon, with the former possibility being overwhelmingly likely. We must emphasize that SNR($\mathbf{r}''$) is defined *at* a point, not over some area about that point. Only the filter $p_f(\mathbf{r}'')$ serves to average adjacent points. It should not be concluded from this result, however, that an unfiltered image is worthless. For example, a photograph of the CRT display of an Anger camera shows each recorded photon as a very small spot and corresponds to a very small value of d_f'' and therefore a small SNR($\mathbf{r}''$). Yet clearly this image is quite useful to a human observer. A good way to reconcile this difference is to ascribe a PSF to the observer, considered as part of the imaging system. The eye has a finite resolution, so that at normal viewing distances the distinct spots on the image may not be resolved. Furthermore, a trained observer must surely unconsciously average the image over some finite area (see Section 10.7). Thus, even if there is no overt filter in the system, a parameter like d_f'' still exists and controls the SNR and hence the clinical usefulness of the image.

The obvious next question is, How should d_f'' be chosen? For best SNR, d_f'' should be very large, but this is a poor choice since d_f'' also controls the system resolution. For a filter in the form of (10.17), the image of a point source is the convolution of the two circ functions $\tilde{g}(\mathbf{r}'')$ and $p_f(\mathbf{r}'')$. From Chapter 4 (especially Fig. 4.17) we know that a cross section of this convolution is approximately trapezoidal with a FWHM of either d_f'' or d_{ph}'', whichever is larger. Scaling back to the image plane as in (4.35), we have for the resolution of the pinhole camera, including the filter,

$$\delta_{ph} \approx \begin{cases} d_{ph}''a/b & \text{if} \quad d_{ph}'' > d_f'' \\ d_f''a/b & \text{if} \quad d_f'' > d_{ph}''. \end{cases} \tag{10.26}$$

Thus, so long as we define resolution as the FWHM of the overall PSF, there is no degradation in resolution until d_f'' exceeds d_{ph}''. [Of course the *shape* of the PSF varies as d_f'' is increased, going from a circ function if $d_f'' = 0$ to the autoconvolution (or autocorrelation) of a circ when $d_f'' = d_{ph}''$. This latter function, plotted in Fig. 4.25, has a nearly triangular profile.] We conclude that the condition $d_f'' = d_{ph}''$ is a good choice for the width of the filter function since it gives the largest SNR that can be achieved without loss of resolution.*

* Strictly speaking, the FWHM resolution is actually slightly *better*, by a factor of 0.808, for the autocorrelation of a circ function than for the circ function itself. This, however, is just a peculiarity of the resolution definition, and probably has very little significance in terms of observer performance or diagnostic accuracy. The real advantage of filtering is the improvement in SNR, not the modest change in the FWHM of the PSF.

Of course, this conclusion is based on $p_f(\mathbf{r}'')$ being a circ function, but qualitatively the same conclusion will hold for other filters; there is no significant image detail in $h(\mathbf{r}'')$ with a scale smaller than d''_{ph}, so we may as well average the noise over this distance.

10.3.2 The Effect of a Finite Detector Resolution

It is straightforward to retrace the derivation in the last section to include a nonideal detector. The detector output is the random process $\mathbf{u}_d(\mathbf{r}'')$, with mean value

$$\langle \mathbf{u}_d(\mathbf{r}'') \rangle = h_d(\mathbf{r}'') = h(\mathbf{r}'') ** d(\mathbf{r}'') = (a/b)^2 C\tilde{f}(\mathbf{r}'') ** \tilde{g}(\mathbf{r}'') ** d(\mathbf{r}'') \quad (10.27)$$

where $d(\mathbf{r}'')$ is the PSF of the detector. The subscripts on $h_d(\mathbf{r}'')$ and $\mathbf{u}_d(\mathbf{r}'')$ indicate that they are measured at the output of the detector. However, as indicated in Section 10.2, if the detector has the effect of mislocating each gamma-ray event instead of blurring it, $\mathbf{u}_d(\mathbf{r}'')$ is still an uncorrelated Poisson random process and $h_d(\mathbf{r}'')$ may be plugged into (10.12) directly. This procedure is valid for Anger cameras but not for screen-film systems.

If the detector has a quantum efficiency η, $d(\mathbf{r}'')$ will be normalized so that

$$\int_\infty d^2r''\, d(\mathbf{r}'') = \eta. \quad (10.28)$$

With this normalization, $h_d(\mathbf{r}'')$ is the mean number of *detected* photons per unit area. The mean total number detected is $\int_\infty h_d(\mathbf{r}'')\, d^2r''$, which is smaller by a factor of η than the mean total number incident, $\int_\infty h(\mathbf{r}'')\, d^2\mathbf{r}''$. [This statement may be proven by application of the central ordinate theorem, (B.96).]

To further characterize the detector, let the FWHM of $d(\mathbf{r}'')$ be denoted by δ''_{det}. We again consider the uniform disk object of (10.15) or (10.16), and assume that $\delta''_{det} \ll d''_{obj}$. Then $h_d(\mathbf{r}'')$ is a disk of approximate diameter d''_{obj} but with a blurred edge. The blur extends over a distance determined by both d''_{ph} and δ''_{det} in some complicated manner. If the FWHM of $\tilde{g}(\mathbf{r}'') ** d(\mathbf{r}'')$ is denoted by δ''_{gd}, then the detected image $h_d(\mathbf{r}'')$ is constant if $\mathbf{r}''$ is removed from the edge by about δ''_{gd}. Equation (10.19) thus becomes

$$h_d(\mathbf{r}'') = \begin{cases} h_o\eta & \text{if } \; r'' \lesssim \frac{1}{2}d''_{obj} - \delta_{gd} \\ 0 & \text{if } \; r'' \gtrsim \frac{1}{2}d''_{obj} + \delta''_{gd}, \end{cases} \quad (10.29)$$

where h_o is still given by (10.20) or (10.21).

Similarly, after convolution with the filter function $p_f(\mathbf{r}'')$, the filtered image $h_d(\mathbf{r}'') ** p_f(\mathbf{r}'')$ is still disklike, but the edge is even more blurred. Let δ''_{tot} denote the FWHM of $\tilde{g}(\mathbf{r}'') ** d(\mathbf{r}'') ** p_f(\mathbf{r}'')$. The arguments that led to

(10.25) now yield

$$\mathrm{SNR}(\mathbf{r}'') \approx \begin{cases} [h_o \eta \pi (d_f'')^2/4]^{1/2} & \text{if} \quad r'' \lesssim \tfrac{1}{2}d_{obj}'' - \delta_{tot}'' \\ 0 & \text{if} \quad r'' \gtrsim \tfrac{1}{2}d_{obj}'' + \delta_{tot}''. \end{cases} \tag{10.30}$$

Although the finite detector resolution has blurred the edge of the image, the most significant difference between (10.25) and (10.30) is the factor of $\sqrt{\eta}$. In contrast to the normalization factor A in $p_f(\mathbf{r}'')$, which does not influence $\mathrm{SNR}(\mathbf{r}'')$, the normalization of $d(\mathbf{r}'')$ is quite important. Basically, this comes about since multiplying $p_f(\mathbf{r}'')$ by a constant merely changes the magnitude with which a photon is recorded. The magnitude of $d(\mathbf{r}'')$, on the other hand, determines *how many* photons are recorded. The normalization of (10.28) is not merely a convenience but is essential if $h_d(\mathbf{r}'')$ is to represent a number of detected events per unit area.

When the finite detector resolution is considered, a reasonable choice for the filter width is $d_f'' \approx \delta_{gd}''$.

10.3.3 More General Objects: The Noise Kernel

In the last two sections, we considered specific forms for $\tilde{f}(\mathbf{r}'')$ and $p_f(\mathbf{r}'')$ in order to obtain analytic results for $\mathrm{SNR}(\mathbf{r}'')$. In this section we consider the general case where the object, aperture, detector, and filter are all described by unspecified functions (Metz and Beck, 1974; Simpson, 1978; Simpson and Barrett, 1980). The only restriction imposed is that the detector output be a sum of delta functions of the form (10.1), so that $h_d(\mathbf{r}'')$ is the mean value of an uncorrelated Poisson random process.

From (10.10) and (10.27), the variance at point $\mathbf{r}''$ in the filtered image is

$$\begin{aligned} \sigma_{u_d^\dagger}^2(\mathbf{r}'') &= [p_f(\mathbf{r}'')]^2 ** h_d(\mathbf{r}'') \\ &= [p_f(\mathbf{r}'')]^2 ** [(a/b)^2 C\tilde{f}(\mathbf{r}'')] ** \tilde{g}(\mathbf{r}'') ** d(\mathbf{r}''), \end{aligned} \tag{10.31}$$

while the mean value of the filtered image is

$$\begin{aligned} \langle \mathbf{u}_d^\dagger(\mathbf{r}'') \rangle &= h_d^\dagger(\mathbf{r}'') = p_f(\mathbf{r}'') ** h_d(\mathbf{r}'') \\ &= p_f(\mathbf{r}'') ** [(a/b)^2 C\tilde{f}(\mathbf{r}'')] ** \tilde{g}(\mathbf{r}'') ** d(\mathbf{r}''). \end{aligned} \tag{10.32}$$

To emphasize the parallel between (10.31) and (10.32), we write

$$\sigma_{u_d^\dagger}^2(\mathbf{r}'') = \tilde{k}(\mathbf{r}'') ** \tilde{f}(\mathbf{r}''), \tag{10.33}$$

$$h_d^\dagger(\mathbf{r}'') = \tilde{p}_{tot}(\mathbf{r}'') ** \tilde{f}(\mathbf{r}''), \tag{10.34}$$

where

$$\tilde{k}(\mathbf{r}'') = (a/b)^2 C[p_f(\mathbf{r}'')]^2 ** \tilde{g}(\mathbf{r}'') ** d(\mathbf{r}''), \tag{10.35}$$

$$\tilde{p}_{tot}(\mathbf{r}'') = (a/b)^2 C p_f(\mathbf{r}'') ** \tilde{g}(\mathbf{r}'') ** d(\mathbf{r}''). \tag{10.36}$$

The quantity $\tilde{k}(\mathbf{r}'')$, called the *noise kernel*, is thus analogous to the overall PSF $\tilde{p}_{\text{tot}}(\mathbf{r}'')$, except that it applies to the variance of the filtered image rather than its mean. [The tildes on $\tilde{k}(\mathbf{r}'')$ and $\tilde{p}_{\text{tot}}(\mathbf{r}'')$ serve as reminders that we are now working in the detector $(\mathbf{r}'')$ plane rather than the original object $(\mathbf{r})$ plane.] Operationally, both $\tilde{p}_{\text{tot}}$ and $\tilde{k}$ depend on the filter, detector, and aperture functions, but not on the object. The only difference is that p_{f}^2 appears in $\tilde{k}$ while p_{f} appears in $\tilde{p}_{\text{tot}}$.

In terms of the noise kernel, the local SNR in the image plane is

$$\text{SNR}(\mathbf{r}'') = \frac{\tilde{f}(\mathbf{r}'') ** \tilde{p}_{\text{tot}}(\mathbf{r}'')}{[\tilde{f}(\mathbf{r}'') ** \tilde{k}(\mathbf{r}'')]^{1/2}}. \tag{10.37}$$

From this equation, the SNR for any object may be determined once the PSF and noise kernel are calculated. Furthermore, if we choose to normalize the filter function such that

$$\int_\infty \tilde{p}_{\text{tot}}(\mathbf{r}'')\, d^2r'' = 1, \tag{10.38}$$

then a further simplification is often possible. If $\tilde{f}(\mathbf{r}'')$ is slowly varying compared to $\tilde{p}_{\text{tot}}(\mathbf{r}'')$ and (10.38) holds, we have

$$\tilde{f}(\mathbf{r}'') ** \tilde{p}_{\text{tot}}(\mathbf{r}'') \approx \tilde{f}(\mathbf{r}''). \tag{10.39}$$

In other words, $\tilde{p}_{\text{tot}}(\mathbf{r}'')$ is like a delta function, and (10.37) becomes

$$\text{SNR}(\mathbf{r}'') \approx \frac{\tilde{f}(\mathbf{r}'')}{[\tilde{f}(\mathbf{r}'') ** \tilde{k}(\mathbf{r}'')]^{1/2}}. \tag{10.40}$$

It may also happen that $\tilde{k}(\mathbf{r}'')$ is sharply peaked and may be treated as a delta function compared to $f(\mathbf{r}'')$. (Basically, this is what we did in Sections 10.3.1 and 10.3.2.) However, it is not possible to simultaneously normalize both $\tilde{p}_{\text{tot}}$ and $\tilde{k}$ to unit area since we have only one free parameter, the magnitude of the filter function [e.g., the parameter A in (10.17)]. The most we can say is that

$$\tilde{f}(\mathbf{r}'') ** \tilde{k}(\mathbf{r}'') \approx \tilde{f}(\mathbf{r}'') \int_\infty \tilde{k}(\mathbf{r}_0'')\, d^2r_0'', \tag{10.41}$$

from which

$$\text{SNR}(\mathbf{r}'') \approx \left(f(\mathbf{r}'') \Big/ \int_\infty \tilde{k}(\mathbf{r}_0'')\, d^2r_0'' \right)^{1/2} = \text{const} \cdot [\tilde{f}(\mathbf{r}'')]^{1/2}. \tag{10.42}$$

Thus, if both $\tilde{p}_{\text{tot}}$ and $\tilde{k}$ are sharply peaked compared to $\tilde{f}$, as in the case of a pinhole camera viewing a large disk object, the SNR is simply a numerical factor times the square root of the scaled object. [One word of caution: A sharply peaked $\tilde{p}_{\text{tot}}$ does not necessarily imply a sharply peaked $\tilde{k}$. The filter $p_{\text{f}}(\mathbf{r}'')$ may be bipolar and hence serve to sharpen the image, but p_{f}^2

which appears in $\tilde{k}$ must be nonnegative. Since nonnegative filters always blur an image, the variance pattern $\sigma^2_{u_d^\dagger}(\mathbf{r}'')$ can only be a blurred version of $h_d(\mathbf{r}'')$.]

To illustrate the use of (10.42), let us repeat the calculation for the pinhole camera and disk object. The integral of $\tilde{k}$ may be determined from the central ordinate theorem (B.96). We find

$$\int_\infty \tilde{k}(\mathbf{r}_0'')\, d^2 r_0'' = \tilde{K}(0) = (a/b)^2 C\tilde{G}(0)D(0)\mathscr{F}_2\{p_f^2\}_{\boldsymbol{\rho}''=0}, \tag{10.43}$$

where, as usual, capital letters denote the Fourier transforms of the corresponding lowercase functions. From (10.28) we know that

$$D(0) = \int_\infty d(\mathbf{r}'')\, d^2 r'' = \eta, \tag{10.44}$$

and it follows from (10.14) that

$$\tilde{G}(0) = \pi (d_{\mathrm{ph}}'')^2/4. \tag{10.45}$$

The remaining factor in (10.43) is

$$\mathscr{F}_2\{p_f^2\}_{\boldsymbol{\rho}''=0} = \int_\infty [p_f(\mathbf{r}'')]^2\, d^2 r''. \tag{10.46}$$

By (10.17) and (10.23),

$$\int_\infty [p_f(\mathbf{r}'')]^2\, d^2 r'' = A \int_\infty p_f(\mathbf{r}'')\, d^2 r'' = \frac{A^2 \pi (d_f'')^2}{4}. \tag{10.47}$$

Combining (10.43)–(10.47) gives

$$\int_\infty \tilde{k}(\mathbf{r}_0'')\, d^2 r_0'' = \left(\frac{a}{b}\right)^2 C \left(\frac{\pi (d_f'')^2}{4}\right)\left(\frac{\pi (d_{\mathrm{ph}}'')^2}{4}\right)\eta A^2. \tag{10.48}$$

But A must be chosen so that (10.38) is satisfied. Again invoking the central ordinate theorem and using (10.36), we must have

$$\begin{aligned}\int_\infty \tilde{p}_{\mathrm{tot}}(\mathbf{r}'')\, d^2\mathbf{r}'' &= \tilde{P}_{\mathrm{tot}}(0) = \left(\frac{a}{b}\right)^2 C P_f(0)\tilde{G}(0)D(0)\\ &= \left(\frac{a}{b}\right)^2 CA \left(\frac{\pi (d_f'')^2}{4}\right)\left(\frac{\pi (d_{\mathrm{ph}}'')^2}{4}\right)\eta = 1.\end{aligned} \tag{10.49}$$

Solving (10.49) for A and inserting it into (10.48) yields

$$\int_\infty \tilde{k}(\mathbf{r}_0'')\, d^2 r_0'' = \left\{\left(\frac{a}{b}\right)^2 C \left(\frac{\pi (d_f'')^2}{4}\right)\left(\frac{\pi (d_{\mathrm{ph}}'')^2}{4}\right)\eta\right\}^{-1}. \tag{10.50}$$

which, with (10.20) and (10.42), essentially reproduces the earlier SNR expression (10.30).

To this point we have considered only planar objects. To generalize, we now consider a three-dimensional object modeled as a stack of planes:

$$f(\mathbf{r}, z) = \sum_i f_i(\mathbf{r})\, \delta(z - z_i), \tag{10.51}$$

where $f_i(\mathbf{r})$ is the two-dimensional source distribution in the plane at distance $z = z_i$ from the aperture. We may still define scaled function $\tilde{f}_i(\mathbf{r}'')$ as usual, but the scale factors a and b are now functions of z_i [see (4.211) and (4.212)]. The calculation of $h_\mathrm{d}(\mathbf{r}'')$ must include an integral over z, which becomes a discrete sum over i by virtue of the delta functions in (10.51). Thus (10.27) becomes (if we neglect attenuation in the object)

$$h_\mathrm{d}(\mathbf{r}'') = \left[\sum_i \left(\frac{a_i}{b_i}\right) C_i \tilde{f}_i(\mathbf{r}'') ** \tilde{g}_i(\mathbf{r}'')\right] ** d(\mathbf{r}'') \equiv \sum_i h_{\mathrm{d,i}}(\mathbf{r}''). \tag{10.52}$$

Each of the functions $h_{\mathrm{d,i}}(\mathbf{r}'')$ is the mean value of an independent Poisson random process. For a sum of independent random variables, the mean of the sum is the sum of the means, and the variance of the sum is the sum of the variances. Thus we can write at once that

$$\mathrm{SNR}(\mathbf{r}'') = \left(\sum_i \tilde{f}_i(\mathbf{r}'') ** \tilde{p}_i(\mathbf{r}'')\right) \Big/ \left(\sum_i \tilde{f}_i(\mathbf{r}'') ** \tilde{k}_i(\mathbf{r}'')\right)^{1/2}, \tag{10.53}$$

where $\tilde{p}_i$ and $\tilde{k}_i$ are, respectively, the PSF and noise kernel appropriate to the ith plane. Equation (10.53) can also readily be generalized to a continuous integral over z rather than a discrete sum.

10.3.4 Collimators

The results of Section 10.3.3 are applicable, with only minor modifications, to a nuclear imaging system consisting of a parallel-hole collimator and an Anger camera detector. In fact, this case is somewhat simpler than the pinhole camera since the magnification is unity, and it is therefore unnecessary to use scaled functions.

In Section 4.5.1 we showed that the average PSF for a parallel-hole collimator is given by (4.140):

$$\bar{p}_{\mathrm{phc}}(\mathbf{r}'') = (4\alpha_{\mathrm{pf}}/\pi D_b^2) C[g_1(b\mathbf{r}'') ** g_1(b\mathbf{r}'')], \tag{10.54}$$

where, according to (4.70),

$$b = L_\mathrm{b}/(L_\mathrm{b} + z), \tag{10.55}$$

and $g_1(\mathbf{r})$ is the circ function describing an individual bore of diameter D_b. In terms of this average PSF, the detector output is given by

$$h_\mathrm{d}(\mathbf{r}'') = f(\mathbf{r}'') ** \bar{p}_{\mathrm{phc}}(\mathbf{r}'') ** d(\mathbf{r}''). \tag{10.56}$$

We also showed in Section 4.5.2 that the use of the average PSF is an excellent approximation if the detected image is passed through a low-pass filter. The detector response $d(\mathbf{r}'')$ may serve as this filter if the fine structure in the exact, space-variant PSF cannot be resolved by the detector. But even if this is not the case, we shall want to pass $h_d(\mathbf{r}'')$ through an additional filter $p_f(\mathbf{r}'')$ for noise smoothing. Furthermore, the width of $p_f(\mathbf{r}'')$ should be comparable to the width of $\overline{p}_{phc}(\mathbf{r}'') ** d(\mathbf{r}'')$, just as in the pinhole case. Thus, even if the fine structure in the exact PSF survives the detector, it will be lost in passing through the last filter, and we may as well ignore it from the outset.

This conclusion is equally valid for calculating the variance pattern $\sigma^2_{u_d^\dagger}(\mathbf{r}'')$ since, by (10.31), the variance is also a filtered version of $h_d(\mathbf{r}'')$ with an effective filter function of $[p_f(\mathbf{r}'')]^2$.

Thus, for the collimator system, (10.33)–(10.36) become

$$\sigma^2_{u_d^\dagger}(\mathbf{r}'') = k(\mathbf{r}'') ** f(\mathbf{r}''), \tag{10.57}$$

$$h_d^\dagger(\mathbf{r}'') = \overline{p}_{tot}(\mathbf{r}'') ** f(\mathbf{r}''), \tag{10.58}$$

where

$$k(\mathbf{r}'') = [p_f(\mathbf{r}'')]^2 ** \overline{p}_{phc}(\mathbf{r}'') ** d(\mathbf{r}''), \tag{10.59}$$

$$\overline{p}_{tot}(\mathbf{r}'') = p_f(\mathbf{r}'') ** \overline{p}_{phc}(\mathbf{r}'') ** d(\mathbf{r}''). \tag{10.60}$$

By following the procedures of Section 10.3.3, it may be shown that these equations again predict an SNR given by the square root of the number of detected photons in an area determined by $[p_f(\mathbf{r}'')]^2$.

10.3.5 Noise, Resolution, and Exposure Time with Nuclear Cameras

Let us return to the pinhole camera and further examine the engineering trade-offs that are available in its design.

From (10.20) and (10.30), the SNR at the center of the disk image is

$$[\mathrm{SNR}(0)]^2 = \left(\frac{s_1}{s_2}\right)^2 \frac{Tf_o}{4\pi(s_1+s_2)^2}\left(\frac{\pi(d''_{ph})^2}{4}\right)\left(\frac{\pi(d''_f)^2}{4}\right). \tag{10.61}$$

We shall assume that s_1/s_2 is chosen to give the desired magnification, while $s_1 + s_2$ is chosen as small as possible consistent with the obliquity considerations presented in Section 4.2.6. The only free parameters are d''_{ph} and the filter width d''_f. We have argued that an optimum value for d''_f is δ''_{gd}, which is the width of $\tilde{g}(\mathbf{r}'') ** d(\mathbf{r}'')$. If the detector has high resolution,

$\delta''_{gd} \approx d''_{\text{ph}} = d'_{\text{ph}}/a$, and (10.61) becomes

$$[\text{SNR}(0)]^2 = \frac{1}{(ab)^2} \frac{Tf_o}{4\pi(s_1 + s_2)^2} \left(\frac{\pi(d'_{\text{ph}})^2}{4} \right)^2. \tag{10.62}$$

To keep the SNR constant as d'_{ph} is varied, the exposure time T must be varied as $(d'_{\text{ph}})^{-4}$. Since, with the assumption of negligible detector blur, the overall resolution δ_{tot} is proportional to d'_{ph}, this means that T must vary as δ_{tot}^{-4}; for example a twofold reduction in δ_{tot} must be accompanied by a 16-fold increase in exposure time to maintain the same SNR.

The situation is even worse when the finite detector resolution is considered, since in that case a twofold decrease in d'_{ph} produces less than a twofold improvement in δ_{tot}. The general equations (10.33)–(10.37) may be used to treat this case, but numerical integrations are generally required.

From the close similarity between the collimator and pinhole cases, as noted in Section 10.3.4, it should be evident that the fourth-power trade-off law between resolution and exposure time also applies to the collimator if resolution is limited by the bore dimensions, and the filter width is chosen optimally.

10.3.6 Scanners

A rectilinear scanner system consists of a collimator, a ratemeter, and a display. As discussed in Section 4.4, each of these elements may be treated as a linear filter and assigned a PSF (MacIntyre *et al.*, 1969).

To analyze the noise properties of a scanner, we must first determine where in the chain the image can be treated as a set of uncorrelated Poisson impulses. Consider a single gamma ray that passes through the collimator and is detected. Assume the scanner head is moving at speed v_s in the x direction. If the ratemeter and display PSFs were very narrow, this gamma ray would be plotted as a small spot for which the x coordinate is a random variable depending on the instantaneous position of the scanner head when the gamma ray happened to be detected. It is a little less obvious, but the y coordinate of the spot is also a random variable, albeit a discrete one since the scanner head moves in discrete steps in the y direction. If the collimator PSF is wide enough to cover many scan lines, then there are many different time intervals during which the gamma ray could be emitted and still be detected. The collimator PSF governs the probability of detection during each of these time intervals, and hence the probability of the spot being located on a particular scan line. We conclude that the detector output consists of a set of randomly located impulses with the x coordinate of each impulse being a continuous random variable and the y coordinate being a discrete one. If the scan lines are close together compared to the final system resolution distance, then we may ignore the discreteness of y and use the detector output as the photon density function $h(\mathbf{r}'')$. Thus,

$$h(\mathbf{r}'') = f(\mathbf{r}'') ** p_c(\mathbf{r}''), \tag{10.63}$$

where $p_c(\mathbf{r}'')$ is the collimator PSF. For a single-bore collimator $p_c(\mathbf{r}'')$ is given by $p_{sb}(\mathbf{r}'')$ in (4.77) or (4.80). For a multibore focused collimator, $p_c(\mathbf{r}'')$ is given by $p_{fc}(\mathbf{r}'')$ in (4.88) or (4.91). (Since the magnification is unity for a scanner, the distinction between $\mathbf{r}''$ and $\mathbf{r}$ is unnecessary and we shall drop the primes.)

The remaining system elements, the ratemeter and display, must be lumped into the processing filter $p_f(\mathbf{r})$ since the noise at the output of these elements is not uncorrelated. The ratemeter introduces correlations in the x direction, while the display, in general, does so in both x and y. We shall consider the simple RC ratemeter of Fig. 4.15. By (4.117) its PSF is

$$p_{rm}(\mathbf{r}) = (v_s\tau)^{-1} \exp(-x/v_s\tau) \operatorname{step}(x)\,\delta(y), \tag{10.64}$$

where $\tau = R_1C_1$ is the time constant.

The display will be modeled here, as in Section 4.4.8, as a square aperture of side ε_a. When only the low-frequency components of the image are of interest, we showed in Section 4.4.8 that the display output can be described by a continuous convolution integral, with a display PSF given by [cf. (4.132)]:

$$p_{dis}(\mathbf{r}) = \varepsilon_a^{-2} \operatorname{rect}(x/\varepsilon_a) \operatorname{rect}(y/\varepsilon_a). \tag{10.65}$$

The overall filter function $p_f(\mathbf{r})$ is

$$p_f(\mathbf{r}) = p_{dis}(\mathbf{r}) ** p_{rm}(\mathbf{r}). \tag{10.66}$$

The overall PSF is

$$p_{tot}(\mathbf{r}) = p_c(\mathbf{r}) ** p_{dis}(\mathbf{r}) ** p_{rm}(\mathbf{r}) = p_c(\mathbf{r}) ** p_f(\mathbf{r}), \tag{10.67}$$

while the noise kernel is

$$k(\mathbf{r}) = p_c(\mathbf{r}) ** [p_f(\mathbf{r})]^2, \tag{10.68}$$

and the SNR is given by (10.37).

We shall now evaluate the SNR for a slowly varying object, first for a single-bore collimator and then for a focused one. If $f(\mathbf{r})$ is nearly constant over the extent of $p_{tot}(\mathbf{r})$, the final filtered image is

$$\begin{aligned} h^\dagger(\mathbf{r}) &= h(\mathbf{r}) ** p_f(\mathbf{r}) = p_{tot}(\mathbf{r}) ** f(\mathbf{r}) \\ &\approx f(\mathbf{r}) \int_\infty p_{tot}(\mathbf{r}_0)\, d^2r_0. \end{aligned} \tag{10.69}$$

By again using the central ordinate theorem as in Section 10.3.3, we have

$$\int_{\infty} p_{\text{tot}}(\mathbf{r}_0)\, d^2 r_0 = P_{\text{tot}}(0) = P_{\text{c}}(0)P_{\text{dis}}(0)P_{\text{rm}}(0). \tag{10.70}$$

But notice that we have normalized p_{rm} and p_{dis} such that

$$\int_{\infty} p_{\text{rm}}(\mathbf{r}_0)\, d^2 r_0 = P_{\text{rm}}(0) = 1, \tag{10.71}$$

$$\int_{\infty} p_{\text{dis}}(\mathbf{r}_0)\, d^2 r_0 = P_{\text{dis}}(0) = 1. \tag{10.72}$$

(With these conditions, p_{tot} is *not* normalized to unit area.) If we use the single-bore expression for p_{c} and assume for simplicity that the object is in contact with the collimator ($z = 0$), we have from (4.77) that

$$\begin{aligned} P_{\text{c}}(0) &= \int_{\infty} p_{\text{c}}(\mathbf{r}_0)\, d^2 r_0 = \int_{\infty} p_{\text{sb}}(\mathbf{r}_0; z = 0)\, d^2 r_0 \\ &= (n_l \dot{C}/v_{\text{s}})[\pi D_{\text{b}}^2/4]^2. \end{aligned} \tag{10.73}$$

Combining (10.69)–(10.73) yields

$$h^{\dagger}(\mathbf{r}) \approx (n_l \dot{C}/v_{\text{s}})[\pi D_{\text{b}}^2/4]^2 f(\mathbf{r}). \tag{10.74}$$

To evaluate the noise kernel we must perform the convolution $p_{\text{rm}}(\mathbf{r}) ** p_{\text{dis}}(\mathbf{r})$ and square it to obtain $[p_{\text{f}}(\mathbf{r})]^2$. The required integral is

$$\begin{aligned} p_{\text{f}}(\mathbf{r}) &= p_{\text{rm}}(\mathbf{r}) ** p_{\text{dis}}(\mathbf{r}) \\ &= \int_{-\infty}^{\infty} dx' \int_{-\infty}^{\infty} dy'\, (v_{\text{s}}\tau)^{-1} \exp\left(-\frac{x'}{v_{\text{s}}\tau}\right) \text{step}(x')\, \delta(y') \\ &\quad \cdot \varepsilon_{\text{a}}^{-2} \operatorname{rect}\left(\frac{x - x'}{\varepsilon_{\text{a}}}\right) \operatorname{rect}\left(\frac{y - y'}{\varepsilon_{\text{a}}}\right) \\ &= (\varepsilon_{\text{a}}^2 v_{\text{s}}\tau)^{-1} \operatorname{rect}\left(\frac{y}{\varepsilon_{\text{a}}}\right) \int_0^{\infty} dx' \exp\left(-\frac{x'}{v_{\text{s}}\tau}\right) \operatorname{rect}\left(\frac{x - x'}{\varepsilon_{\text{a}}}\right). \end{aligned} \tag{10.75}$$

The remaining integral is elementary but a little cumbersome. However, the essential features of the result can be seen if we assume that $v_{\text{s}}\tau \gg \varepsilon_{\text{a}}$. [This simplifying assumption is not altogether unrealistic. In practice v_{s} and τ may be selected by the operator of the scanner, while ε_{a} is usually fixed by the manufacturer. The operator should adjust $v_{\text{s}}\tau$ to be comparable to the width of $p_{\text{c}}(\mathbf{r})$, which in turn is usually substantially larger than ε_{a}.] With this assumption we may approximate the rect function as

$$\varepsilon_{\text{a}}^{-1} \operatorname{rect}[(x - x')/\varepsilon_{\text{a}}] \approx \delta(x - x'), \tag{10.76}$$

and (10.75) becomes

$$p_{\text{f}}(\mathbf{r}) = (\varepsilon_{\text{a}} v_{\text{s}}\tau)^{-1} \exp(-x/v_{\text{s}}\tau)\, \text{step}(x) \operatorname{rect}(y/\varepsilon_{\text{a}}). \tag{10.77}$$

Since both the step and rect functions are unchanged by squaring, we have

$$[p_{\mathrm{f}}(\mathbf{r})]^2 = (\varepsilon_{\mathrm{a}} v_{\mathrm{s}} \tau)^{-2} \exp(-2x/v_{\mathrm{s}}\tau)\, \mathrm{step}(x)\, \mathrm{rect}(y/\varepsilon_{\mathrm{a}}) \tag{10.78}$$

and a simple integration gives

$$\int_\infty [p_{\mathrm{f}}(\mathbf{r})]^2\, d^2r = (2\varepsilon_{\mathrm{a}} v_{\mathrm{s}} \tau)^{-1}. \tag{10.79}$$

Thus the area under the noise kernel is

$$\begin{aligned}\int_\infty k(\mathbf{r})\, d^2r &= \int_\infty \{p_{\mathrm{c}}(\mathbf{r}) ** [p_{\mathrm{f}}(\mathbf{r})]^2\}\, d^2r \\ &= K(0) = P_{\mathrm{c}}(0)\mathscr{F}_2\{p_{\mathrm{f}}^2\}_{\rho=0} \\ &= \left(\int_\infty p_{\mathrm{c}}(\mathbf{r})\, d^2r\right)\left(\int_\infty [p_{\mathrm{f}}(\mathbf{r})]^2\, d^2r\right) \\ &= (n_l \dot{C}/v_{\mathrm{s}})(\pi D_{\mathrm{b}}^2/4)^2 (2\varepsilon_{\mathrm{a}} v_{\mathrm{s}} \tau)^{-1},\end{aligned} \tag{10.80}$$

where we have used the central ordinate theorem and (10.73) and (10.79).

For a slowly varying $f(\mathbf{r})$, we may write

$$\sigma_{u\dagger}^2(\mathbf{r}) = f(\mathbf{r}) ** k(\mathbf{r}) \approx f(\mathbf{r}) \int_\infty k(\mathbf{r}_0)\, d^2r_0. \tag{10.81}$$

Combining (10.74), (10.80), and (10.81) yields

$$[\mathrm{SNR}(\mathbf{r})]^2 = \frac{[h^\dagger(\mathbf{r})]^2}{\sigma_{u\dagger}^2(\mathbf{r})} \approx (n_l \dot{C}/v_{\mathrm{s}})(\pi D_{\mathrm{b}}^2/4)^2 (2\varepsilon_{\mathrm{a}} v_{\mathrm{s}} \tau) f(\mathbf{r}). \tag{10.82}$$

We remind the reader that this result applies to a scanner with a single-bore collimator in near contact with a slowly varying object $[p_{\mathrm{c}}(\mathbf{r}) = p_{\mathrm{sb}}(\mathbf{r}; z = 0)]$, and assumes that $v_{\mathrm{s}}\tau \gg \varepsilon_{\mathrm{a}}$.

To obtain the SNR for a multibore collimator or for $z \neq 0$, the only quantity that needs to be changed in this analysis is $\int_\infty p_{\mathrm{c}}(\mathbf{r}_0)\, d^2r_0$ in (10.73). The general expression for the SNR of any scanner is

$$[\mathrm{SNR}(\mathbf{r})]^2 = \left(\int_\infty p_{\mathrm{c}}(\mathbf{r}_0)\, d^2r_0\right)(2\varepsilon_{\mathrm{a}} v_{\mathrm{s}} \tau) f(\mathbf{r}), \tag{10.83}$$

where the assumptions that $v_{\mathrm{s}}\tau \gg \varepsilon_{\mathrm{a}}$ and that $f(\mathbf{r})$ is slowly varying are still required. The integral of $p_{\mathrm{c}}(\mathbf{r})$ may be evaluated using the appropriate expressions from Section 4.4.

Equation (10.83) should be compared to (10.30), which gives the SNR for a pinhole camera. In both cases, the SNR is the square root of the number of detected photons in an area determined by the filter function. In (10.83) the factor of $f(\mathbf{r}) \int_\infty p_{\mathrm{c}}(\mathbf{r}_0)\, d^2r_0$, which is an approximation to $f(\mathbf{r}) ** p_{\mathrm{c}}(\mathbf{r})$, is the number of counts per unit area at the input to the filter (ratemeter plus display). The effective averaging area for the filter is just $(2\varepsilon_{\mathrm{a}} v_{\mathrm{s}} \tau)$. To be more general still, the factor of $2\varepsilon_a v_s \tau$ in (10.83) should be replaced by an effective noise-averaging area A_{eff} defined by

$$\left[\int_\infty p_f(\mathbf{r})\, d^2r\right]^2 \Big/ \left\{\int_\infty [p_f(\mathbf{r})]^2\, d^2r\right\}. \tag{10.84}$$

Then the approximation $v_s \tau \gg \varepsilon_a$ would not be required and (10.83) would hold for any ratemeter and display. However, the assumption that $f(\mathbf{r})$ is slowly varying compared to $p_{\text{tot}}(\mathbf{r})$ and $k(\mathbf{r})$ is still necessary.

10.3.7 Noise, Resolution, and Exposure Time with Scanners

If a scanner must cover a square area of side L, the total scan time T_s is given by

$$T_s = n_l L^2 / v_s. \tag{10.85}$$

The scan speed v_s is adjustable by the operator, but n_l, the number of scan lines per unit length, is assumed to be set by the manufacturer.

The parameter v_s in the combination $v_s \tau$ determines the degree of noise smoothing in the x direction. Just as in the pinhole case (see the discussion at the end of Section 10.3.1), the filter width $v_s \tau$ should be chosen comparable to the resolution distance δ_c determined by the collimator. If $v_s \tau \gg \delta_c$, the overall resolution (in the x direction) is determined by the ratemeter, and the collimator is unnecessarily inefficient. On the other hand, if $v_s \tau \ll \delta_c$, the image is unnecessarily noisy. Thus we assume that $v_s \tau$ is kept more or less equal to δ_c. Since δ_c is proportional to the bore diameter D_b in any collimator, we may write $v_s \tau = \beta D_b$, where β is the proverbial factor of order unity.

With these considerations the SNR for the single-bore collimator, (10.82), becomes

$$[\text{SNR}(\mathbf{r})]^2 = (\pi\beta/32 L^2 L_b^2) D_b^5 \varepsilon_a T_s f(\mathbf{r}), \tag{10.86}$$

where we are still assuming $z = 0$, so that $C = (4\pi L_b^2)^{-1}$, with L_b being the length of the bore. If the object $f(\mathbf{r})$ and the geometric parameters L, L_b, and ε_a are fixed, so that D_b and T_s are the only variables, we see that T_s must vary as D_b^{-5} for the SNR to remain constant. This result may seem to be at odds with the sixth-power law deduced in Section 4.4.6, but that is just a consequence of the present assumption that ε_a is constant, as indeed it is in most commercial scanners. Optimally, however, one should change ε_a with every change in collimators and keep $\varepsilon_a \propto D_b$. If this were done, (10.86) would predict $T_s \propto D_b^{-6}$ for constant SNR. Furthermore, if there is an implicit filter in the system—the observer's eye or brain—then it is reasonable to assume that the averaging distances in both x and y are proportional to D_b, again leading to the sixth-power law.

Of course, single-bore collimators are not really used in modern nuclear medicine, but the more practical case of a multibore focused collimator is a simple extension of this analysis. For an object in the focal plane ($z = z_f$), we have from (4.92), (4.95), and (4.99) that

$$\int_\infty p_{fc}(\mathbf{r}; z_f)\, d^2 r = \left(\frac{n_l}{v_s}\right)\left(\frac{\pi}{64L_b^2}\right) M_b D_1^2 D_2^2, \tag{10.87}$$

where M_b is the total number of bores in the collimator, and D_1 and D_2 are the lower and upper diameter, respectively, of each tapered bore. From (4.105),

$$M_b = \alpha_{pf}(D_{det}/D_2)^2, \tag{10.88}$$

where D_{det} is the detector diameter and α_{pf} is the packing fraction.

Using (10.87) and (10.88) in (10.83) gives

$$[\mathrm{SNR}(\mathbf{r})]^2 = (\pi\beta/32L_b^2)\alpha_{pf} D_{det}^2 D_1^3 \varepsilon_a T_s f(\mathbf{r}), \tag{10.89}$$

where now $v_s \tau = \beta D_1$, and the total scan time T_s is still given by (10.85).

For constant SNR, (10.89) requires that $T_s \propto D_1^{-3}$ if ε_a is fixed, or $T_s \propto D_1^{-4}$ if $\varepsilon_a \propto D_1$. Since, by (4.103), the collimator resolution is given by

$$\delta_{fc} = 0.808 D_1 [1 + (z_f/L_b)], \tag{10.90}$$

the scan time must vary inversely as the third or fourth power of δ_{fc}. Again, the fourth-power law is the more nearly optimal situation where ε_a is varied in proportion to the bore diameters.

10.4 TRANSMISSION IMAGING

10.4.1 The Wiener Spectrum with a Film–Screen Detector

The distribution of x-ray quanta in a spatially modulated beam is one sample function of a two-dimensional random process. The expectation value of the random process is, of course, the two-dimensional distribution corresponding to the projection of the object.

With a film–screen detector, each x-ray photon absorbed by the phosphor screen is converted to a flash of low-energy (optical) photons in the film plane. This is equivalent to spatially filtering the two-dimensional input random process with a filter whose impulse response is the distribution of optical energy in the film plane caused by a single absorbed x-ray photon. The exposure received by the film is thus a filtered random process, and, as a consequence, so is the density distribution of the developed film. For now, we shall consider only stationary processes; that is, it is assumed that the x-ray exposure has an average flux density that is constant over the area of the screen. With this assumption, we may describe the fluctuations in film exposure and film density by their power spectral densities or *Wiener spectra* (see Section 3.1.4) (Doi, 1969; Rossmann, 1963; Wagner, 1977). The Wiener spectrum of the density fluctuations is often called, somewhat loosely, the "Wiener spectrum of the film–screen system." This is incorrect because the film–screen system is not a random process. It is a piece of hardware. Only random processes may be described by Wiener spectra. However, we too shall use this casual terminology since there is no real danger of confusion.

In this section we shall calculate from first principles the noise transfer properties of the film–screen system. It must be realized that the actual filtering operation takes place by the spreading of light from a point source where the x-ray is absorbed to the emulsion where the film is exposed. The observable and measurable input and output processes are not distributions of film exposure. The input is an x-ray photon flux distribution and the output is a fluctuating density distribution. The overall system response is thus determined by (i) converting from x rays to an input irradiance distribution, (ii) performing the filtering, and (iii) converting the filtered exposure fluctuations to density fluctuations.

We consider a screen of area A irradiated with a stationary x-ray beam whose average fluence is Φ_0 photons/unit area. The input is described by the random process $\mathbf{u}_{\text{in}}(\mathbf{r})$, given by [see (3.128) and Fig. 10.2]

$$\mathbf{u}_{\text{in}}(\mathbf{r}) = \sum_{j=1}^{\mathbf{K}} \delta(\mathbf{r} - \mathbf{r}_j), \tag{10.91}$$

with an ensemble average of

$$\langle \mathbf{u}_{\text{in}}(\mathbf{r}) \rangle = \langle \mathbf{K} \rangle / A \equiv \Phi_0 = \text{const.} \tag{10.92}$$

We consider the phosphor screen to be divided into M elemental slabs of thickness Δz. The absorption events of each layer are statistically independent of each other,* so we proceed by calculating the screen properties due to one thin layer and then summing (actually integrating) over the layers.

The mean number of x-ray photons per unit area absorbed within the mth slab located at $z = z_m$ is given by the product of the incident x-ray fluence $\Phi_0 \exp(-\mu_p z_m)$ and the probability of absorption $\mu_p \Delta z$:

$$\Phi_m = \Phi_0 \mu_p \Delta z \exp(-\mu_p z_m), \tag{10.93}$$

* There is one possible type of interaction that would introduce a degree of statistical dependence between layers. If a photon is Compton scattered in one layer and then either rescattered or absorbed in another layer, then the events in the two layers are not independent. We can ignore this scenario if photoelectric events predominate in the phosphor.

where μ_p is the x-ray attenuation coefficient of the phosphor. The random process corresponding to this absorption is

$$\mathbf{u}_m(\mathbf{r}) = \sum_{j=1}^{\mathbf{K}_m} \delta(\mathbf{r} - \mathbf{r}_j), \tag{10.94}$$

where

$$\langle \mathbf{u}_m(\mathbf{r}) \rangle = \langle \mathbf{K}_m \rangle / A = \Phi_m. \tag{10.95}$$

Each absorption event creates a flash of optical energy $\mathscr{E}$. The optical energy density (energy per unit area) in the mth layer is thus described by the random process $\mathbf{E}_m(\mathbf{r})$, defined by

$$\mathbf{E}_m(\mathbf{r}) = \mathscr{E}\mathbf{u}_m(\mathbf{r}), \tag{10.96}$$

with an average value of

$$\langle \mathbf{E}_m(\mathbf{r}) \rangle = \mathscr{E}\Phi_m. \tag{10.97}$$

The autocorrelation function of $\mathbf{E}_m(\mathbf{r})$ is

$$R_{E_m}(\mathbf{L}) = \langle \mathbf{E}_m(\mathbf{r})\mathbf{E}_m(\mathbf{r} + \mathbf{L}) \rangle = \mathscr{E}^2[\Phi_m \delta(\mathbf{L}) + \Phi_m^2]. \tag{10.98}$$

Note that we are treating the total energy per flash $\mathscr{E}$ as a deterministic constant rather than a random variable. This is an approximation, but it causes no serious error; the variability in optical pulse height, as shown in Section 5.5.1, will increase the noise variance by perhaps 10–20%.

Next, we consider the filtering action produced by propagation of the light from the mth layer of the phosphor to the film plane. Of the total energy $\mathscr{E}$ released in the flash, only a fraction α_m reaches the film. This fraction is usually about $\frac{1}{2}$, but it can be higher if a reflective backing is used or lower if the phosphor contains an absorbing dye. The spreading of the light during propagation is described by the point spread function $p_m(\mathbf{r})$, which will be normalized as follows:

$$\int_\infty p_m(\mathbf{r})\, d^2r = 1. \tag{10.99}$$

The film exposure (energy per unit area) is the filtered random process $\mathbf{E}_m^\dagger(\mathbf{r})$, given by

$$\mathbf{E}_m^\dagger(\mathbf{r}) = \alpha_m \mathbf{E}_m(\mathbf{r}) ** p_m(\mathbf{r}). \tag{10.100}$$

The mean exposure is $\alpha_m \mathscr{E}\Phi_m$. By use of (10.98) and (3.199), the autocorrelation function of the exposure is found to be

$$\begin{aligned} R_{E_m^\dagger}(\mathbf{L}) &= \langle \mathbf{E}_m^\dagger(\mathbf{r})\mathbf{E}_m^\dagger(\mathbf{r} + \mathbf{L}) \rangle \\ &= \alpha_m^2[R_{E_m}(\mathbf{L}) ** p_m(\mathbf{L}) \star\star p_m(\mathbf{L})] \\ &= \mathscr{E}_m^2 \Phi_m p_m(\mathbf{L}) \star\star p_m(\mathbf{L}) + \mathscr{E}_m^2 \Phi_m^2, \end{aligned} \tag{10.101}$$

where $\mathscr{E}_m \equiv \alpha_m \mathscr{E}$.

The term $\mathscr{E}_m^2\Phi_m^2$ in (10.101) is simply the square of the mean exposure. The autocorrelation function of the fluctuations in exposure is given by

$$R_{\Delta E_m^\dagger}(\mathbf{L}) = \mathscr{E}_m^2\Phi_m p_m(\mathbf{L}) \star\star\, p_m(\mathbf{L}). \tag{10.102}$$

The Wiener spectrum $S_{\Delta E_m^\dagger}(\boldsymbol{\rho})$ is given by the Fourier transform of $R_{\Delta E_m^\dagger}(\mathbf{L})$:

$$S_{\Delta E_m^\dagger}(\boldsymbol{\rho}) = \mathscr{E}_m^2\Phi_m|P_m(\boldsymbol{\rho})|^2, \tag{10.103}$$

where $P_m(\boldsymbol{\rho})$, being the Fourier transform of $p_m(\mathbf{r})$, is simply the optical transfer function associated with the mth layer.

The autocorrelation function and Wiener spectrum for the whole screen are given by summing over all layers:

$$R_{\Delta E^\dagger}(\mathbf{L}) = \sum_{m=1}^{M} \mathscr{E}_m^2\Phi_m[p_m(\mathbf{L}) \star\star\, p_m(\mathbf{L})], \tag{10.104}$$

$$S_{\Delta E^\dagger}(\boldsymbol{\rho}) = \sum_{m=1}^{M} \mathscr{E}_m^2\Phi_m|P_m(\boldsymbol{\rho})|^2. \tag{10.105}$$

In the limit of $M \to \infty$, with $M\,\Delta z \to d_s$, the screen thickness, we have

$$R_{\Delta E^\dagger}(\mathbf{L}) = \int_0^{d_s} [\mathscr{E}(z)]^2\Phi'(z)[p_z(\mathbf{L}) \star\star\, p_z(\mathbf{L})]\,dz, \tag{10.106}$$

$$S_{\Delta E^\dagger}(\boldsymbol{\rho}) = \int_0^{d_s} [\mathscr{E}(z)]^2\Phi'(z)|P_z(\boldsymbol{\rho})|^2\,dz \tag{10.107}$$

where

$$\Phi'(z) = \Phi_0\mu_p \exp(-\mu_p z). \tag{10.108}$$

[Note that $\Phi'(z)$ has dimensions of (length)$^{-3}$, so that $\Phi'(z)\,dz$ is a number per unit area. On the other hand, $\mathscr{E}(z)$ has the same dimensions as $\mathscr{E}_m$, namely, energy.] Equations (10.106) and (10.107) are the fundamental relationships expressing the noise imaging properties of the screen system in terms of deterministic quantities.

It remains still to convert the exposure fluctuations to measurable density fluctuations. Small fluctuations in exposure ΔE and the corresponding density fluctuations ΔD are related by

$$\Delta D = 0.434\gamma\,\Delta E/E_{\text{avg}}, \tag{10.109}$$

where γ is the slope of the H–D curve (see Section 5.2.3) at the average exposure E_{avg}. Thus we can write the expression for the Wiener spectrum of the (small) density fluctuations:

$$S_{\Delta D}(\boldsymbol{\rho}) = \left[\frac{0.434\gamma}{E_{\text{avg}}}\right]^2 S_{\Delta E^\dagger}(\boldsymbol{\rho}). \tag{10.110}$$

The average exposure is given by the integrated light arriving from all levels within the screen:

$$E_{\text{avg}} = \int_0^{d_s} \mathscr{E}(z)\Phi'(z)\,dz. \tag{10.111}$$

We now have the desired expression for the system Wiener spectrum:

$$S_{\Delta D}(\boldsymbol{\rho}) = \frac{(0.434\gamma)^2}{\left(\int_0^{d_s} \mathscr{E}(z)\Phi'(z)\,dz\right)^2} \int_0^{d_s} [\mathscr{E}(z)]^2 \Phi'(z) |P_z(\boldsymbol{\rho})|^2\,dz. \tag{10.112}$$

10.4.2 Example of Wiener Spectrum Calculations

To evaluate (10.112) we have to model the functions $\mathscr{E}(z)$ and $P_z(\boldsymbol{\rho})$. As in Section 5.3, we consider the full screen thickness d_s to be made up of an active layer of thickness d_1 and an inactive protective cover layer of thickness d_2 (see Fig. 10.4). For simplicity, we shall assume that the screen is optically nonabsorbing so that $\mathscr{E}(z)$ is independent of z within the active layer. In addition, we shall assume that the screen is sufficiently thin that $\exp(-\mu_p z)$ can be replaced by unity for all z values lying inside the screen.

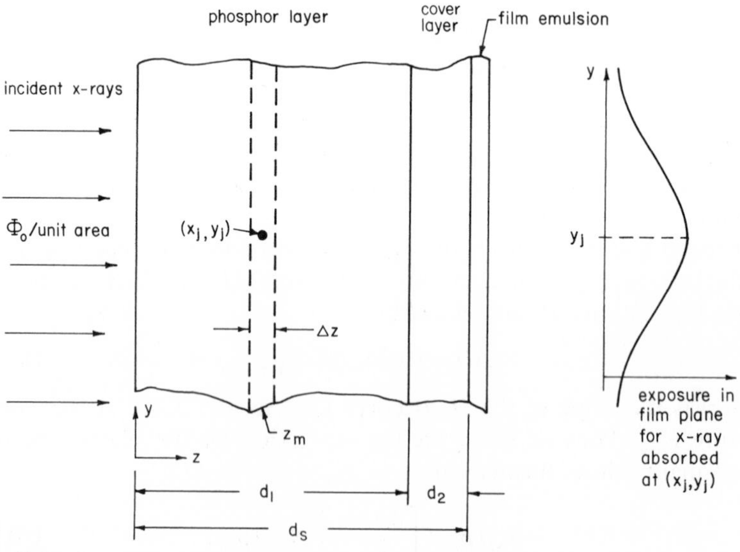

Fig. 10.4 Geometry used for calculation of the Wiener spectrum of a film–screen system.

Equation (10.112) then simplifies to

$$S_{\Delta D}(\boldsymbol{\rho}) = \frac{(0.434\gamma)^2}{\mu_p \Phi_0 d_1^2} \int_0^{d_1} |P_z(\boldsymbol{\rho})|^2 \, dz. \tag{10.113}$$

A reasonable point spread function for nonabsorbing phosphor layers is found by assuming that the irradiance at the film decreases as the inverse square of the distance from the point of scintillation and also as the cosine of the angle between the local normal to the emulsion and the direction of scintillation. This gives rise to a rotationally symmetrical point spread function [cf. (5.130)],

$$p_z(x, y) = \frac{d_s - z}{2\pi} [(d_s - z)^2 + x^2 + y^2]^{-3/2}, \tag{10.114}$$

which, as required, satisfies (10.99). The corresponding MTF is the Fourier transform of $p_z(x, y)$ (Gaskill, 1978, p. 324),

$$P_z(\boldsymbol{\rho}) = \mathscr{F}_2\{p_z(x, y)\} = \exp[-2\pi(d_s - z)\rho]. \tag{10.115}$$

Substituting (10.115) into (10.113) gives

$$S_{\Delta D}(\boldsymbol{\rho}) = \frac{(0.434\gamma)^2}{\mu_p \Phi_0 d_1^2} \left\{ \frac{\exp(-4\pi\rho d_2)[1 - \exp(-4\pi\rho d_1)]}{4\pi\rho} \right\}. \tag{10.116}$$

This function is plotted in Fig. 10.5.

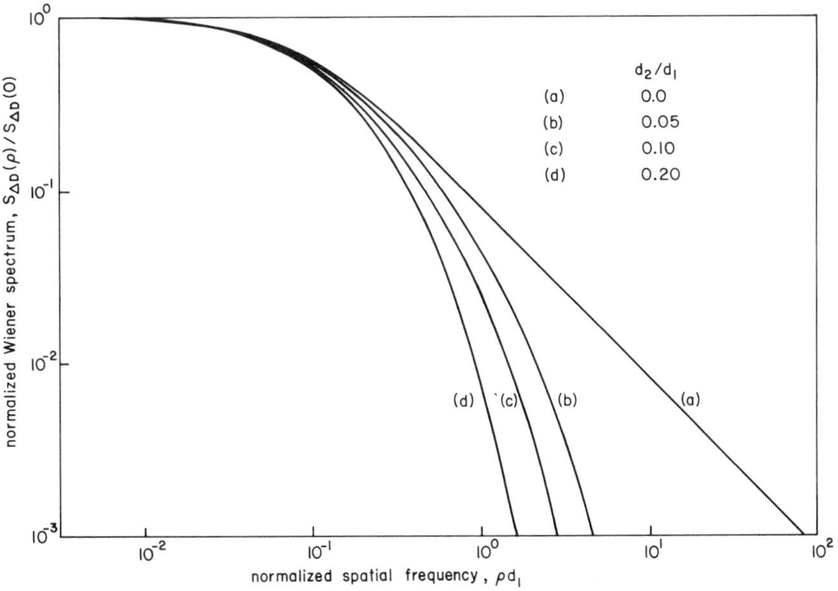

Fig. 10.5 Theoretical Wiener spectrum for a film–screen system.

The value of $S_{\Delta D}(0)$ has an interesting interpretation. With the substitution of $\boldsymbol{\rho} = 0$ in (10.112) the following expression is obtained:

$$S_{\Delta D}(0) = \frac{(0.434\gamma)^2}{\Phi_{\text{abs}}} \frac{e_0 e_2}{e_1^2}, \tag{10.117}$$

where

$$e_0 = \int_0^{d_s} \Phi'(z)\,dz \equiv \Phi_{\text{abs}}, \quad e_1 = \int_0^{d_s} \mathscr{E}(z)\Phi'(z)\,dz, \quad e_2 = \int_0^{d_s} [\mathscr{E}(z)]^2\Phi'(z)\,dz, \tag{10.118}$$

and Φ_{abs} is the x-ray photon fluence absorbed by the screen. For most screens $\Phi_{\text{abs}} = k\Phi_0$ where constant k is less than but close to unity. If there is no optical absorption, i.e., $\mathscr{E}(z) = \text{const}$, the term $e_0 e_2/e_1^2$ is unity and we have

$$S_{\Delta D}(0) = (0.434\gamma)^2/\Phi_{\text{abs}} \approx 1/\Phi_0 \tag{10.119}$$

where for the last part of (10.119) we have used the approximations $k = 1$ and $0.434\gamma = 1$. With this degree of approximation, $S_{\Delta D}(0)$ may be thus interpreted as an absolute measure of the speed of the system.

The ratio of moments $e_0 e_2/e_1^2$ in (10.117) is analogous to the Swank factor of Section 5.5.1 [cf. (5.243)]. In both cases, it accounts for the additional randomness due to a variable amount of light in each flash. In Section 5.5.1, the origin of that randomness was the basic physics of the scintillation process; here it is the random depth in the phosphor at which the x ray is absorbed.

10.4.3 Relation between Wiener Spectrum and MTF

We have already seen that with some systems the Wiener spectrum is directly proportional to the square of the MTF [cf. (3.200)]. With film–screen systems this is not the case since the point spread function is not really a deterministic quantity. The distribution of irradiance in the film plane depends strongly upon the (random) depth at which the x-ray quantum is absorbed. In Section 5.3 we computed the system response for a film–screen detector by averaging the exposure contribution from various layers in a linear fashion [see (5.129)]. Equivalently, we could have obtained an expression for the system MTF by performing an integration of the kind:

$$\text{MTF}(\boldsymbol{\rho}) = d_s^{-1} \int_0^{d_s} \text{MTF}_z(\boldsymbol{\rho})\,dz. \tag{10.120}$$

From (10.113) we see that the Wiener spectrum is given by

$$S_{\Delta D}(\boldsymbol{\rho}) \propto \int_0^{d_s} |\text{MTF}_z(\boldsymbol{\rho})|^2\,dz. \tag{10.121}$$

From (10.120) and (10.121) it is apparent that

$$S_{\Delta D}(\boldsymbol{\rho}) \neq \text{const} \cdot |\text{MTF}(\boldsymbol{\rho})|^2. \tag{10.122}$$

Thus, it is incorrect, in spite of frequent assertions in the literature to the contrary, to determine $S_{\Delta D}(\boldsymbol{\rho})$ for film–screen systems by squaring the measured MTF, or to determine the MTF by the converse analysis of the measured Wiener spectrum. Compare for example (10.116) and (5.137).

Wiener spectra are usually determined by taking the Fourier transform of the one-dimensional autocorrelation function of a series of one-dimensional scans. This process was described in Section 5.2.11. When the results are displayed as a one-dimensional power spectrum, with dimensions of length, the length of the scanning aperture l must be known before the absolute value of the two-dimensional spectrum can be determined by means of (5.90).

In practice, the measurement of Wiener spectra is a tricky task. The reader is cautioned to consult a treatise such as Wagner and Sandrik (1979) if the precise data-gathering and data-reduction techniques are required.

10.4.4 Film Grain Noise

In addition to the noise associated with the x-ray flux, there is also some noise due to the film itself. We have tacitly assumed so far that the film is a grainless recording medium. In fact, the granular structure of the film adds to the noise in the observed images. The autocorrelation function of a uniformly exposed piece of film has a very sharp central peak whose width is given by the characteristic dimension of the halide grains. This function rapidly falls to a constant value as the relative shift increases beyond about one grain diameter. The corresponding Wiener spectrum of the density fluctuations is given by the Fourier transform of the central peak, which is a relatively flat curve from low frequency up to a frequency given approximately by the reciprocal of the grain diameter. The number of optical quanta striking the film is many times greater than the number of x rays interacting within the phosphor. Even though it takes typically four absorbed optical quanta to expose a grain, and many of the optical quanta present do not contribute to forming the latent image, there are still many grains exposed for each incident absorbed x-ray photon. With regard to the absolute value of the Wiener spectrum at $\boldsymbol{\rho} = 0$, similar considerations apply to film as they do to the screen as exemplified by (10.119). However, due to the greatly increased number of "information areas" per unit area, the zero-frequency value of the Wiener spectrum for film grain noise is correspondingly much smaller than that caused by the x-ray flux.

Since the distribution of grains in the film emulsion and the distribution of x-ray events in the phosphor screen are statistically independent, at least

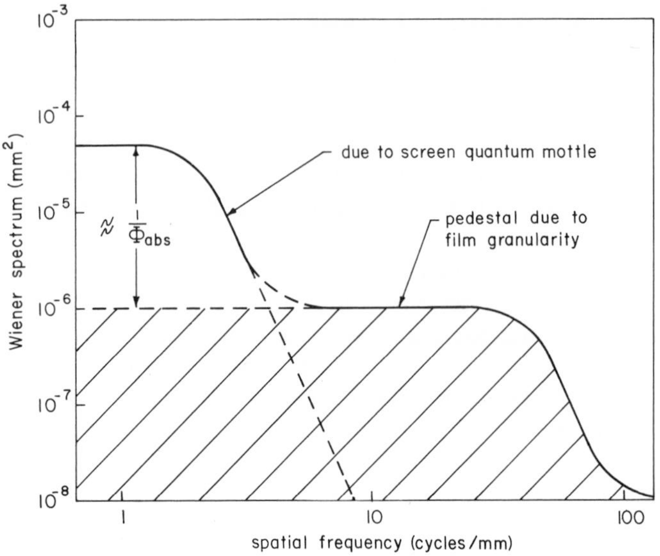

Fig. 10.6 Schematic Wiener spectrum for a film–screen system. The low-amplitude component extending to high spatial frequencies is the film grain noise.

when the density fluctuations due to x-ray quantum mottle are small, the total system power spectrum may be obtained by summing the power spectra of its components. As illustrated in Fig. 10.6, the total power spectrum is dominated by x-ray quantum noise at low frequencies, and by film grain noise at high frequencies. Since the radiographic image information is confined to the low frequencies, we are justified in ignoring the film grain noise. There can also be a contribution to the Wiener spectrum from the grain structure of the screen itself, but this is usually negligible.

10.4.5 Nonstationary Quantum Noise

Although the Wiener spectrum is the most common noise description in the literature on transmission radiography, it is instructive to reconsider transmission imaging in terms of the nonstationary methods used in Section 10.3.

Consider a nonstationary x-ray flux incident on a film–screen detector. The mean number of incident quanta per unit area is $h(\mathbf{r})$. As in Section 10.4.1, consider the screen to be divided up into M slabs, each of thickness Δz. The mean number of x-ray quanta per unit area absorbed in the mth slab is [cf. (10.93), where Φ_m is the stationary counterpart of $h_m(\mathbf{r})$]

$$h_m(\mathbf{r}) = h(\mathbf{r})\mu_p \, \Delta z \exp(-\mu_p z_m). \tag{10.123}$$

As before, the filter function is $p_m(\mathbf{r})$, and the mean and variance of the film exposure are

$$\langle \mathsf{E}^{\dagger}(\mathbf{r}) \rangle = \sum_{m=1}^{M} \mathscr{E}_m h_m(\mathbf{r}) ** p_m(\mathbf{r}), \tag{10.124}$$

$$\sigma_{E\dagger}^2(\mathbf{r}) = \sum_{m=1}^{M} \mathscr{E}_m^2 h_m(\mathbf{r}) ** [p_m(\mathbf{r})]^2. \tag{10.125}$$

These results agree with the previous ones if $h_m(\mathbf{r})$ is equal to the constant Φ_m. In that case,

$$\begin{aligned} h_m(\mathbf{r}) ** [p_m(\mathbf{r})]^2 &\to \Phi_m \int_{\infty} [p_m(\mathbf{r})]^2 \, d^2 r \\ &= \Phi_m [p_m(\mathbf{L}) \star\star p_m(\mathbf{L})]_{\mathbf{L}=0}. \end{aligned} \tag{10.126}$$

Equation (10.125) is a special case of (10.104) since

$$R_{\Delta E\dagger}(0) = \sigma_{E\dagger}^2. \tag{10.127}$$

The stationary results are therefore applicable whenever $h(\mathbf{r})$ is slowly varying compared to $p_m(\mathbf{r})$ for all m. However, in order to maintain a parallel to Section 10.3, we shall use the nonstationary formulation in Section 10.4.6.

10.4.6 Effect of Further Filtering

In discussing nuclear imaging in Section 10.3, we saw that the SNR could be improved by deliberately degrading the resolution with a smoothing filter. Can the same thing be accomplished in transmission radiography?

In transmission imaging, the resolution is governed by the x-ray focal spot, the MTF of the screen, and any postfilter that is used, including the observer's eye. The focal spot size does not enter into the noise averaging area, any more than the pinhole diameter did in Section 10.3. Of course, a larger focal spot may emit more photons, just as a larger pinhole collects more, but this just influences the number of detected photons per unit area rather than the area over which they are averaged.

On the other hand, there is an important difference between nuclear medicine and transmission radiography when the noise properties of the detector are considered. An Anger camera does not produce any noise smoothing since its output is still uncorrelated (or has a flat Wiener spectrum, if a stationary description is allowable). A phosphor screen, however, does provide a degree of noise smoothing since each x-ray photon produces a film exposure that is spread out over some area. Thus a thicker screen will produce more noise smoothing (and, as a side benefit, have a larger quantum efficiency) at the expense of spatial resolution.

A complication arises if we want to include a postfilter, with PSF $p_{\mathrm{pf}}(\mathbf{r})$, in the system. The difficulty is that we have a nonlinear element (the film) between one filter (the screen) and another (the postfilter). The input to the film is the exposure pattern, but the output may be taken as either the density or the transmittance of the developed film. If the postfilter is implemented digitally, the film is first scanned with a microdensitometer, and either a density or a transmittance readout may be chosen as the input to the post-filter. If the postfilter is the observer's eye, density is a better description since the human eye responds more or less logarithmically to irradiance changes. Therefore, we shall consider the film output to be a density pattern. Futher-more, we shall consider only low-contrast patterns so that the density changes are small. (If the density changes are large, noise is of little concern.) This allows us to treat the film as being approximately a linear element.

Equation (10.109), originally stated for density fluctuations due to x-ray photon noise, is equally valid for "signal" variations due to small changes in object attenuation. The output of the postfilter, due to photons absorbed in the mth layer of the screen, is the random process $\delta\mathbf{D}_m^\dagger(\mathbf{r})$, given by

$$\delta\mathbf{D}_m^\dagger(\mathbf{r}) = (0.434\gamma/E_{\mathrm{avg}})\,\delta\mathbf{E}_m^\dagger(\mathbf{r}) ** p_{\mathrm{pf}}(\mathbf{r}), \tag{10.128}$$

where lowercase deltas in front of random variables denote deviations from the local *spatial*-average (rather than ensemble-average) values, and the dagger on $\delta\mathbf{D}_m^\dagger(\mathbf{r})$ denotes a filtered version of $\delta\mathbf{D}_m(\mathbf{r})$.

The total density variation due to all layers is

$$\delta\mathbf{D}^\dagger(\mathbf{r}) = \sum_{m=1}^{M} \delta\mathbf{D}_m^\dagger(\mathbf{r}), \tag{10.129}$$

which is still assumed to be a small quantity. Since the absorption events in each layer are statistically independent, the mean and variance of $\delta\mathbf{D}^\dagger(\mathbf{r})$ are [cf. (10.124) and (10.125)]

$$\langle\delta\mathbf{D}^\dagger(\mathbf{r})\rangle = \sum_{m=1}^{M} \left(\frac{0.434\gamma\mathscr{E}_m}{E_{\mathrm{avg}}}\right) \Delta h_m(\mathbf{r}) ** p_m(\mathbf{r}) * p_{\mathrm{pf}}(\mathbf{r}), \tag{10.130}$$

$$\sigma_{D^\dagger}^2(\mathbf{r}) = \sum_{m=1}^{M} \left[\frac{0.434\gamma\mathscr{E}_m}{E_{\mathrm{avg}}}\right]^2 h_m(\mathbf{r}) ** [p_m(\mathbf{r}) ** p_{\mathrm{pf}}(\mathbf{r})]^2. \tag{10.131}$$

Note that $\Delta h_m(\mathbf{r})$, which describes the spatial variation of photon density due to variations in object attenuation, appears in (10.130) but $h_m(\mathbf{r})$ must be used in (10.131).

We now make two more approximations that should help clarify these rather complicated equations. First, we assume that the screen is optically nonabsorbing so that $\mathscr{E}_m$ has the same value, $\mathscr{E}_0$, for all layers. Second, we assume that $p_m(\mathbf{r})$ is very narrow compared to $p_{pf}(\mathbf{r})$. Since $p_m(\mathbf{r})$ is normalized to unit area by (10.99), it may be replaced by $\delta(\mathbf{r})$ in (10.130) and (10.131), yielding

$$\langle \delta \mathbf{D}^\dagger(\mathbf{r}) \rangle = \sum_{m=1}^{M} \left(\frac{0.434\gamma \mathscr{E}_0}{E_{avg}} \right) \Delta h_m(\mathbf{r}) ** p_{pf}(\mathbf{r})$$

$$= \left(\frac{0.434\gamma \mathscr{E}_0}{E_{avg}} \right) \eta\, \Delta h(\mathbf{r}) ** p_{pf}(\mathbf{r}), \tag{10.132}$$

$$\sigma_{D^\dagger}^2(\mathbf{r}) = \left(\frac{0.434\gamma \mathscr{E}_0}{E_{avg}} \right)^2 \eta h(\mathbf{r}) ** [p_{pf}(\mathbf{r})]^2, \tag{10.133}$$

where

$$\eta h(\mathbf{r}) \equiv \sum_{m=1}^{M} h_m(\mathbf{r}), \tag{10.134}$$

with η being the quantum efficiency of the screen.

The interpretation of (10.133) is straightforward. The factor $\eta h(\mathbf{r})$ is the total number of absorbed photons per unit area, and the convolution with $(p_{pf})^2$ serves to integrate $\eta h(\mathbf{r})$ over an area determined by $[p_{pf}(\mathbf{r})]^2$. The remaining factors in (10.133) merely serve to convert from photons per unit area to density.

If $h(\mathbf{r})$ is slowly varying compared to $p_{pf}(\mathbf{r})$, (10.132) and (10.133) reduce to

$$\langle \delta \mathbf{D}^\dagger(\mathbf{r}) \rangle \approx \left[\frac{0.434\gamma \mathscr{E}_0}{E_{avg}} \right] \eta \Delta h(\mathbf{r}) \int_\infty p_{pf}(\mathbf{r}_0)\, d^2 r_0, \tag{10.135}$$

$$\sigma_{D^\dagger}^2(\mathbf{r}) \approx \left[\frac{0.434\gamma \mathscr{E}_0}{E_{avg}} \right]^2 \eta h(\mathbf{r}) \int_\infty [p_{pf}(\mathbf{r}_0)]^2\, d^2 r_0. \tag{10.136}$$

10.4.7 Connection with Stationary Statistics

If $h(\mathbf{r}) = \Phi_0 = \text{const}$, then (10.136) simplifies further. The average exposure E_{avg} is given by

$$E_{avg} = \eta \Phi_0 \mathscr{E}_0 = \Phi_{abs} \mathscr{E}_0, \tag{10.137}$$

where, as in (10.118), Φ_{abs} is the number of absorbed x-ray quanta per unit area. Combining (10.136) and (10.137) yields

$$\sigma_{D^\dagger}^2 = \frac{(0.434\gamma)^2}{\Phi_{abs}} \int_\infty [p_f(\mathbf{r}_0)]^2\, d^2 r_0. \tag{10.138}$$

We shall now show that precisely this same result can be obtained from the Wiener spectrum.

The variance of the filtered density pattern is given by

$$\sigma_{D^\dagger}^2 = R_{\Delta D^\dagger}(0) = \int_\infty d^2\rho\, S_{\Delta D^\dagger}(\boldsymbol{\rho}). \tag{10.139}$$

However, by (3.200),

$$S_{\Delta D^\dagger}(\boldsymbol{\rho}) = |P_{\mathrm{pf}}(\boldsymbol{\rho})|^2 S_{\Delta D}(\boldsymbol{\rho}). \tag{10.140}$$

But we have been assuming that $p_{\mathrm{pf}}(\mathbf{r})$ is much broader than $p_m(\mathbf{r})$ for all m. This is equivalent to assuming that $S_{\Delta D}(\boldsymbol{\rho})$ is essentially flat over the frequency range where $|P_{\mathrm{pf}}(\boldsymbol{\rho})|^2$ is appreciable. Therefore (10.139) becomes

$$\begin{aligned}\sigma_{D^\dagger}^2 &= \int_\infty d^2\rho\, |P_{\mathrm{pf}}(\boldsymbol{\rho})|^2 S_{\Delta D}(\boldsymbol{\rho}) \\ &\approx S_{\Delta D}(0) \int_\infty |P_{\mathrm{pf}}(\boldsymbol{\rho})|^2\, d^2\rho.\end{aligned} \tag{10.141}$$

If we use (10.119) for $S_{\Delta D}(0)$ and apply Parseval's theorem (B.19) to the integral, we again obtain (10.138).

10.4.8 Noise, Resolution, and Exposure

Although we have written expressions for the mean and variance of the density pattern $\mathbf{D}(\mathbf{r})$ and its filtered counterpart $\mathbf{D}^\dagger(\mathbf{r})$, we have refrained from stating the results in the form of a signal-to-noise ratio. The difficulty is that it is not obvious what we should call "signal." We could, of course,

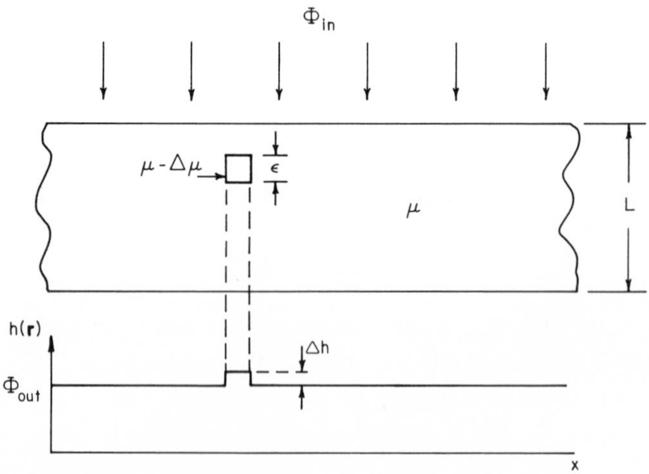

Fig. 10.7 Illustration of a transmission radiography problem in which a small cube of attenuation coefficient $\mu - \Delta\mu$ is embedded in a slab of attenuation coefficient μ.

define the SNR for the filtered density pattern by

$$\mathrm{SNR}(\mathbf{r}) = \langle \delta \mathbf{D}^{\dagger}(\mathbf{r}) \rangle / \sigma_{D^{\dagger}}(\mathbf{r}), \tag{10.142}$$

which, by use of (10.132) and (10.133), becomes

$$\mathrm{SNR}(\mathbf{r}) = \frac{\sqrt{\eta}\,\Delta h(\mathbf{r}) ** p_{\mathrm{pf}}(\mathbf{r})}{\{h(\mathbf{r}) ** [p_{\mathrm{pf}}(\mathbf{r})]^2\}^{1/2}}, \tag{10.143}$$

but this does not really solve the problem since $\Delta h(\mathbf{r})$ is some unspecified small change in x-ray fluence.

To proceed, we must pose a specific detection task. Consider the situation illustrated in Fig. 10.7, where a uniform slab of material of thickness L and attenuation coefficient μ has imbedded in it a small cube (with side ε) of a material with a slightly smaller attenuation coefficient $\mu - \Delta\mu$. Assume the slab is irradiated with an essentially parallel x-ray beam, with an incident photon fluence given by the constant Φ_{in}. The mean image $h(\mathbf{r})$ at the detector is given by

$$\begin{aligned} h(\mathbf{r}) &= \Phi_{\mathrm{in}} \exp\left(-\int_0^L \mu(\mathbf{r}, z)\, dz \right) \\ &= \Phi_{\mathrm{in}} \exp(-\mu L)[1 - \mathrm{rect}(\mathbf{r}/\varepsilon)] \\ &\quad + \Phi_{\mathrm{in}} \exp(-\mu L) \exp(\Delta\mu\varepsilon)\, \mathrm{rect}(\mathbf{r}/\varepsilon), \end{aligned} \tag{10.144}$$

where $\mathrm{rect}(\mathbf{r}/\varepsilon) = \mathrm{rect}(x/\varepsilon)\,\mathrm{rect}(y/\varepsilon)$. If we are trying to detect the small cube, the variation in photon density produced by it is the appropriate $\Delta h(\mathbf{r})$ to use in (10.143). Thus, if $\Delta\mu\varepsilon$ is small,

$$\begin{aligned} \Delta h(\mathbf{r}) &= h(\mathbf{r}) - \Phi_{\mathrm{in}} \exp(-\mu L) \\ &= \Phi_{\mathrm{in}} \exp(-\mu L)\, \Delta\mu\varepsilon\, \mathrm{rect}(\mathbf{r}/\varepsilon) \\ &= \Phi_{\mathrm{out}}\, \Delta\mu\varepsilon\, \mathrm{rect}(\mathbf{r}/\varepsilon), \end{aligned} \tag{10.145}$$

where $\Phi_{\mathrm{out}} \equiv \Phi_{\mathrm{in}} \exp(-\mu L)$ is the fluence emerging from the slab.

To optimally detect the cube, we should make the postfilter a matched filter for the image of the cube, i.e., we should take

$$p_{\mathrm{pf}}(\mathbf{r}) = \mathrm{rect}(\mathbf{r}/\varepsilon), \tag{10.146}$$

where we are still assuming that $p_m(\mathbf{r})$ is much narrower than $p_{\mathrm{pf}}(\mathbf{r})$.

In evaluating the denominator of (10.143), we note that $[p_{\mathrm{pf}}(\mathbf{r})]^2 = p_{\mathrm{pf}}(\mathbf{r})$, and that, since $\Delta\mu\varepsilon$ is small, it is a good approximation to set $h(\mathbf{r}) \approx \Phi_{\mathrm{out}}$. Equation (10.143) then becomes

$$\mathrm{SNR}(\mathbf{r}) = \sqrt{\eta \Phi_{\mathrm{out}}}\, \Delta\mu\, p_{\mathrm{pf}}(\mathbf{r}) ** \mathrm{rect}(\mathbf{r}/\varepsilon). \tag{10.147}$$

The SNR is proportional to the autoconvolution of the function $\mathrm{rect}(\mathbf{r}/\varepsilon)$. [We do not write $\mathrm{rect}(\mathbf{r}/\varepsilon) ** \mathrm{rect}(\mathbf{r}/\varepsilon)$, because, by our shorthand conventions, this would have to be interpreted as rect($\mathbf{r}'$) ** rect($\mathbf{r}'$) evaluated at $\mathbf{r}' = \mathbf{r}/\varepsilon$, which is not what we mean. See Section B.5 in Appendix B.] In any event, the maximum SNR occurs at $\mathbf{r} = 0$, where the convolution in (10.147) has the value ε^2. This leaves

$$\mathrm{SNR}(0) = \sqrt{\eta\Phi_{\mathrm{out}}}\,\Delta\mu\varepsilon^2. \tag{10.148}$$

In other words, with optimal filtering, the photon fluence required to detect a small cube must vary as the inverse fourth power of the cube dimension: $\Phi_{\mathrm{out}} \propto \varepsilon^{-4}$ for constant SNR. Of course, for a constant-strength x-ray source Φ_{out} is also proportional to the exposure time T, so we must also have $T \propto \varepsilon^{-4}$ for constant SNR. The fourth-power law that was so common in nuclear medicine has occurred again.

There is one important distinction between the transmission and emission cases. In a pinhole camera, for example, we saw that halving the pinhole diameter requires a 16-fold increase in exposure time for the same SNR, i.e., $T \propto d_{\mathrm{ph}}^{-4}$. However, the radiation dose to the patient is unchanged. A certain amount of isotope is in the body, decaying with a half-life $T_{1/2}$ which is almost always long compared to the exposure time T. Thus, T does not necessarily have anything to do with dose, although we can choose to decrease T by correspondingly increasing the dose and keeping everything else constant. In transmission radiography, on the other hand, the only photons that impinge on the detector are those that have passed through the object. An increase in Φ_{out}, whether by using a stronger x-ray tube or a longer exposure time *always* increases the dose. Thus, for our cube problem, we have dose proportional to ε^{-4}.

Finally, we should note that the fourth-power law came about since we chose to vary all dimensions of the object and the filter function at once. The situation is very different if we consider a rectangular parallelepiped of side ε in the x and y directions but side ε' in the z direction. Then (10.148) becomes

$$\mathrm{SNR}(0) = \sqrt{\eta\Phi_{\mathrm{out}}}\,\Delta\mu\varepsilon'\varepsilon \tag{10.149}$$

The product $\Delta\mu\varepsilon'$ is a measure of the radiographic contrast of the object. If the contrast is fixed, we see that $\Phi_{\mathrm{out}} \propto \varepsilon^{-2}$ for constant SNR.

More generally, for any fixed object we should expect the required photon fluence to vary as the inverse square of some resolution distance. The easiest way to prove this contention is to use (10.135) and (10.136), which are valid if $\Delta h(\mathbf{r})$ and $h(\mathbf{r})$ are slowly varying compared to $p_{\mathrm{pf}}(\mathbf{r})$. From those equations, along with (10.142), we have

$$\mathrm{SNR}(\mathbf{r}) = \sqrt{\eta A_{\mathrm{eff}}}\,\Delta h(\mathbf{r})/\sqrt{h(\mathbf{r})}, \tag{10.150}$$

where A_{eff} is the effective noise-averaging area defined by

$$A_{\text{eff}} = \left(\int_{\infty} p_{\text{pf}}(\mathbf{r}_0)\, d^2 r_0 \right)^2 \Big/ \int_{\infty} [p_{\text{pf}}(\mathbf{r}_0)]^2\, d^2 r_0 . \qquad (10.151)$$

Since both $\Delta h(\mathbf{r})$ and $h(\mathbf{r})$ vary linearly with the fluence Φ_{out}, constant SNR requires that $\Phi_{\text{out}} \propto A_{\text{eff}}^{-1}$. Also, for a constant-strength source, $T \propto A_{\text{eff}}^{-1}$. Furthermore, since $p_{\text{pf}}(\mathbf{r})$ dominates the system resolution by our previous assumptions, we must also have $\Phi_{\text{out}} \propto \delta_{\text{tot}}^{-2}$ or $T \propto \delta_{\text{tot}}^{-2}$. The same conclusions, of course, also apply to the input fluence Φ_{in} if the slab thickness L is constant.

10.5 COMPUTED TOMOGRAPHY

10.5.1 Statistical Description of the Projection Data

The basic geometry for transmission computed tomography is shown in Fig. 7.2. The object is irradiated with a parallel x-ray beam making an angle $\phi = \phi_l$ (for the lth projection) with the x axis. A rotated coordinate system $(x_{\text{r}}, y_{\text{r}}, z)$ is defined such that the x-ray beam travels parallel to the y_{r} axis, producing a two-dimensional flux distribution on a linear detector array in the x_{r}–z plane. The mean photon density at point (x_{r}, z) in the lth projection is $h_l(x_{\text{r}}, z)$. The jth detector in the array is centered at $(x_{\text{r}} = x_{\text{r}j}, z = 0)$, and has width Δx and height Δz. During the exposure time for one projection, it detects a mean number of photons $\bar{N}_{lj}$ given by

$$\bar{N}_{lj} = \eta \int_{x_{\text{r}j} - \Delta x/2}^{x_{\text{r}j} + \Delta x/2} dx_{\text{r}} \int_{-\Delta z/2}^{\Delta z/2} dz\, h_l(x_{\text{r}}, z), \qquad (10.152)$$

where η is the quantum efficiency of the detector. The number $\bar{N}_{lj}$ is the mean value of a random variable $\mathbf{N}_{lj}$, which, by the discussion in Section 3.4.8, must obey Poisson statistics if the x-ray source is stable (i.e., has a constant mean output).

The first step in any reconstruction algorithm is to take the logarithm of the measured x-ray transmission. This yields the projection $\lambda_{\phi}(x_{\text{r}})$ as defined in (7.11). For the present discussion, the projection for the lth angle and the jth detector is the random variable $\boldsymbol{\lambda}_{\phi_l}(x_{\text{r}j})$, or simply $\boldsymbol{\lambda}_{lj}$ for short, given by

$$\boldsymbol{\lambda}_{lj} = -\ln(\mathbf{N}_{lj}/N_0). \qquad (10.153)$$

Strictly speaking, the normalizing constant N_0, which is the number of photons that would be detected in the absence of an absorbing object, should also be a random variable. This point will be considered in more detail in Section 10.5.6; for now we take N_0 to be a deterministic constant.

Since we are concerned with the fluctuation of $\mathbf{N}_{lj}$, it is convenient to define a zero-mean random variable $\Delta\mathbf{N}_{lj}$ by

$$\Delta\mathbf{N}_{lj} = \mathbf{N}_{lj} - \bar{N}_{lj}. \tag{10.154}$$

From the discussion in Section 3.4.7 we know that counts from two distinct detectors, or from one detector at two nonoverlapping time intervals, are statistically independent Poisson random variables. Therefore

$$\langle \Delta\mathbf{N}_{lj} \Delta\mathbf{N}_{l'j'} \rangle = \bar{N}_{lj} \delta_{ll'} \delta_{jj'}, \tag{10.155}$$

where δ_{mn} is the Kronecker symbol defined by

$$\delta_{mn} = \begin{cases} 1 & \text{if} \quad m = n \\ 0 & \text{if} \quad m \neq n. \end{cases} \tag{10.156}$$

When $j = j'$ and $l = l'$, (10.155) merely states that the variance of $\mathbf{N}_{lj}$ equals its mean as required by Poisson statistics.

In order to discuss the statistics of the projection $\boldsymbol{\lambda}_{lj}$, we expand (10.153) in a Taylor series around its value when $\Delta\mathbf{N}_{lj} = 0$:

$$\boldsymbol{\lambda}_{lj} = -\ln(\bar{N}_{lj}/N_0) - (\Delta\mathbf{N}_{lj}/\bar{N}_{lj}) + (\Delta\mathbf{N}_{lj})^2/(2\bar{N}_{lj}^2) + \cdots. \tag{10.157}$$

Since the logarithm is a nonlinear function, the mean value of the logarithm of a random variable is not, in general, equal to the logarithm of the mean value of the variable. From (10.157) and (10.155) we have

$$\langle \boldsymbol{\lambda}_{lj} \rangle = -\ln(\bar{N}_{lj}/N_0) + 1/(2\bar{N}_{lj}) + \cdots, \tag{10.158}$$

where we have also used the fact that $\langle \Delta\mathbf{N}_{lj} \rangle = 0$.

For medical applications in the diagnostic energy range, the x-ray beam is usually attenuated by a factor of 20–1000. Therefore, the first term in (10.158) is in the range of 3–7 since $\ln(\frac{1}{20}) \approx -3$ and $\ln(\frac{1}{1000}) \approx -7$. Furthermore, the mean number of photons detected in an individual measurement $\bar{N}_{lj}$ is always large compared to unity in practice. The second term and all higher terms in (10.158) are therefore negligible compared to the first term, leaving

$$\langle \boldsymbol{\lambda}_{lj} \rangle \approx -\ln(\bar{N}_{lj}/N_0). \tag{10.159}$$

In this particular case, it is indeed a good approximation to replace the mean of the logarithm with the logarithm of the mean.

The second-order statistics of the projection data now follow readily. The only problem is to be sure we have included all necessary terms. We first define another zero-mean random variable by

$$\Delta\boldsymbol{\lambda}_{lj} = \boldsymbol{\lambda}_{lj} - \langle \boldsymbol{\lambda}_{lj} \rangle \approx \boldsymbol{\lambda}_{lj} + \ln(\bar{N}_{lj}/N_0) - 1/(2\bar{N}_{lj}). \tag{10.160}$$

The necessity of again including the term $1/(2\bar{N}_{lj})$ in $\boldsymbol{\lambda}_{lj}$ will become apparent shortly.

From (10.157) and (10.160), we have

$$\langle \Delta\boldsymbol{\lambda}_{lj}\,\Delta\boldsymbol{\lambda}_{l'j'}\rangle = \left\langle\left(-\frac{\Delta\mathbf{N}_{lj}}{\bar{N}_{lj}} - \frac{1}{2\bar{N}_{lj}} + \frac{(\Delta\mathbf{N}_{lj})^2}{2\bar{N}_{lj}^2}\right)\left(-\frac{\Delta\mathbf{N}_{l'j'}}{\bar{N}_{l'j'}} - \frac{1}{2\bar{N}_{l'j'}} + \frac{(\Delta\mathbf{N}_{l'j'})^2}{2\bar{N}_{l'j'}^2}\right)\right\rangle. \tag{10.161}$$

To simplify the notation, we temporarily let $\Delta\mathbf{N}_{lj} \equiv \Delta\mathbf{N}$, $\Delta\mathbf{N}_{l'j'} \equiv \Delta\mathbf{N}'$, $\bar{N}_{lj} \equiv \bar{N}$, $\bar{N}_{l'j'} \equiv \bar{N}'$. Then (10.161) becomes

$$\begin{aligned}\langle \Delta\boldsymbol{\lambda}_{lj}\,\Delta\boldsymbol{\lambda}_{l'j'}\rangle &= \frac{\langle \Delta\mathbf{N}\,\Delta\mathbf{N}'\rangle}{\bar{N}\bar{N}'} + \frac{1}{4\bar{N}\bar{N}'} \\ &\quad + \frac{\langle(\Delta\mathbf{N})^2(\Delta\mathbf{N}')^2\rangle}{4\bar{N}^2\bar{N}'^2} - \frac{\langle(\Delta\mathbf{N})(\Delta\mathbf{N}')^2\rangle}{2\bar{N}\bar{N}'^2} \\ &\quad - \frac{\langle(\Delta\mathbf{N}')^2\rangle}{4\bar{N}\bar{N}'^2} - \frac{\langle(\Delta\mathbf{N})^2(\Delta\mathbf{N}')\rangle}{2\bar{N}^2\bar{N}'} - \frac{\langle(\Delta\mathbf{N})^2\rangle}{4\bar{N}^2\bar{N}'},\end{aligned} \tag{10.162}$$

where we have used $\langle\Delta\mathbf{N}\rangle = \langle\Delta\mathbf{N}'\rangle = 0$ to eliminate two terms. If $j \neq j'$ or $l \neq l'$, then we also have $\langle(\Delta\mathbf{N})(\Delta\mathbf{N}')\rangle = \langle(\Delta\mathbf{N})\rangle\langle\Delta\mathbf{N}'\rangle = 0$. Similarly,

$$\langle(\Delta\mathbf{N})^2(\Delta\mathbf{N}')\rangle = \langle(\Delta\mathbf{N}')^2(\Delta\mathbf{N})\rangle = 0,$$

while

$$\langle(\Delta\mathbf{N})^2(\Delta\mathbf{N}')^2\rangle = \langle(\Delta\mathbf{N})^2\rangle\langle(\Delta\mathbf{N}')^2\rangle = \bar{N}\bar{N}'.$$

These results and a little algebra show that the remaining terms cancel, so that

$$\langle\Delta\boldsymbol{\lambda}_{lj}\Delta\boldsymbol{\lambda}_{l'j'}\rangle = 0 \qquad \text{if} \quad l \neq l' \quad \text{or} \quad j \neq j'. \tag{10.163}$$

This cancellation of terms is physically reasonable since fluctuations in the projections from different detectors or different projection angles cannot be correlated for a Poisson source. However, complete cancellation would not have occurred without all three terms from (10.160).

When $j = j'$ *and* $l = l'$, all seven terms in (10.162) are nonzero. By use of (3.111) for $\langle(\Delta\mathbf{N})^3\rangle$ and $\langle(\Delta\mathbf{N})^4\rangle$, and some more algebra, we find

$$\langle(\Delta\boldsymbol{\lambda}_{lj})^2\rangle = \frac{1}{\bar{N}_{lj}} - \frac{1}{2\bar{N}_{lj}^2} + \frac{1}{4\bar{N}_{lj}^3}. \tag{10.164}$$

By our previous assumption that $\bar{N}_{lj} \gg 1$, the first term in this equation dominates. Combining (10.163) and (10.164), we are left with

$$\langle\Delta\boldsymbol{\lambda}_{lj}\,\Delta\boldsymbol{\lambda}_{l'j'}\rangle \approx \delta_{jj'}\,\delta_{ll'}/\bar{N}_{lj}. \tag{10.165}$$

Since the assumption that $\bar{N}_{lj} \gg 1$ was so crucial to the above discussion, each detector must have sufficient area to collect a large number of photons.

The problem is inherently discrete. Nevertheless, it is often useful to approximate the discrete projection data set by a continuous one. This allows us to describe the filtering and back-projection operations by continuous integrals rather than discrete sums, and also allows us to concentrate on the effects of statistical fluctuations unfettered by sampling errors or reconstruction artifacts peculiar to discrete data.

To go over a continuous formulation, the Kronecker deltas must somehow be replaced with Dirac deltas. For a set of points $x_j = j\,\Delta x$, the equivalence is

$$\delta_{jj'} \Leftrightarrow \delta(x_j - x_{j'})\,\Delta x \approx \delta(x_j - x_{j'})\,dx_j \tag{10.166}$$

in the sense that a discrete sum over the left-hand side gives the same result as an integral over the right-hand side, i.e.,

$$\sum_{j=-\infty}^{\infty} f(x_j)\,\delta_{jj'} = \int_{\infty} f(x_j)\,\delta(x_j - x_{j'})\,dx_j = f(x_{j'}). \tag{10.167}$$

Similarly, in the sum over projection angles,

$$\delta_{ll'} \Leftrightarrow \delta(\phi_l - \phi_{l'})\,\Delta\phi. \tag{10.168}$$

If a total of M projections are recorded over a range of π radians,

$$\Delta\phi = \pi/M. \tag{10.169}$$

With these correspondences, (10.159) and (10.165) become

$$\langle \boldsymbol{\lambda}_\phi(x_r) \rangle = -\ln[\bar{n}_\phi(x_r)/n_0] \tag{10.170}$$

$$\langle \Delta\boldsymbol{\lambda}_\phi(x_r)\,\Delta\boldsymbol{\lambda}_{\phi'}(x_r + X) \rangle = \frac{\pi}{M}\,\frac{\delta(X)\,\delta(\phi - \phi')}{\bar{n}_\phi(x_r)}, \tag{10.171}$$

where $\bar{n}_\phi(x_r)$ and n_0 are linear count densities (photons per unit length) defined by

$$\bar{n}_{\phi_l}(x_{rj}) \equiv \bar{N}_{lj}/\Delta x, \tag{10.172}$$

$$n_0 \equiv N_0/\Delta x. \tag{10.173}$$

The implicit assumption here is that the detector width Δx and angular increment $\Delta\phi$ are so small that $\bar{n}_\phi(x_r)$ may be treated as a continuous function of x_r and ϕ even though it is defined at a discrete set of points.

10.5.2 Noise Propagation through the Convolution Algorithm

From (7.40) the reconstructed image $\hat{\boldsymbol{\mu}}(r, \theta)$, now a random variable, is given by

$$\hat{\boldsymbol{\mu}}(r, \theta) = \frac{M}{\pi} \int_0^{\pi} d\phi\,[\boldsymbol{\lambda}_\phi(x_r) * q_1(x_r)]_{x_r = r\cos(\theta - \phi)}, \tag{10.174}$$

where $q_1(x_r)$ is the impulse response of the one-dimensional filter. Note that (10.174) differs from (7.40) by a factor of M since here we are defining $\hat{\mu}(r,\theta)$ as the sum rather than the average of the filtered back projections. By use of (10.170) and (3.201), we have

$$\langle \hat{\boldsymbol{\mu}}(r,\theta)\rangle = \frac{-M}{\pi}\int_0^\pi d\phi \left\{ \ln\left(\frac{\overline{n}_\phi(x_r)}{n_0}\right) * q_1(x_r)\right\}_{x_r = r\cos(\theta-\phi)}. \tag{10.175}$$

We define a zero-mean random variable by

$$\begin{aligned}\Delta\hat{\boldsymbol{\mu}}(r,\theta) &= \hat{\boldsymbol{\mu}}(r,\theta) - \langle\hat{\boldsymbol{\mu}}(r,\theta)\rangle \\ &= \frac{M}{\pi}\int_0^\pi d\phi\,[\Delta\boldsymbol{\lambda}_\phi(x_r) * q_1(x_r)]_{x_r = r\cos(\theta-\phi)} \\ &= \frac{M}{\pi}\int_0^\pi d\phi \int_{-\infty}^{\infty} dx_r\,\Delta\boldsymbol{\lambda}_\phi(x_r) q_1[r\cos(\theta-\phi) - x_r].\end{aligned} \tag{10.176}$$

The variance of $\hat{\boldsymbol{\mu}}(r,\theta)$ is given by

$$\begin{aligned}\sigma_{\hat{\mu}}^2(r,\theta) &= \langle[\Delta\hat{\boldsymbol{\mu}}(r,\theta)]^2\rangle \\ &= \left\langle \frac{M^2}{\pi^2}\int_0^\pi d\phi \int_0^\pi d\phi' \int_{-\infty}^{\infty} dx_r\,\Delta\boldsymbol{\lambda}_\phi(x_r) q_1[r\cos(\theta-\phi) - x_r] \right. \\ &\quad \left. \cdot \int_{-\infty}^{\infty} dx_r'\,\Delta\boldsymbol{\lambda}_{\phi'}(x_r') q_1[r\cos(\theta-\phi') - x_r'] \right\rangle.\end{aligned} \tag{10.177}$$

Interchanging the order of statistical averaging and integration and invoking (10.171), we have

$$\begin{aligned}\sigma_{\hat{\mu}}^2(r,\theta) &= \frac{M}{\pi}\int_0^\pi d\phi \int_0^\pi d\phi'\,\delta(\phi-\phi') \\ &\quad \cdot \int_{-\infty}^{\infty} dx_r \int_{-\infty}^{\infty} dx_r'\,\delta(x_r - x_r')\left(\frac{1}{\overline{n}_\phi(x_r)}\right) \\ &\quad \cdot q_1[r\cos(\theta-\phi) - x_r] q_1[r\cos(\theta-\phi') - x_r'] \\ &= \frac{M}{\pi}\int_0^\pi d\phi \int_{-\infty}^{\infty} dx_r \left(\frac{1}{\overline{n}_\phi(x_r)}\right)\{q_1[r\cos(\theta-\phi) - x_r]\}^2 \\ &= \frac{M}{\pi}\int_0^\pi d\phi \left\{\left(\frac{1}{\overline{n}_\phi(x_r)}\right) * q_1^2(x_r)\right\}_{x_r = r\cos(\theta-\phi)}.\end{aligned} \tag{10.178}$$

Thus, to find the variance at point (r,θ) in the reconstruction, one must convolve the *reciprocal* of the *linear* photon density with the square of the filter function, back project, and sum (integrate) over all projection angles. The situation is reminiscent of the noise kernel [see (10.35)], but the quantity being convolved with q_1^2 is not the object or even its projection, but rather $1/\bar{n}_\phi(x_r)$.

As usual, we define an SNR by

$$\mathrm{SNR}(r,\theta) = \langle \hat{\mu}(r,\theta) \rangle / \sigma_{\hat{\mu}}(r,\theta). \tag{10.179}$$

The implications of this equation are developed in Sections 10.5.3 and 10.5.4.

The discrete formalism can be recovered by regarding the asterisk in (10.178) as denoting a discrete convolution, and replacing the integral over ϕ by a sum.

10.5.3 SNR for a Disk Object

We shall illustrate the use of (10.178) and (10.179) by calculating the SNR for a uniform disk object specified by

$$\mu(r,\theta) = \mu_0 \,\mathrm{circ}(r/R_{\mathrm{obj}}). \tag{10.180}$$

Because of the symmetry of the object, its mean projection is the same for all projection angles:

$$\langle \lambda_\phi(x_r) \rangle = \int_{-\infty}^{\infty} \mu(r,\theta)\,dy_r = 2\mu_0(R_{\mathrm{obj}}^2 - x_r^2)^{1/2}\,\mathrm{rect}(x_r/2R_{\mathrm{obj}}). \tag{10.181}$$

The mean linear photon density is given by

$$\bar{n}_\phi(x_r) = n_0 \exp[-2\mu_0(R_{\mathrm{obj}}^2 - x_r^2)^{1/2}\,\mathrm{rect}(x_r/2R_{\mathrm{obj}})]. \tag{10.182}$$

According to (10.178), the noise variance is given by

$$\sigma_{\hat{\mu}}^2(r,\theta) = \frac{M}{\pi n_0}\int_0^{\pi} d\phi \int_{-\infty}^{\infty} dx_r \exp[2\mu_0(R_{\mathrm{obj}}^2 - x_r^2)^{1/2}\mathrm{rect}(x_r/2R_{\mathrm{obj}})]$$
$$\cdot\, q_1^2[r\cos(\theta-\phi) - x_r]. \tag{10.183}$$

But $q_1^2(x_r)$ is an all-positive function that has appreciable value only near $x_r = 0$. [The sidelobes of $q_1^2(x_r)$ fall off as x_r^{-4}.] Therefore it is a good approximation to treat $q_1^2(x_r)$ as a delta function of appropriate weight, i.e.,

$$q_1^2(x_r) \approx \delta(x_r)\int_{-\infty}^{\infty} q_1^2(x_r')\,dx_r'. \tag{10.184}$$

With this approximation, (10.183) becomes

$$\sigma_{\hat{\mu}}^2(r,\theta) = \frac{M}{\pi n_0}\int_{-\infty}^{\infty} q_1^2(x_r')\,dx_r'$$
$$\cdot \int_0^{\pi} d\phi \exp\{2\mu_0[R_{\mathrm{obj}}^2 - r^2\cos^2(\theta-\phi)]^{1/2}\} \quad (r < R_{\mathrm{obj}}). \tag{10.185}$$

Rather than attempting to evaluate this integral in general, we shall be content with finding the variance at the center of the image, $r = 0$. The ϕ integral is then trivial, and we obtain

$$\sigma_{\hat{\mu}}^2(0,0) = \frac{M}{n_0}\left(\int_{-\infty}^{\infty} q_1^2(x_r')\,dx_r'\right)\exp(2\mu_0 R_{\text{obj}}). \tag{10.186}$$

The mean signal (the numerator of the SNR expression) is just the object convolved with the system PSF:

$$\langle \hat{\boldsymbol{\mu}}(r,\theta)\rangle = \mu(r,\theta) ** p(r,\theta), \tag{10.187}$$

where $p(r,\theta)$ is given by (7.42) as the summation image of $q_1(x_r)$. For the present discussion, we are concerned with the convolution in (10.187) evaluated at zero shift. If the disk radius R_{obj} is large compared to the system resolution, the convolution is given by

$$\langle \hat{\boldsymbol{\mu}}(0,0)\rangle = \mu_0 \int_{\infty} p(r,\theta) d^2 r = \mu_0, \tag{10.188}$$

where the last form is valid if $p(r,\theta)$ is normalized to unit area. We then have

$$\text{SNR}(0,0) = \frac{\mu_0}{\left[(M/n_0)\left(\int_{-\infty}^{\infty} q_1^2(x_r')\,dx_r'\right)\exp(2\mu_0 R_{\text{obj}})\right]^{1/2}}. \tag{10.189}$$

To be specific, we consider the abrupt-cutoff filter given by

$$Q_1(\xi_r) = \begin{cases} (\pi/M)|\xi_r| & \text{for} \quad |\xi| < \xi_m \\ 0 & \text{for} \quad |\xi| > \xi_m. \end{cases} \tag{10.190}$$

The integral in (10.189) may be evaluated by Parseval's rule (B.19) as

$$\int_{-\infty}^{\infty} [q_1(x_r')]^2\,dx_r' = \int_{-\infty}^{\infty} |Q_1(\xi_r)|^2\,d\xi_r = \left[\frac{\pi\xi_m^2}{M}\right]^2 \cdot \frac{2}{3\xi_m}. \tag{10.191}$$

The SNR at the center of the disk is thus

$$\text{SNR}(0,0) = (3/2\pi^2)^{1/2} \mu_0 \xi_m^{-3/2} [M n_0 \exp(-2\mu_0 R_{\text{obj}})]^{1/2}. \tag{10.192}$$

We can recast this result in terms of the spatial resolution δ, defined as usual as the FWHM of the PSF and given by $\delta = 0.70/\xi_m$, which leads to

$$\text{SNR}(0,0) = 0.665 \mu_0 \delta^{3/2} [M n_0 \exp(-2\mu_0 R_{\text{obj}})]^{1/2}. \tag{10.193}$$

Note that $n_0 \exp(-2\mu_0 R_{\text{obj}})$ is just the linear density of detected photons at the center of each projection, while $M n_0 \exp(-2\mu_0 R_{\text{obj}})$ is this quantity summed over all projections.

10.5.4 Dose, Resolution, and SNR

Equation (10.193) relates the SNR and resolution to the transmitted x-ray fluence. For practical purposes, it is more desirable to express the result in terms of the absorbed dose in rads. (See Appendix D for a discussion of radiation units.) Basically, 1 rad corresponds to 100 ergs of absorbed energy per gram of tissue.

A rigorous dose calculation is actually quite difficult. The main problem is relating the photon density, n_0 or h, to the absorbed dose. For photon energies of interest in diagnostic CT, the dominant attenuation mechanism is Compton scattering in which a small fraction ($\sim$10-20%) of the photon energy is transferred to an electron, while the rest is carried off by a scattered photon. This scattered photon could have several fates. It could be scattered again outside the layer of interest, it could be scattered back into the layer, it could be photoelectrically absorbed, or it could escape the body altogether. Accounting for all these processes analytically is not possible in general. The best approach would be a Monte Carlo calculation in which a computer is used to trace the fate of a large number of photons with random interactions. However, we shall be content to indicate the general nature of the problem by a simple calculation that should be valid for finding the dose at the center of a disk object when only a thin slab is irradiated (Barrett *et al.*, 1976). Specifically, the beam height Δz must satisfy $\mu_0 \Delta z \ll 1$.

The photon fluence (photons per unit area) at the center of the disk in each projection is given by

$$h_c = (\Delta z)^{-1}(n_0/\eta)\exp(-\mu_0 R_{\text{obj}}). \tag{10.194}$$

If the incident x-ray energy $\mathscr{E}_x$ were completely absorbed in each interaction, the dose at the center would be $\mu_0 h_c \mathscr{E}_x/\rho$, where ρ is the mass density of the object. However, only a fraction of the photon energy is transferred to the scattering electron. This fraction is given by μ_{en}/μ_0, where μ_{en}/ρ is the mass *energy* transfer coefficient (see Appendices C and D). This fraction of the energy is dissipated within the slab of interest if the range of the scattered electron is small compared to Δz, which is almost always the case. On the other hand, the rest of the energy, the part carried off by the scattered photon, is most likely *not* dissipated within the layer if $\mu_0 \Delta z \ll 1$, which is also usually valid in practice. Under these conditions, the dose for one projection is $(\mu_{\text{en}}/\mu_0)\mu_0 h_c \mathscr{E}_x/\rho$. For all M projections, the dose is M times as large and is given by

$$D = (\mu_{\text{en}}\mathscr{E}_x/\eta\rho\,\Delta z)Mn_0\exp(-\mu_0 R_{\text{obj}}). \tag{10.195}$$

Combining (10.193) and (10.195) yields

$$D = \frac{2.26\mu_{\text{en}}\mathscr{E}_x\exp(\mu_0 R_{\text{obj}})[\text{SNR}(0,0)]^2}{\eta\rho\,\Delta z\mu_0^2\delta^3}. \tag{10.196}$$

Note that $D \propto 1/\Delta z$, which is just a result of dose being defined on a per-unit-mass basis. If the same number of photons are directed through a thinner layer, the total absorbed energy remains the same but the energy per unit mass increases.

The dependence of dose on object size is a severe one: $D \propto \exp(\mu_0 R_{\text{obj}})$. As the object radius increases, the dose required to maintain constant resolution and SNR increases exponentially.

If the geometrical parameters and the x-ray energy remain constant, we have

$$D \propto \delta^{-3}(\text{SNR})^2. \tag{10.197}$$

Thus, if the SNR is to remain constant, the dose must vary as δ^{-3} as the resolution is varied. A twofold improvement in resolution can be obtained at the expense of an eightfold increase in dose. Furthermore, if we choose to vary the beam height Δz in proportion to δ, we have

$$D \propto (\Delta z)^{-1}\,\delta^{-3}(\text{SNR})^2 \propto \delta^{-4}(\text{SNR})^2, \tag{10.198}$$

which is again the ubiquitous fourth-power trade-off law.

We should emphasize that the results of this section were predicated on a continuous model for the projection data as expressed in (10.170) and (10.171). If the finite width Δx of the detectors cannot be neglected, then there is an additional contribution to δ, unrelated to the width of the filter function, and (10.197) or (10.198) no longer apply.

10.5.5 Effect of a Two-Dimensional ρ Filter: Autocorrelation Function and Wiener Spectrum of the Reconstruction

So far, the discussion of noise in computed tomography has been based on the convolution algorithm—one-dimensional filtering followed by back projection and summation as described in Section 7.2.6. We showed in Chapter 7 that the other analytic (noniterative) algorithms are equivalent to this one, so our results must apply to them also. It is instructive, however, to specifically examine the noise propagation in the filtered-summation-image algorithm (see Section 7.2.5) where the filtering occurs after back-projection and is therefore two dimensional (Riederer *et al.*, 1978).

An immediate difficulty with this analysis is that the noise at the input to the filter is not uncorrelated. As shown below, back-projection introduces correlations. Equation (10.9) and (10.10) are therefore not valid, and we must resort to the more general form (10.5).

From (7.22), the unfiltered summation image is given by

$$\mathbf{b}(\mathbf{r}) = \frac{M}{\pi}\int_0^{\pi} d\phi\, \boldsymbol{\lambda}_\phi[r\cos(\theta - \phi)], \tag{10.199}$$

where $\mathbf{r} = (r, \theta) = [x, y]$. The autocorrelation function for the zero-mean process $\Delta\mathbf{b}(\mathbf{r})$ is

$$R_{\Delta b}(\mathbf{r}, \mathbf{r}') = \left(\frac{M}{\pi}\right)^2 \int_0^\pi d\phi \int_0^\pi d\phi' \langle \Delta\boldsymbol{\lambda}_\phi[r\cos(\theta - \phi)] \cdot \Delta\boldsymbol{\lambda}_{\phi'}[r'\cos(\theta' - \phi')]\rangle, \tag{10.200}$$

where $\mathbf{r}' = (r', \theta')$. Use of (10.171) yields

$$R_{\Delta b}(\mathbf{r}, \mathbf{r}') = \frac{M}{\pi} \int_0^\pi d\phi \, \{\bar{n}_\phi[r\cos(\theta - \phi)]\}^{-1} \cdot \delta[r\cos(\theta - \phi) - r'\cos(\theta' - \phi)]. \tag{10.201}$$

If we define

$$\mathbf{L} = \mathbf{r}' - \mathbf{r}, \tag{10.202}$$

then, by the construction of Fig. 10.8, we see that the argument of the delta function in (10.201) is just $(\mathbf{L} \cdot \hat{\mathbf{x}}_r)$, where $\hat{\mathbf{x}}_r$ is a unit vector in the x_r direction. We can also write

$$\delta(\mathbf{L} \cdot \hat{\mathbf{x}}_r) = \delta[L\cos(\theta_L - \phi)], \tag{10.203}$$

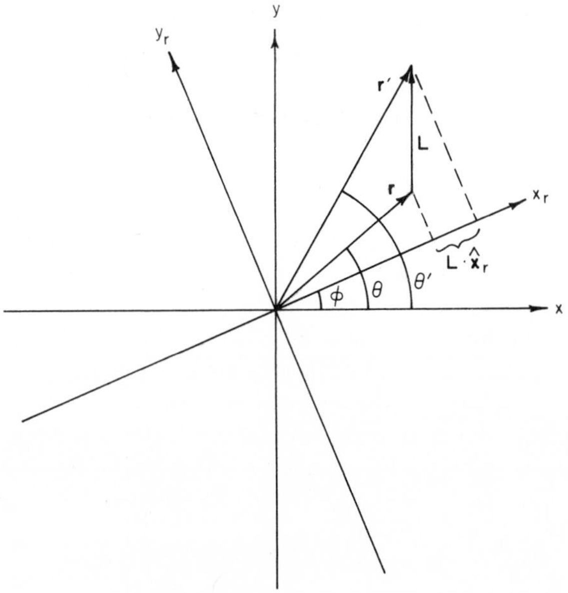

Fig. 10.8 Geometry needed in calculation of the autocorrelation function in a reconstructed CT image.

where $\mathbf{L} = (L, \theta_L)$. The remaining integral in (10.201) may now be performed with the aid of (A.23), yielding

$$R_{\Delta b}(\mathbf{r}, \mathbf{r} + \mathbf{L}) = (M/\pi L)\{\bar{n}_{\theta_L + \pi/2}[r\cos(\theta - \theta_L)]\}^{-1}. \tag{10.204}$$

This is the basic result we need to calculate either the autocorrelation function or the variance in the filtered image by means of (10.5). Note that only a single projection, the one at angle $\theta_L + \pi/2$, contributes to $R_{\Delta b}(\mathbf{r}, \mathbf{r} + \mathbf{L})$.

An interesting special case of (10.204) occurs for large, low-contrast objects for which

$$\bar{n}_\phi(x_r) \approx \bar{n} = \text{const.} \tag{10.205}$$

Then

$$R_{\Delta b}(\mathbf{r}, \mathbf{r} + \mathbf{L}) = M/(\pi \bar{n} L). \tag{10.206}$$

The statistics of the unfiltered summation image are thus stationary in this case, and we may write $R_{\Delta b}(\mathbf{r}, \mathbf{r} + \mathbf{L}) \equiv R_{\Delta b}(\mathbf{L})$. The power spectral density for $\Delta \mathbf{b}(\mathbf{r})$ is given by

$$S_{\Delta b}(\boldsymbol{\rho}) = \mathscr{F}_2\{R_{\Delta b}(\mathbf{L})\} = M/(\pi \bar{n} \rho), \tag{10.207}$$

since $\mathscr{F}_2\{1/L\} = 1/\rho$.

If we now filter $b(\mathbf{r})$ with a two-dimensional filter of impulse response $q_2(\mathbf{r})$, we obtain a reasonable estimate of $\mu(\mathbf{r})$, i.e.,

$$\hat{\mu}(\mathbf{r}) = \mathbf{b}(\mathbf{r}) ** q_2(\mathbf{r}). \tag{10.208}$$

The power spectral density of the zero-mean process $\Delta\hat{\mu}(\mathbf{r})$ is given by [cf. (3.200)]

$$S_{\Delta\hat{\mu}}(\boldsymbol{\rho}) = |Q_2(\boldsymbol{\rho})|^2 S_{\Delta b}(\boldsymbol{\rho}) = (\pi M/\bar{n})\rho\,|A_2(\boldsymbol{\rho})|^2, \tag{10.209}$$

where, by (7.31),

$$Q_2(\boldsymbol{\rho}) = \pi\rho A_2(\rho), \tag{10.210}$$

with $A_2(\boldsymbol{\rho})$ being the apodizing function.

The important conclusion here is that the noise in the filtered image is not white, but is concentrated at high frequencies. In contrast, the noise in the *unfiltered* image is concentrated at low frequencies since $S_{\Delta b}(\boldsymbol{\rho}) \propto (1/\rho)$. The factor of ρ^2 in $|Q_2(\boldsymbol{\rho})|^2$ more than compensates for the $(1/\rho)$ in $S_{\Delta b}(\boldsymbol{\rho})$.

Since $A_2(\boldsymbol{\rho})$ is also the MTF of the system if the resolution loss due to the finite detector size is unimportant, a measurement of the Wiener spectrum of the reconstruction can be used to determine the MTF (or vice versa).

10.5.6 Normalization Errors

We now return to a point glossed over in Section 10.5.1, viz., the normalizing constant N_0 in (10.153) (or, equivalently, n_0 in the continuous formulation). In any real CT system, N_0 is the result of a measurement and is hence a random variable ($\mathbf{N}_0$). We must account for the fluctuations of $\mathbf{N}_0$ in the statistical description of the projection data.

We assume that an auxiliary detector is used to continuously monitor the output of the x-ray source. The various $\mathbf{N}_{lj}$ can be measured sequentially, as in a translate–rotate system, or some subset of them can be measured simultaneously as in a fan–beam system. In either case, for each measurement $\mathbf{N}_{lj}$ there is a corresponding simultaneous measurement of $\mathbf{N}_0$, which we shall denote by $\mathbf{N}_{0lj}$, that can be used for normalization. The projection for the lth angle and the jth detector is the random variable $\boldsymbol{\lambda}_{lj}$, now given by [cf. (10.153)]

$$\boldsymbol{\lambda}_{lj} = -\ln(\mathbf{N}_{lj}/\mathbf{N}_{0lj}). \tag{10.211}$$

We expect that this normalization will be successful in eliminating any excess (non-Poisson) fluctuations of the source. To demonstrate this point, we shall retrace the derivation of $\langle \Delta\boldsymbol{\lambda}_{lj} \Delta\boldsymbol{\lambda}_{l'j'} \rangle$ in Section 10.5.1, making use of results from Section 3.4.

The x-ray source, which now is *not* assumed to obey Poisson statistics, emits $\mathbf{N}_{slj}$ photons during the measurement time in which $\mathbf{N}_{0lj}$ and $\mathbf{N}_{lj}$ are measured. The average value of $\mathbf{N}_{slj}$ is $\bar{N}_s$ and its variance is $\sigma^2_{N_s}$. We do not need subscripts l and j on $\bar{N}_s$ and $\sigma^2_{N_s}$ if the source statistics are temporally stationary. But the same token, we may assume that $\langle \mathbf{N}_{0lj} \rangle = \bar{N}_0$, again independent of l and j.

On the average, a fraction f_0 of the emitted photons are detected by the auxiliary detector and a fraction f_{lj} are detected by the primary detector. Hence

$$\bar{N}_{lj} = f_{lj}\bar{N}_s; \qquad \bar{N}_0 = f_0\bar{N}_s. \tag{10.212}$$

If $\bar{N}_{lj} \gg 1$ and $\bar{N}_0 \gg 1$, then

$$\langle \boldsymbol{\lambda}_{lj} \rangle \approx -\ln(\bar{N}_{lj}/\bar{N}_0), \tag{10.213}$$

an approximation that was justified in Section 10.5.1. The zero-mean process $\Delta\boldsymbol{\lambda}_{lj}$ is given by

$$\Delta\boldsymbol{\lambda}_{lj} = -\frac{\Delta\mathbf{N}_{lj}}{\bar{N}_{lj}} + \frac{\Delta\mathbf{N}_{0lj}}{\bar{N}_0} + \cdots. \tag{10.214}$$

Higher-order terms in (10.214) are negligible just as they were in Section 10.5.1.

The autocorrelation of $\Delta\boldsymbol{\lambda}_{lj}$ is given by

$$\langle \Delta\boldsymbol{\lambda}_{lj}\Delta\boldsymbol{\lambda}_{l'j'}\rangle = \frac{\langle \Delta\mathbf{N}_{lj}\Delta\mathbf{N}_{l'j'}\rangle}{\bar{N}_{lj}\bar{N}_{l'j'}} + \frac{\langle \Delta\mathbf{N}_{0lj}\Delta\mathbf{N}_{0l'j'}\rangle}{\bar{N}_0^2} - \frac{\langle \Delta\mathbf{N}_{lj}\Delta\mathbf{N}_{0l'j'}\rangle}{\bar{N}_{lj}\bar{N}_0} - \frac{\langle \Delta\mathbf{N}_{l'j'}\Delta\mathbf{N}_{0lj}\rangle}{\bar{N}_{l'j'}\bar{N}_0}. \tag{10.215}$$

At this point, we must distinguish two cases, depending on how strongly correlated $\Delta\mathbf{N}_{0lj}$ and $\Delta\mathbf{N}_{0l'j'}$ are. At one extreme, they might be the same quantity, as when the measurements of $\mathbf{N}_{lj}$ and $\mathbf{N}_{l'j'}$ are taken simultaneously. Then even if $j \neq j'$ or $l \neq l'$, the same measurement of $\mathbf{N}_0$ is used to normalize both $\mathbf{N}_{lj}$ and $\mathbf{N}_{l'j'}$. The opposite extreme is when the measurements of $\mathbf{N}_{0lj}$ and $\mathbf{N}_{0l'j'}$ are taken far enough apart in time that there is no correlation of the source fluctuations in the two measurements. In the latter case we have at once that $\langle \Delta\boldsymbol{\lambda}_{lj}\Delta\boldsymbol{\lambda}_{l'j'}\rangle = 0$, just as we had earlier in (10.163). The more interesting case is the former one where $\Delta\mathbf{N}_{0lj}$ and $\Delta\mathbf{N}_{0l'j'}$ are identical, or at least very highly correlated. In that case, (10.215) becomes

$$\langle \Delta\boldsymbol{\lambda}_{lj}\Delta\boldsymbol{\lambda}_{l'j'}\rangle = \frac{\langle \Delta\mathbf{N}_{lj}\Delta\mathbf{N}_{l'j'}\rangle}{\bar{N}_{lj}\bar{N}_{l'j'}} + \frac{\sigma_{N0}^2}{\bar{N}_0^2} - \frac{\langle \Delta\mathbf{N}_{lj}\Delta\mathbf{N}_{0}\rangle}{\bar{N}_{lj}\bar{N}_0} - \frac{\langle \Delta\mathbf{N}_{l'j'}\Delta\mathbf{N}_{0}\rangle}{\bar{N}_{l'j'}\bar{N}_0}, \tag{10.216}$$

where the subscripts lj and $l'j'$ are no longer necessary on $\mathbf{N}_0$ since all four measurements ($\mathbf{N}_{lj}$, $\mathbf{N}_{l'j'}$, $\mathbf{N}_{0lj}$, and $\mathbf{N}_{0l'j'}$) are essentially simultaneous.

The expectation values in (10.216) may be evaluated in terms of properties of the source by use of (3.190) and (3.174), which give

$$\begin{aligned} \langle \Delta\mathbf{N}_{lj}\Delta\mathbf{N}_{l'j'}\rangle &= f_{lj}f_{l'j'}(\sigma_{N_s}^2 - \bar{N}_s) \qquad \text{if} \quad l \neq l' \quad \text{or} \quad j \neq j', \\ \langle \Delta\mathbf{N}_{lj}\Delta\mathbf{N}_{0}\rangle &= f_{lj}f_0(\sigma_{N_s}^2 - \bar{N}_s), \\ \sigma_{N0}^2 &= \bar{N}_0 + f_0^2(\sigma_{N_s}^2 - \bar{N}_s). \end{aligned} \tag{10.217}$$

Combining (10.212), (10.216), (10.217), and a dollop of algebra then shows that

$$\langle \Delta\boldsymbol{\lambda}_{lj}\Delta\boldsymbol{\lambda}_{l'j'}\rangle = \bar{N}_0^{-1} \qquad \text{if} \quad l \neq l' \quad \text{or} \quad j \neq j'. \tag{10.218}$$

In other words, in the limit of large $\bar{N}_0$, the different projections are independent in spite of the fluctuations of the source. (It is not difficult to have $\bar{N}_0$ large compared to the $\bar{N}_{lj}$ since the radiation reaching the reference detector is not attenuated by passing through the patient.) Without normalization the projections would not be independent, as can be seen from (3.190). But with proper normalization, any source is as good as a stable, Poisson one.

We still must consider the case where $l = l'$ *and* $j = j'$. In other words we must determine the variance of $\boldsymbol{\lambda}_{lj}$. In this case, (10.216) reads

$$\langle(\Delta\boldsymbol{\lambda}_{lj})^2\rangle = \frac{\langle(\Delta\mathbf{N}_{lj})^2\rangle}{\bar{N}_{lj}^2} + \frac{\sigma_{N_0}^2}{\bar{N}_0^2} - \frac{2\langle\Delta\mathbf{N}_{lj}\,\Delta\mathbf{N}_0\rangle}{\bar{N}_{lj}\bar{N}_0}, \tag{10.219}$$

which, by use of (10.217), (10.212), and (3.174) becomes

$$\langle(\Delta\boldsymbol{\lambda}_{lj})^2\rangle = 1/\bar{N}_{lj} + 1/\bar{N}_0. \tag{10.220}$$

Comparing this equation to our previous result, (10.164) or (10.165), we see that normalization has introduced the new term $1/\bar{N}_0$. This term results from *the Poisson part* of the fluctuations in $\mathbf{N}_s$. The non-Poisson part $\sigma_{N_s}^2 - \bar{N}_s$ fluctuates the same way for both $\mathbf{N}_0$ and $\mathbf{N}_{lj}$ and cancels out of their ratio. However, as discussed in Section 3.4.7, if the source were pure Poisson, $\mathbf{N}_0$ and $\mathbf{N}_{lj}$ would be independent Poisson random variables and (10.220) would follow easily.

Clearly, if $\bar{N}_0 \gg \bar{N}_{lj}$, the new term is negligible.

10.6 CODED APERTURES

We have actually already solved the problem of noise in coded-aperture imaging. The general equations (10.33), (10.34), and (10.37), which express the signal and noise in terms of the object, the overall PSF, and the noise kernel, are just as valid for coded apertures as for pinholes. However, some of the subsequent approximations used in pinhole imaging do not often apply in the coded-aperture case. In particular, we frequently assumed, as in (10.41), that the noise kernel was strongly peaked compared to the object and could be approximated by a delta function. This approximation is almost never valid with coded apertures where the aperture function $g(\mathbf{r})$, the filter function $p_f(\mathbf{r})$, and the noise kernel $k(\mathbf{r})$ are all very broad functions. The large spatial extent of the noise kernel allows distant object points to contribute to the noise at the reconstructed image of a given object point. The noise in the image is decidedly nonlocal.

Although many different aperture codes and decoding schemes have been proposed in the literature, the same basic principles apply to all of them. There is, however, a qualitative difference between filled and dilute apertures as defined in Section 8.1.2. Therefore, we shall illustrate the noise properties of coded-aperture systems by discussing one dilute aperture—the annulus—and one filled aperture—the uniformly redundant array (Simpson, 1978; Simpson and Barrett, 1980).

10.6.1 SNR for a Dilute Aperture—The Annulus

Figure 10.9a shows the coded image for an annular coded aperture and a point source. Suppose this image is to be decoded by matched filtering or template matching as described in Section 8.2.2. The template is an annulus identical in scale to the annular shadow. When it is exactly centered over the shadow, all N recorded photons are visible through the template. For this one point in the reconstructed image, the noise must be the same as if the detector itself were shaped like an annulus. Therefore the SNR at this point is just $\sqrt{N}$.

This result is quite general. For *any* binary aperture [where $g(\mathbf{r}')$ can be only zero or one] and matched-filter decoding, the peak SNR for a point object is always the square root of the number of recorded photons. Hence, if the coded aperture has an open area of $\mathscr{A}_{ca}$ it will collect $\mathscr{A}_{ca}/\mathscr{A}_{ph}$ times as

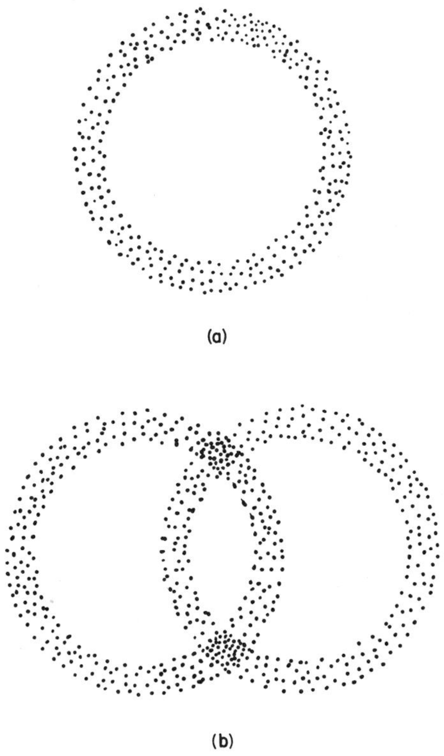

Fig. 10.9 (a) Illustration of a coded image obtained with a single point source and an annular coded aperture. Each dot represents a detected gamma ray. (b) Same, except that two point sources are present.

many photons as a pinhole of area $\mathscr{A}_{\text{ph}}$ in the same plane, and will have an SNR that is better by a factor of $(\mathscr{A}_{\text{ca}}/\mathscr{A}_{\text{ph}})^{1/2}$.

We must emphasize that this conclusion holds only for a single point object. In Fig. 10.9b we show a coded image when two point objects are present. Now when the template is centered over one of the annular shadows, it picks up not only the photons from the point source that produced that shadow, but also some of the photons from the other point, namely the photons in the region where the two shadows overlap. The total number of photons viewed through the template is now N', which is greater than N. The noise variance is thus increased by the presence of the second source, and the SNR is reduced. As more and more points are added to the source, the SNR advantage for the coded aperture progressively diminishes and eventually becomes a net disadvantage.

To make this discussion more quantitative, we shall calculate the noise kernel. For this purpose, let us assume that the decoding is carried out not by matched filtering alone, which we know from Section 8.2.2 to give poor imagery, but by matched filtering followed by ρ filtering. The overall filter function $p_{\text{f}}(\mathbf{r}'')$ is given by

$$p_{\text{f}}(\mathbf{r}'') = q_{\text{ann}}(\mathbf{r}'') ** \mathscr{F}_2^{-1}\{\rho'' A(\rho'')\}, \qquad (10.221)$$

where $q_{\text{ann}}(\mathbf{r}'')$ is the annular template or matched filter given by (8.21). In general, this filter function must be evaluated numerically (Simpson, 1978). An example is shown in Fig. 8.17.

However, it is very useful to have an analytic expression for the SNR, even if it is only approximate, in order to identify trends and trade-offs. One way to accomplish this goal is to recognize from Fig. 8.17 that $[p_{\text{f}}(\mathbf{r}'')]^2$ is rather like an annulus itself, having appreciable value only when $r'' \approx \bar{r}''$, where $\bar{r}'' \equiv \bar{r}'/a$. Therefore, we may approximate p_{f}^2 by a ring delta function,

$$[p_{\text{f}}(\mathbf{r}'')]^2 \approx \alpha\, \delta(r'' - \bar{r}''), \qquad (10.222)$$

where, as usual, $r'' = |\mathbf{r}''|$. The weight α must be adjusted so that both sides of (10.222) have the same area integral, i.e.,

$$\int_\infty [p_{\text{f}}(\mathbf{r}'')]^2\, d^2r'' = \int_\infty \alpha\, \delta(r'' - \bar{r}'')\, d^2r''$$
$$= 2\pi\alpha \int_0^\infty \delta(r'' - \bar{r}'') r''\, dr'' = 2\pi\alpha\bar{r}''. \qquad (10.223)$$

The integral of p_{f}^2 may be found by use of Parseval's theorem (B.19):

$$\int_\infty [p_{\text{f}}(\mathbf{r}'')]^2\, d^2r'' = \int_\infty [P_{\text{f}}(\boldsymbol{\rho}'')]^2\, d^2\rho''$$
$$= 2\pi \int_0^\infty [Q_{\text{ann}}(\boldsymbol{\rho}'')\rho'' A(\rho'')]^2 \rho''\, d\rho''. \qquad (10.224)$$

If we use a ring delta function for $q_{\text{ann}}(\mathbf{r}'')$, its Fourier transform is, by (8.12), (8.19), and (8.21),

$$Q_{\text{ann}}(\boldsymbol{\rho}'') = J_0(2\pi\rho''\bar{r}''). \tag{10.225}$$

If we further approximate the Bessel function by (8.33) and take $A(\rho'') = \text{rect}(\rho''/2\rho''_m)$, we have

$$\begin{aligned}\int_\infty [p_f(r'')]^2\, d^2r'' &\approx \frac{2}{\pi\bar{r}''}\int_0^{\rho''_m} \cos^2\left(2\pi\rho''\bar{r} - \frac{\pi}{4}\right)\rho''^2\, d\rho'' \\ &\approx \rho_m''^3/3\pi\bar{r}''.\end{aligned} \tag{10.226}$$

The easiest way to see that the last step is valid is to replace the rapidly oscillating $\cos^2$ factor by its average value of $\frac{1}{2}$. Combining (10.222), (10.223), and (10.226) yields

$$[p_f(\mathbf{r}'')]^2 \approx (\rho_m''^3/6\pi^2\bar{r}''^2)\,\delta(r'' - \bar{r}''). \tag{10.227}$$

From (8.6), (8.12), and (10.35), the noise kernel is now given by

$$\tilde{k}(\mathbf{r}'') = (a/b)^2 C(\rho_m''^3/6\pi^2\bar{r}''^2)(\Delta r'/a)\;\delta(r'' - \bar{r}'') ** \delta(r'' - \bar{r}''), \tag{10.228}$$

where we have assumed that the detector is ideal so that $d(\mathbf{r}'') = \delta(\mathbf{r}'')$. With these approximations, $\tilde{k}(\mathbf{r}'')$ is proportional to the autocorrelation of a ring delta function, which is evaluated in Appendix A and plotted in Fig. 8.9. By use of (A.46), we may write

$$\tilde{k}(\mathbf{r}'') = (a/b)^2 C(\rho_m''^3/6\pi^2\bar{r}''^2)(\Delta r'/a)\cdot\frac{4\bar{r}''^2}{r''[4(\bar{r}'')^2 - (r'')^2]^{1/2}}, \qquad (r'' < \bar{r}''). \tag{10.229}$$

We shall now use this noise kernel to evaluate the SNR for a uniform disk object of radius R_{obj} as in (10.15). We assume that R_{obj} is larger than the width of the PSF, but much smaller than $\bar{r}'/b$ so that the disk can be properly imaged without any degradation due to the glitch (see Sections 8.2.2 and 8.2.3). Furthermore, we shall consider only the SNR at the center of the reconstruction, which is actually a worst case since the noise is highest at that point.

The noise variance for this object is given by [cf. (10.33)]

$$\begin{aligned}\sigma_{\hat{h}\dagger\dagger}^2(\mathbf{r}'' = 0) &= [\tilde{k}(\mathbf{r}) ** \tilde{f}(\mathbf{r})]_{\mathbf{r}''=0} \\ &= f_0 2\pi\int_0^{R''_{\text{obj}}} \tilde{k}(r'')r''\, dr'',\end{aligned} \tag{10.230}$$

where the double dagger on $h^{\dagger\dagger}$ indicates that both correlation decoding and ρ filtering have been performed [cf. (8.35)]. If R''_{obj} (or bR_{obj}/a) is small compared to $\bar{r}''$ (or $\bar{r}'/a$), then the square-root factor in the denominator of (10.229) may be approximated by $2\bar{r}''$, so that $\tilde{k}(\mathbf{r}'') = \text{const}/r''$. Then (10.230) becomes

$$\sigma^2_{\hat{h}\dagger\dagger}(0) = (a/b)^2 C(\rho''^3_m/6\pi^2\bar{r}'')(\Delta r'')4\pi f_0 R''_{\text{obj}}, \tag{10.231}$$

where $\Delta r'' = \Delta r'/a$. The important feature of this result is that *the noise variance increases linearly with the radius of the object*. Very large objects generate a lot of noise in the reconstruction.

The signal part of the SNR equation is given by [cf. (10.34)]

$$\begin{aligned} h^{\dagger\dagger}(0) &= [\tilde{p}_{\text{rfa}}(\mathbf{r}'') ** \tilde{f}(\mathbf{r}'')]_{\mathbf{r}''=0} \\ &= 2\pi f_0 \int_0^{R''_{\text{obj}}} \tilde{p}_{\text{rfa}}(\mathbf{r}'')r''\,dr'', \end{aligned} \tag{10.232}$$

where, by comparison with (10.36) and (10.221),

$$\begin{aligned} \tilde{p}_{\text{rfa}}(\mathbf{r}'') &= (a/b)^2 C p_{\text{f}}(\mathbf{r}'') ** \tilde{g}_{\text{ann}}(\mathbf{r}'') \\ &= (a/b)^2 C[2\pi r'\,\Delta r'/a^2]^{-1}\tilde{g}_{\text{ann}}(\mathbf{r}'') ** \tilde{g}_{\text{ann}}(\mathbf{r}'') ** \mathscr{F}_2^{-1}\{\rho'' A(\rho'')\}. \end{aligned} \tag{10.233}$$

Basically, the integral in (10.232) extends over the central core of the PSF, excluding the glitch region if R''_{obj} is small enough for glitch-free imaging. Excluding the glitch is equivalent to replacing the $\cos^2$ factor in (8.34) by $\frac{1}{2}$. With this approximation, the integral in (10.232) can be extended to infinity and evaluated by means of the central ordinate theorem (B.96). We find

$$\begin{aligned} 2\pi \int_0^\infty \tilde{p}_{\text{rfa}}(\mathbf{r}'')r''\,dr'' &= \left(\frac{a}{b}\right)^2 C[2\pi\bar{r}''\,\Delta r'']^{-1}[|\tilde{G}_{\text{ann}}(\boldsymbol{\rho}'')|^2\rho'' A(\rho'')]_{\rho''=0} \\ &\approx (a/b)^2 C\,\Delta r''/\pi, \end{aligned} \tag{10.234}$$

where the last step holds *only* in the approximation of excluding the glitch. If the glitch is included, the integral of $\tilde{p}_{\text{rfa}}$ vanishes identically since the filter function has zero value at $\rho'' = 0$.

The SNR at the center of the image is now given by

$$\text{SNR}_{\text{ann}}(0) = \frac{[(a/b)^2 C\bar{r}''\,\Delta r'' f_0]^{1/2}}{[\frac{2}{3}\pi(\rho''_m)^3 R''_{\text{obj}}]^{1/2}}. \tag{10.235}$$

It is interesting to compare this equation to the corresponding result for a pinhole. In order to make a fair comparison, both systems should give the same resolution δ'' (FWHM of the PSF measured in the r'' plane). From (10.192) $\delta'' = 0.70/\rho''_m$ for the abrupt-cutoff filter used with the annulus, while for the pinhole $\delta'' \approx d''_{\text{ph}} \approx d''_{\text{f}}$. Thus (10.61) may be rewritten

$$[\text{SNR}_{\text{ph}}(0)]^2 = (a/b)^2 C f_0 \mathscr{A}''_{\text{ph}}(\pi\delta''^2/4), \tag{10.236}$$

where $\mathscr{A}''_{\text{ph}} = \pi d''^2_{\text{ph}}/4$ is the projected area of the pinhole. By the same token,

$$[\text{SNR}_{\text{ann}}(0)]^2 = 0.56\left(\frac{a}{b}\right)^2 C f_0 \mathscr{A}''_{\text{ann}} \frac{\pi\delta''^2}{4}\frac{\delta''}{2R''_{\text{obj}}}, \tag{10.237}$$

where $\mathscr{A}''_{\text{ann}} = 2\pi\bar{r}''\,\Delta r''$ is the projected area of the annulus. Therefore

$$\frac{[\text{SNR}_{\text{ann}}(0)]^2}{[\text{SNR}_{\text{ph}}(0)]^2} = \frac{0.56\mathscr{A}''_{\text{ann}}}{\mathscr{A}''_{\text{ph}}} \cdot \frac{\delta''}{2R''_{\text{obj}}}. \tag{10.238}$$

The factor $\mathscr{A}''_{\text{ann}}/\mathscr{A}''_{\text{ph}}$ is the relative geometric efficiency of the annulus. The annulus will collect more photons by this factor than will a pinhole of the same resolution, spacings (s_1 and s_2), and exposure time. The factor $\delta''/2R''_{\text{obj}}$ is the square root of the area of one resolution cell divided by the area of the object, i.e.,

$$\frac{\delta''}{2R''_{\text{obj}}} = \left(\frac{\pi\delta''^2/4}{\pi R''^2_{\text{obj}}}\right)^{1/2} = \left(\frac{\mathscr{A}''_{\text{rc}}}{\mathscr{A}''_{\text{obj}}}\right)^{1/2}. \tag{10.239}$$

Thus, since $\text{SNR}_{\text{ann}}(0) \propto \mathscr{A}''^{-1/4}_{\text{obj}}$, the advantage of the annulus steadily decreases as $\mathscr{A}_{\text{obj}}$ increases. The situation is illustrated in Fig. 10.10, which is based on a numerical evaluation of the noise kernel and PSF (Simpson,

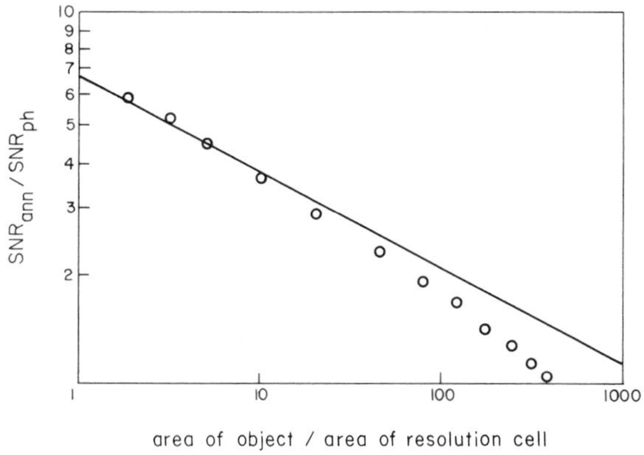

Fig. 10.10 Relative SNR for an annulus compared to a pinhole. The solid line is a plot of Eq. (10.238), while the points are the result of a numerical calculation carried out by Simpson (1978). For this comparison, $\mathscr{A}''_{\text{ann}}/\mathscr{A}''_{\text{ph}} = 80$.

1978) rather than the elaborately nested approximations used in this section. Perhaps surprisingly, (10.238) turns out to be in good accord with these numerical results, at least for values of $\mathscr{A}''_{\text{obj}}/\mathscr{A}''_{\text{rc}}$ up to about 100. For larger objects, (10.238) is somewhat high, primarily because of the approximation that $\tilde{k}(\mathbf{r}'') \propto 1/r''$, which appeared in (10.231). Use of the more exact expression (10.229) for $\tilde{k}(\mathbf{r}'')$ would predict a smaller SNR for large objects.

10.6.2 SNR for a Filled Aperture—The Uniformly Redundant Array

In the discussion of the uniformly redundant array (URA) in Section 8.4.3, we noted that the decoding function should be a cyclically repeated version of the code. As an example, consider the seven-element one-dimensional code specified by the sequence

$$1010011. \tag{10.240}$$

The cyclically repeated version of this sequence is

$$\ldots 101001110100111010011 \ldots, \tag{10.241}$$

and the cross correlation of the code and the decoding function is

$$\ldots 2242222224222222422 \ldots . \tag{10.242}$$

To get rid of the background level of 2, we may modify the decoding function to a bipolar sequence by replacing every 0 with -1, yielding

$$\ldots 1\bar{1}1\bar{1}\bar{1}111\bar{1}1\bar{1}\bar{1}111\bar{1}1\bar{1}\bar{1}11 \ldots, \tag{10.243}$$

where $\bar{1} \equiv -1$. The cross correlation of this new decoding function with the original code is

$$\ldots 0040000004000000400 \ldots . \tag{10.244}$$

Similar considerations apply in two dimensions. As illustrated in Fig. 8.42, the basic two-dimensional code is a matrix of square subapertures, each being either transparent or opaque according to the code. The two-dimensional bipolar decoding function $p_{\text{f}}(\mathbf{r}'')$ is obtained by cyclically repeating the basic code in all directions and assigning a weight $+1$ to initially transparent subapertures and -1 to opaque ones.

In terms of continuous variables, the scaled aperture function for a code with $L_x \times L_y$ elements is

$$\tilde{g}_{\text{URA}}(\mathbf{r}'') = \sum_{j=1}^{L_x} \sum_{k=1}^{L_y} \beta_{jk} \operatorname{rect}\left(\frac{x'' - j\varepsilon''}{\varepsilon''}\right) \operatorname{rect}\left(\frac{y'' - k\varepsilon''}{\varepsilon''}\right), \tag{10.245}$$

where ε'' is the length of the side of each subaperture as projected to the image plane, and $\beta_{jk} = 0$ or 1 according to the code. The indefinitely repeated decoding function is given by

$$p_f(r'') = \sum_{m=-\infty}^{\infty} \sum_{n=-\infty}^{\infty} \sum_{j=1}^{L_x} \sum_{k=1}^{L_y} (2\beta_{jk} - 1) \cdot \operatorname{rect}\left(\frac{x'' - j\varepsilon'' - mL_x\varepsilon''}{\varepsilon''}\right) \operatorname{rect}\left(\frac{y'' - k\varepsilon'' - nL_y\varepsilon''}{\varepsilon''}\right), \quad (10.246)$$

where $2\beta_{jk} - 1 = \pm 1$.

The PSF is proportional to the autocorrelation of $\tilde{g}_{\mathrm{URA}}(\mathbf{r}'')$ and $p_f(\mathbf{r}'')$. If the object is sufficiently small that we may ignore the various replicas of the central core, we have

$$\tilde{g}_{\mathrm{URA}}(\mathbf{r}'') ** p_f(\mathbf{r}'') = M\tilde{g}_{\mathrm{sa}}(\mathbf{r}'') ** \tilde{g}_{\mathrm{sa}}(\mathbf{r}''), \quad (10.247)$$

where M is the number of transparent subapertures in the code (in practice, $M \approx \frac{1}{2}L_x L_y$), and $\tilde{g}_{\mathrm{sa}}(\mathbf{r}'')$ is the scaled transmission function for each subaperture,

$$\tilde{g}_{\mathrm{sa}}(\mathbf{r}'') = \operatorname{rect}(\mathbf{r}''/\varepsilon''). \quad (10.248)$$

The noise kernel for this particular code and decoding function is very simple since $[p_f(\mathbf{r}'')]^2 = 1$ everywhere. Therefore, from (10.34),

$$\begin{aligned} \tilde{k}(\mathbf{r}'') &= (a/b)^2 C[p_f(\mathbf{r}'')]^2 ** \tilde{g}(\mathbf{r}'') \\ &= \left(\frac{a}{b}\right)^2 C \int_\infty d^2r''\, \tilde{g}(\mathbf{r}'') \\ &= (a/b)^2 CM(\varepsilon'')^2 = \text{const.} \end{aligned} \quad (10.249)$$

For a uniform object with emission density f_0 and projected area $\mathscr{A}''_{\mathrm{obj}}$, we have

$$\begin{aligned} \sigma^2_{\tilde{h}^\dagger}(\mathbf{r}'') &= \tilde{k}(\mathbf{r}'') ** \tilde{f}(\mathbf{r}'') \\ &= \left(\frac{a}{b}\right)^2 CM(\varepsilon'')^2 \int_\infty \tilde{f}(\mathbf{r}'')\, d^2r'' \\ &= \left(\frac{a}{b}\right)^2 CM(\varepsilon'')^2 \mathscr{A}''_{\mathrm{obj}} f_0. \end{aligned} \quad (10.250)$$

The mean signal for this object is

$$\begin{aligned} h^\dagger(\mathbf{r}'') &= (a/b)^2 C p_f(\mathbf{r}'') ** \tilde{g}(\mathbf{r}'') ** \tilde{f}(\mathbf{r}'') \\ &= (a/b)^2 CM(\varepsilon'')^2 f_0, \end{aligned} \quad (10.251)$$

where we have assumed that $\mathscr{A}''_{\text{obj}} > \varepsilon''^2$ and have used the fact that $\int_\infty [\tilde{g}_{\text{sa}}(\mathbf{r}'') ** \tilde{g}_{\text{sa}}(\mathbf{r}'')]\, d^2r'' = \varepsilon''^2$. Equation (10.251) is valid for all points except those within ε'' of the boundary of $\tilde{f}(\mathbf{r}'')$, while (10.250) is valid for all $\mathbf{r}''$.

Combining (10.250) and (10.251), we find for the SNR within the image of the disk

$$[\text{SNR}_{\text{URA}}(\mathbf{r}'')]^2 = (a/b)^2 C(\varepsilon'')^2 M f_0 / \mathscr{A}''_{\text{obj}}. \tag{10.252}$$

Comparing this result to the corresponding result for a pinhole with $\pi(\delta'')^2/4 = (\varepsilon'')^2$ (which is almost fair), we see from (10.235) that

$$\left[\frac{\text{SNR}_{\text{URA}}}{\text{SNR}_{\text{ph}}}\right]^2 = M\mathscr{A}''_{\text{ph}}/\mathscr{A}''_{\text{obj}}. \tag{10.253}$$

Just as with the dilute aperture, the SNR advantage for the filled aperture, the URA, decreases as the object size is increased. The initial advantage for a filled aperture is larger since M is very large, but the advantage decreases faster since (10.252) varies as $1/\mathscr{A}''_{\text{obj}}$, while its counterpart for a dilute aperture, (10.238), varies only as $(1/\mathscr{A}''_{\text{obj}})^{1/2}$.

As a final note, the dependence indicated in (10.253) applies whenever $\tilde{k}(\mathbf{r}'')$ is constant or nearly so, which is almost always a good approximation for a filled aperture. For example, the zone plate with optical decoding has $p_f(\mathbf{r}'') \propto \exp(i\alpha r''^2)$, and hence $|p_f(\mathbf{r}'')|^2 \equiv 1$ and $\tilde{k}(\mathbf{r}'') \equiv \text{const}$ (Barrett and DeMeester, 1974).

10.7 NOISE AND IMAGE QUALITY

The process by which a physician perceives a blurred, noisy image and arrives at a diagnosis is an enormously complicated one. Broadly speaking, the steps in the process are *detection*, *localization*, and *classification*. For simple detection of a lesion, the system resolution must be just good enough to barely resolve the lesion, but the SNR should be as large as possible. Localization of the lesion with respect to other anatomical structures and classification of it as either a normal structure or some particular pathology places an increased burden on the resolution.

The psychology of localization and classification is relatively poorly understood and will not be pursued here. However, a great deal of work has been done on the detection problem and how it relates to the resolution and SNR of the imaging system. This work, which falls within a branch of psychology known as psychophysics (Green and Swets, 1974), will be briefly reviewed in this section.

10.7.1 SNR and Detectability

DeVries (1943) was apparently the first to postulate that there is an intimate relationship between an observer's ability to detect an abnormality in an image and the SNR associated with that abnormality. This conjecture was verified by Rose (1948a,b) and many workers since then. A fairly recent review is found in the volume edited by Biberman (1973). In particular, Rosell and Willson (1973) present in that volume an enormous amount of data relating detectability to SNR.

To illustrate the general outcome of such studies, consider a simple detection task in nuclear imaging. A scintillation camera viewing a uniform flood source produces an image with a mean count density of $\bar{h}$ counts per unit area. There may or may not be a disk area of diameter D and reduced count density $\bar{h} - \Delta h$ within the field. A series of such images is presented to a number of observers whose ability to detect the disk is studied as a function of $\bar{h}$, Δh, and D. Studies of this kind usually show that the disk is detectable some reasonable percentage of the time if

$$\frac{\Delta h}{\bar{h}} > \frac{K}{(\bar{h}\pi D^2/4)^{1/2}}, \tag{10.254}$$

where K is the range of 2–5. This result has a simple interpretation. The quantity $\bar{h}\pi D^2/4$ is the mean number of counts within a background region the same size as the disk. Its square root is just the RMS fluctuation in this number. Hence $(\bar{h}\pi D^2/4)^{1/2}$ is the SNR that would be achieved by an ideal matched filter that integrated over the disk area. Equation (10.254) expresses the result that a human observer behaves as an ideal filter and can detect the disk when its filtered image differs from the background by K standard deviations. Schnitzler (1973) puts it this way:

> It seems clear . . . that the visual system functions like an adaptive areal matched filter (of course, limited in range) with an adaptive decision-making device at the output. The visual system automatically adjusts the summation area of the photoreceptor field to match the area of the image of the target and automatically adjusts the decision threshold . . . to be two to three times the standard deviation of the background fluctuations within the area of the target image.

Of course, there are limits to the abilities of a human observer. If the the disk is very large, the observer cannot deal with the whole image at once, and the effective integration area is less than $\pi D^2/4$ (Rose, 1948a; Blackwell, 1946). Similarly, if the disk is very small, such that its image is blurred and reduced in contrast by either the primary imaging system or the observer's eye, then again (10.254) is an overly optimistic estimate of performance. There is also an intrinsic contrast threshold. Even when the SNR is arbitrarily high, the human observer cannot detect contrast differences less than about 4% (Blackwell, 1946; Snyder, 1973; Whitehead, 1977). Finally, the detectability of an object can be significantly degraded by "clutter"—other objects in the scene, nonuniform background, TV raster lines, etc. Results obtained in highly idealized experiments, such as detection of a disk against a uniform noisy background, must be treated with caution. It is very difficult to establish that these results are applicable to real clinical images.

10.7.2 Quantitative Measures of Detectability

The important result quoted in Section 10.7.1, (10.254), was actually rather vague. What does it mean to say that the disk is "detected"? Indeed, a canny observer could always have a 100% probability of detection simply by saying that there was a disk in every image presented to him, whether or not he actually saw one. Of course, he would also often be wrong and would have a high *false-alarm rate*, but he would certainly not miss any disks that were actually present. Even if the observer is not deliberately biasing the results in this way, the threshold for deciding whether or not the disk is present is always a variable, depending on the observer, time of day, viewing conditions, penalties for a wrong answer, and a host of other parameters.

		Is the object really present?	
		Yes	No
Does the observer say the object is present?	Yes	True Positive (TP)	False Positive (FP)
	No	False Negative (FN)	True Negative (TN)

Fig. 10.11 2 × 2 decision matrix.

For a simply binary decision, such as whether an object is present or absent in an image, it is convenient to use a 2 × 2 *decision matrix* as shown in Fig. 10.11. The possible outcomes of the observation are *true positive* (TP) and *true negative* (TN), when the observer correctly determines the presence or absence of the object, *false positive* (FP), when he incorrectly decides that the object is present, and *false negative* (FN), when he incorrectly decides that the object is absent.

Suppose that N_{tot} observations are made, with N_{TP} of them being true positives, N_{TN} true negatives, N_{FP} false positives, and N_{FN} false negatives. Then we may define various performance indices as follows (Metz, 1978; Patton, 1978):

$$\begin{aligned}\text{True positive fraction} &= \text{TPF}\\ &\equiv \frac{(\text{Number of true positive decisions})}{(\text{Number of actually positive cases})}\\ &= \frac{N_{\text{TP}}}{N_{\text{TP}} + N_{\text{FN}}},\end{aligned} \tag{10.255}$$

$$\begin{aligned}\text{True negative fraction} &= \text{TNF}\\ &\equiv \frac{(\text{Number of true negative decisions})}{(\text{Number of actually negative cases})}\\ &= \frac{N_{\text{TN}}}{N_{\text{TN}} + N_{\text{FP}}},\end{aligned} \tag{10.256}$$

$$\begin{aligned}\text{False positive fraction} &= \text{FPF}\\ &\equiv \frac{(\text{Number of false positive decisions})}{(\text{Number of actually negative cases})}\\ &= \frac{N_{\text{FP}}}{N_{\text{TN}} + N_{\text{FP}}},\end{aligned} \tag{10.257}$$

$$\begin{aligned}\text{False negative fraction} &= \text{FNF}\\ &\equiv \frac{(\text{Number of false negative decisions})}{(\text{Number of actually positive cases})}\\ &= \frac{N_{\text{FN}}}{N_{\text{TP}} + N_{\text{FN}}},\end{aligned} \tag{10.258}$$

It follows readily that

$$\text{TPF} + \text{FNF} = 1, \tag{10.259}$$

$$\text{TNF} + \text{FPF} = 1. \tag{10.260}$$

The TPF is also called the *sensitivity*, while TNF is the *specificity*. Another important measure is the *accuracy*, or fraction of the cases that are correctly decided. It is given by

$$\text{Accuracy} = \frac{(\text{Number of correct decisions})}{(\text{total number of cases})}$$

$$= \frac{N_{\text{TP}} + N_{\text{TN}}}{N_{\text{tot}}}. \qquad (10.261)$$

None of these measures should be regarded as an absolute. As previously mentioned, the observer can vary his TPF simply by varying his decision threshold. If he calls every image positive, his TPF will be unity since there will be no negatives, false or otherwise, and $N_{\text{FN}} = 0$. However, his FPF will also be unity. Similarly, if he calls every image negative, he will have both TPF and FPF equal zero. Neither extreme is a particularly intelligent choice, and in practice the observer will adopt some intermediate threshold.

In fact, for a given set of input stimuli (images), the observer can be instructed to vary his threshold and thereby generate not single numbers for TPF and FPF, but a whole family of values. A convenient way of representing these results is in terms of a *receiver operating characteristic* or ROC curve (Lusted, 1968; Egan and Clarke, 1966; Goodenough, 1972; Goodenough *et al.*, 1972, 1973, 1974), as illustrated in Fig. 10.12. This curve is a plot of TPF vs FPF, with various points along the curve obtained simply by varying the decision threshold. The imaging system, the input object,

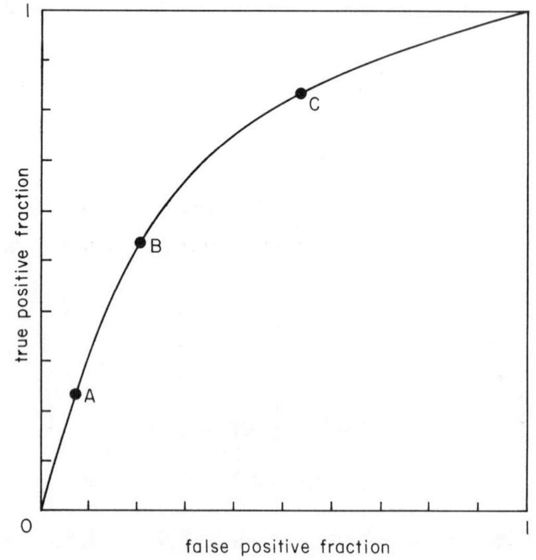

Fig. 10.12 Receiver operating characteristic curve for some particular imaging system. Points *A*, *B*, and *C* correspond to different decision thresholds.

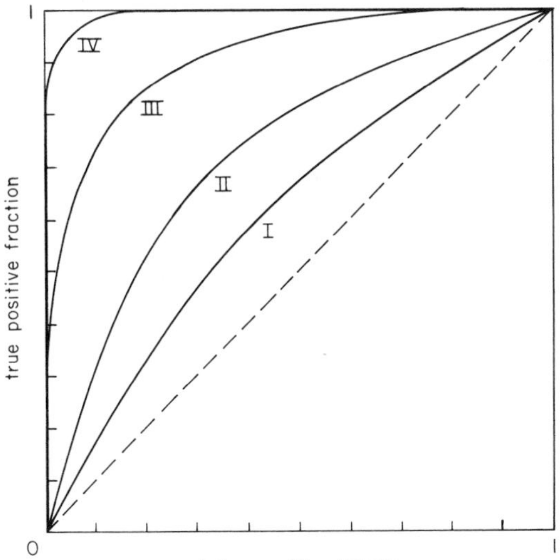

Fig. 10.13 ROC curves for four different imaging systems. System IV is the best, system I the worst for this detection task.

and the viewing conditions should all be held constant for a particular curve.

ROC curves can be used to compare different systems as illustrated in Fig. 10.13. An ideal system would give no false positives unless the observer insisted on calling everything positive. Its ROC curve would therefore hug the left and top edges of the graph, something like Curve IV in Fig. 10.13. On the other hand, if the image conveyed no information at all to the observer and he simply guessed whether the object was present, the resulting ROC curve would be the diagonal line from lower left to upper right. Thus the amount by which the ROC curve bows away from the diagonal and towards the upper left-hand corner is a measure of the usefulness of the system, at least for the simple binary detection experiment for which the ROC curve was constructed. The report by Swets and Pickett (1979) is a practical how-to-do-it book on ROC analysis.

10.7.3 Elementary Decision Theory

If the total number of observations N_{tot} is large, the various ratios defined by (10.255)–(10.258) may be interpreted as conditional probabilities. For example, the TPF is the probability that the observation will be positive when it is known that the object is actually present in the input. We may write

$$\lim_{N_{\text{tot}}\to\infty} \text{TPF} = \Pr(O+\,|\,I+), \tag{10.262}$$

where O stands for the observation or output of the system and I stands for the input. Similarly,

$$\lim_{N_{\text{tot}}\to\infty} \text{TNF} = \Pr(O-|I-), \tag{10.263}$$

$$\lim_{N_{\text{tot}}\to\infty} \text{FPF} = \Pr(O+|I-), \tag{10.264}$$

$$\lim_{N_{\text{tot}}\to\infty} \text{FNF} = \Pr(O-|I+), \tag{10.265}$$

In order to relate these probabilities to a decision threshold, we introduce the concept of the ideal observer (Egan and Clarke, 1966; Egan, 1975). This mythical being perceives an image $\mathbf{w}(r)$, which may consist of just noise $\mathbf{n}(\mathbf{r})$ or may also contain a signal $s(\mathbf{r})$. He then performs a matched filtering operation, yielding a new image $\mathbf{y}(\mathbf{r})$ given by

$$\mathbf{y}(\mathbf{r}) = \mathbf{w}(\mathbf{r}) \star\star\, s(\mathbf{r}). \tag{10.266}$$

If $s(\mathbf{r})$ is a positive-definite deterministic quantity, the probability density for $\mathbf{y}(\mathbf{r})$ will be shifted upward whenever the signal is present in $\mathbf{w}(\mathbf{r})$ (see Fig. 10.14). The ideal observer then sets some decision threshold such that whenever $\mathbf{y}(\mathbf{r})$ exceeds the threshold at some point $\mathbf{r}$, he asserts that a signal is present and centered at that point.

It must be emphasized that $\mathbf{y}(\mathbf{r})$ is a psychological variable, not a real physical one. We seldom have direct access to $\mathbf{y}(\mathbf{r})$ but can only postulate that some such variable exists and is the basis for detection decisions by real human observers.

Let $\text{pr}(y|n)$ denote the probability density for $\mathbf{y}(\mathbf{r})$ at some point $\mathbf{r}$ when $\mathbf{w}(\mathbf{r})$ contains only noise, and let $\text{pr}(y|s+n)$ be the corresponding quantity when $\mathbf{w}(\mathbf{r})$ contains both signal and noise. If the decision threshold is y_t, and

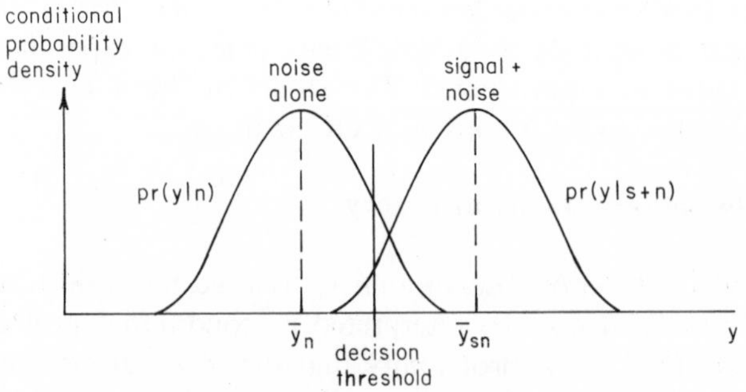

Fig. 10.14 Probability density functions for noise alone and signal plus noise. See text for a discussion of the meaning of **y**.

the ideal observer asserts that the object is present whenever $\mathbf{y} > y_t$, then the TPF is given by

$$\mathrm{TPF} = \int_{y_t}^{\infty} dy\, \mathrm{pr}(y|s+n). \tag{10.267}$$

(The limit $N_{\mathrm{tot}} \to \infty$ is to be understood from here on.) Similarly

$$\mathrm{TNF} = \int_{-\infty}^{y_t} dy\, \mathrm{pr}(y|n), \tag{10.268}$$

$$\mathrm{FPF} = \int_{y_t}^{\infty} dy\, \mathrm{pr}(y|n), \tag{10.269}$$

$$\mathrm{FNF} = \int_{-\infty}^{y_t} dy\, \mathrm{pr}(y|s+n). \tag{10.270}$$

The TPF and FPF as functions of y_t are shown in Fig. 10.15. If $\mathbf{y}$ is a Gaussian random variable, as it often will be in light of the central limit theorem, then these curves are complementary error functions. A single point on an ROC curve is generated by taking a particular y_t and reading off the corresponding TPF and FPF from Fig. 10.15.

As we have set up the problem, $\mathrm{pr}(y|n)$ and $\mathrm{pr}(y|s+n)$ are identical functions except for a horizontal shift because $s(\mathbf{r})$ is not a random variable but rather a deterministic quantity. If the mean values of $\mathbf{y}$ for these two distributions are $\bar{y}_n$ and $\bar{y}_{sn}$, and their common standard deviation is σ_y, a measure of the separation between them is

$$d' \equiv (\bar{y}_{sn} - \bar{y}_n)/\sigma_y. \tag{10.271}$$

A family of ROC curves for different d' is shown in Fig. 10.16 (Goodenough, 1975). It should be noted that all these curves are symmetric about the diagonal from upper left to lower right. ROC curves from real observers are often asymmetric, showing the limitations of the ideal-observer model.

The parameter d' is easily related back to a calculable SNR. For the problem in Section 10.7.1 of detecting an area of reduced count density

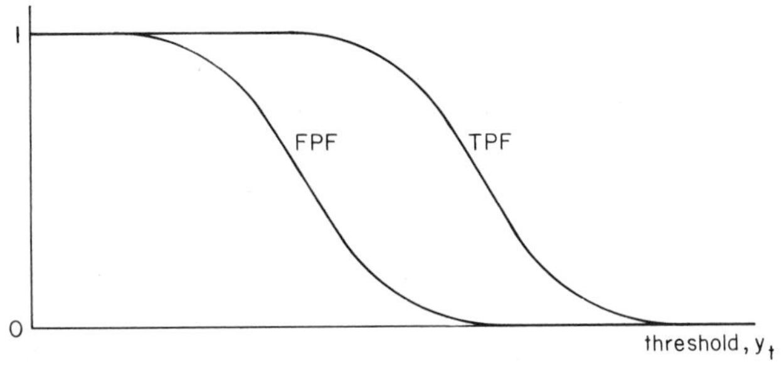

Fig. 10.15 True positive fraction and false positive fraction as a function of threshold.

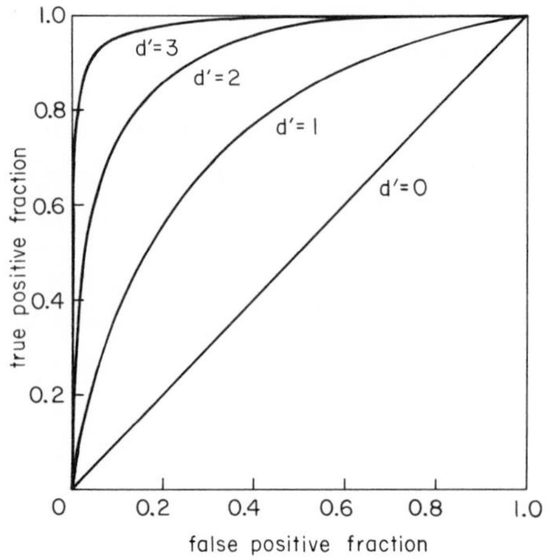

Fig. 10.16 Family of ROC curves for different values of the SNR parameter d'.

$\bar{h} - \Delta\bar{h}$ in a scintigram, we have

$$\bar{y}_{sn} - \bar{y}_n = \Delta h(\pi D^2/4), \tag{10.272}$$

$$\sigma_y = [\bar{h}(\pi D^2/4)]^{1/2}, \tag{10.273}$$

$$d' = (\Delta h/\bar{h})[\bar{h}(\pi D^2/4)]^{1/2}, \tag{10.274}$$

so that (10.254) becomes simply

$$d' > K. \tag{10.275}$$

Comparison with Fig. 10.16 shows that $d' = 3$ (or $K = 3$) will force the ROC curve well into the upper left-hand corner.

10.7.4 The Search Problem

The discussion to this point has assumed that the observer knows where in the image to look for the object and also what the object looks like. The latter condition is satisfied in many psychophysical experiments in which, for example, the observer is told to look for a disk of a certain size. However, he will usually have to search over a large image and determine if the object is present anywhere in it.

The ideal observer would approach this problem by optimally filtering the image as before, and then applying the decision threshold to $\mathbf{y}(\mathbf{r})$ at a matrix of points $\mathbf{r} = \mathbf{r}_i$, $i = 1, \ldots, M$, where M is the number of resolution cells in the filtered image. Real observers are probably not so systematic, but some sort of search over the image does occur, and the general nature of the problem can be seen from consideration of the ideal observer.

The ideal observer will assert that there is no object present anywhere in the scene only if he determines that there is no object in each of the M independent resolution cells tested. We define TNF_M to be the overall true negative fraction when M cells are tested. That is, TNF_M is the conditional probability that no object is found anywhere in the scene when it is known that, in fact, no object is present. (Similar notation will be used for the other three fractions as well.) TNF_M is readily related to TNF_1 if we assume that all M cells are independent (Goodenough, 1975). In that case, the overall probability of a negative response is just the product of the M probabilities that apply to the individual tests, i.e.,

$$\mathrm{TNF}_M = (\mathrm{TNF}_1)^M. \tag{10.276}$$

Using (10.260), we have

$$\mathrm{FPF}_M = 1 - \mathrm{TNF}_M = 1 - (\mathrm{TNF}_1)^M = 1 - [1 - \mathrm{FPF}_1]^M. \tag{10.277}$$

Next, consider the case where the object is really present in one of the M cells, but the observer still fails to detect it. This situation gives FNF_M, which is the product of the $M - 1$ probabilities TNF_1, and one factor of FNF_1 for the one cell in which the object was present. Therefore,

$$\mathrm{FNF}_M = \mathrm{FNF}_1 \cdot \mathrm{TNF}_{M-1} = (\mathrm{FNF}_1/\mathrm{TNF}_1)\mathrm{TNF}_M. \tag{10.278}$$

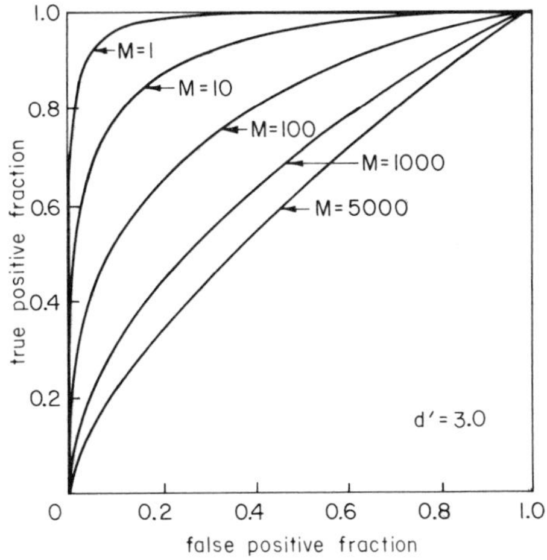

Fig. 10.17 Family of ROC curves parameterized by M, the number of resolvable cells in the image. (After Goodenough, 1975.)

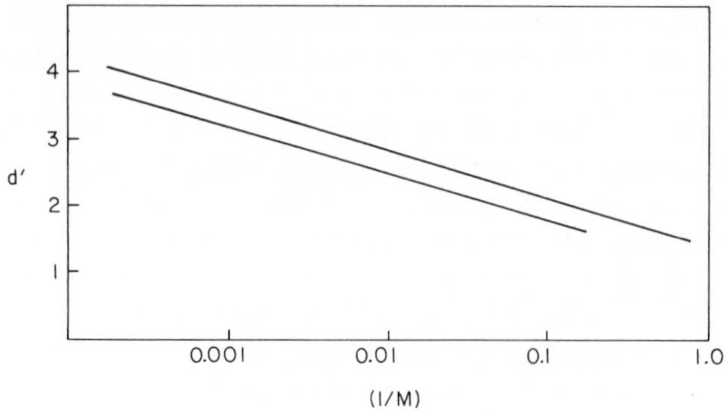

Fig. 10.18 Required values of d' vs M^{-1}. The upper curve assumes that the ROC curve passes through the point TPF = 0.5, FPF = 0.1, while the lower curve assumes it passes through TPF = 0.5, FPF = 0.2. (After Goodenough, 1975.)

Using (10.259) and (10.276), we find

$$\mathrm{TPF}_M = 1 - \mathrm{FNF}_M = 1 - (\mathrm{FNF}_1/\mathrm{TNF}_1)(\mathrm{TNF}_1)^M. \qquad (10.279)$$

Equations (10.277) and (10.279) can be used to construct an M-cell ROC curve from a one-cell curve. Some examples from the work of Goodenough are shown in Fig. 10.17 and 10.18. The general conclusion is that larger images require larger SNR. However, from Fig. 10.18, we see that even $M = 10{,}000$ requires a d' of only 4–5. This again justifies the empirical observation that the value of K in (10.254) need not exceed 5 for reliable detection.

11

Scattered Radiation

11.1 INTRODUCTION

We have largely ignored the effects of scattered radiation in the preceding chapters. For example, in discussing transmission imaging in Chapter 4 we considered a planar absorbing object described by a transmission function $g(\mathbf{r})$, and assumed that all x-ray photons travel in straight lines from source to detector. The interaction that caused $g(\mathbf{r})$ to be less than one was tacitly assumed to completely destroy the photon rather than redirect it to some other point on the detector. Similarly, in discussing emission imaging in Chapter 4, we again assumed only straight-line propagation. In Section 4.6.4 we somewhat superficially accounted for the attenuation of the gamma rays by interactions occurring in the portions of the patient's body lying between the radioactive organ and the detector, but paid no attention to the eventual fate of the scattered rays.

Neglect of scattered radiation can be an egregious error. From Fig. C.15 in Appendix C, we see that Compton scattering is the dominant interaction in soft tissue (essentially water) for photons in the energy range from about 40 keV to over 10 meV. Thus, contrary to our models, photons in this large energy range are *not* completely absorbed when they interact, but in fact may still contribute to the image after scattering. As we shall see in more detail later in this chapter, the detected scattered photons do not contribute much *useful* information to the image, but merely reduce its contrast and increase its noise level. In fact, scatter is often the *most* important factor limiting image quality and diagnostic accuracy. For this reason considerable effort has gone into the elimination of scattered radiation through geometrical or electronic means. These efforts are described in Section 11.4.

On the other hand, a few researchers have been able to make good use of scattered and fluorescent radiation with imaging systems based on deliberate detection of scattered rather than unscattered radiation. This work is briefly treated in Section 11.5.

11.2 METHODS OF ANALYSIS FOR SCATTER PROBLEMS

11.2.1 Three Energy Regimes

The character of the Compton scattering process changes significantly as the photon energy is increased (see Appendix C). Although the boundaries are somewhat subjective, we may distinguish three separate energy regimes with properties summarized in Table 11.1. The low-energy regime below about 40 keV is of interest for mammography, radiography of the extremities, and nuclear scans with a few low-energy isotopes, notably ^{125}I. In this regime, photoelectric interactions predominate and scattering may be negligible. What scattering there is is elastic (small energy loss $\Delta\mathscr{E}$) and relatively isotropic $[d\sigma^C/d\Omega \propto (1 + \cos^2\theta)]$ (see Figs. C.10 and C.11).

In the important intermediate energy range, say 40–150 keV, Compton scattering dominates. It is usually a reasonable approximation to still use the low-energy form for $d\sigma^C/d\Omega$, but the energy loss $\Delta\mathscr{E}$ may well be signifi-

TABLE 11.1

Characteristics of Compton Scattering

Energy range	Dominant interaction in soft tissue	Angular dependence of differential scattering cross section	Photon energy loss on scattering
Low $\lesssim 40$ keV	Photoelectric	$\frac{d\sigma^C}{d\Omega} \propto (1 + \cos^2\theta)$	$\Delta\mathscr{E}$ very small
Medium approx. 40–150 keV	Compton	$\frac{d\sigma^C}{d\Omega} \propto (1 + \cos^2\theta)^a$	$\Delta\mathscr{E}$ may be significant
High 150 keV to 10 meV	Compton	Forward peaked	$\Delta\mathscr{E}$ large

[a] This approximation works best for $\theta \lesssim 90°$ at the higher energies in this range (see Figs. C.10 and C.11).

cant. For example, at 150 keV the average $\Delta\mathscr{E}$ is 27 keV or 18% of the photon energy (Evans, 1968). At such energies it is therefore beginning to be possible to discriminate against scattered photons on the basis of their energies.

At energies above 150 keV, usually of interest only in nuclear medicine, the differential scattering cross section is definitely forward peaked, and the energy loss is large. For example, for a 511-keV gamma ray produced by positron annihilation, forward scattering is about five times more probable than backward scattering, and the average ΔE is 170 keV or 34% of the incident energy.

The other trend to be noted is that the total scattering cross section gradually decreases as the photon energy is increased (Fig. C.8).

These differences in scattering behavior influence the validity of various approximations that can be used to analyze the effects of scattered radiation, as well as the means available to control scatter in imaging systems.

11.2.2 The Single-Scatter Approximation

The simplest way to analyze scatter problems is to assume that none of the detected photons has undergone more than one scattering event. This would be a valid approximation if a typical dimension d of the body were small enough that $\mu^{\mathrm{C}} d \lesssim 1$, where μ^{C} is the total Compton linear attenuation coefficient as defined in Appendix C. Unfortunately this condition is seldom satisfied in radiographic imaging since it requires that d be less than 5–10 cm. Alternatively, single scatter may still be a useful approximation in nuclear medicine systems with energy discrimination if, on the average, multiple scattering results in sufficient energy loss to place the photon well below the energy window. In any case, consideration of this approximation can still give useful qualitative insights even when it is not quantitatively justified.

To illustrate the use of the single-scatter approximation, let us consider the simple transmission imaging geometry shown in Fig. 11.1. A uniform slab of scattering medium of thickness L is irradiated by a very distant point source so that the incident beam is essentially collimated. We consider a thin pencil of rays of cross-sectional area $\mathscr{A}$; the scatter pattern for the whole beam may be found by superposing the patterns for many such pencils. We shall assume that the beam is monoenergetic and of sufficiently low energy that we may write [see (C.34)]

$$\frac{d\sigma^{\mathrm{C}}}{d\Omega} = \frac{r_0^2}{2}(1 + \cos^2\theta), \tag{11.1}$$

where r_0 is the classical electron radius.

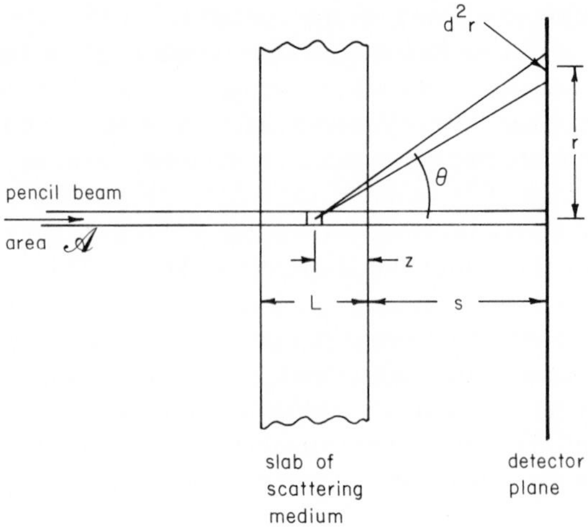

Fig. 11.1 Simple transmission-imaging arrangement in which a uniform slab is irradiated with a thin pencil beam.

If we consider a volume element $\mathscr{A}\ dz$ situated along the pencil at a distance z from the *exit* face of the slab, it receives an unscattered x-ray fluence of

$$\Phi(z) = \Phi_0 \exp[-\mu^{\text{tot}}(L - z)], \tag{11.2}$$

where μ^{tot} is the total linear attenuation coefficient and Φ_0 is the incident fluence. (Both $\Phi(z)$ and Φ_0 are measured in photons per unit area.) Of course, this element may also receive and rescatter photons that have already been scattered one or more times, but these photons are neglected in the single-scatter approximation.

The element $\mathscr{A}\ dz$ contains $n_e\ \mathscr{A}\ dz$ electrons, where n_e is the electron density (electrons per unit volume). The total number of photons per unit solid angle scattered by the volume element is

$$\Phi(z)\left(\frac{d\sigma^{\text{C}}}{d\Omega}\right) n_e \mathscr{A}\ dz. \tag{11.3}$$

A detector element of area d^2r located a distance r from the axis of the pencil subtends a differential solid angle (see Section 4.1) of

$$d\Omega = \frac{d^2r}{(s + z)^2} \cos^3 \theta, \tag{11.4}$$

where

$$\theta = \tan^{-1}[r/(z + s)]. \tag{11.5}$$

The number of photons scattered in the direction of this detector element by the volume element $\mathscr{A}\,dz$ is obtained by multiplying (11.3) and (11.4). However, some of these photons may be attenuated before they emerge from the body. Since they must travel a distance $z \sec\theta$ from the scattering point to the exit face of the slab, the appropriate attenuation factor is

$$\exp(-\mu^{\text{tot}} z \sec\theta). \tag{11.6}$$

The total number of scattered photons received by the detector element d^2r is denoted by $h_s(\mathbf{r})\,d^2r$, where, as in previous chapters, the notation $h(\mathbf{r})$ expresses a number of photons per unit area in the detector plane. Combining (11.1), (11.4), and (11.6) and integrating over z to account for all scattering elements along the pencil, we have

$$h_s(\mathbf{r}) = \tfrac{1}{2} r_0^2 n_e \mathscr{A} \Phi_0 \int_0^L \exp[-\mu^{\text{tot}}(L - z)]$$
$$\cdot \exp[-\mu^{\text{tot}} z \sec\theta](1 + \cos^2\theta) \frac{\cos^3\theta}{(s + z)^2}\, dz. \tag{11.7}$$

In general, θ is a function of z through (11.5). However, if the air gap s is at least as large as L, then $\cos\theta$ varies very little with z. It is then an excellent approximation to set

$$\theta \approx \bar{\theta} \equiv \tan^{-1}[r/(s + \tfrac{1}{2}L)] \tag{11.8}$$

everywhere in the integrand. To the same order of approximation

$$(s + z)^2 \approx (s + \tfrac{1}{2}L)^2. \tag{11.9}$$

The integral in (11.7) is now trivial, and we have

$$h_s(\mathbf{r}) = \tfrac{1}{2} r_0^2 n_e \mathscr{A} \Phi_0 \exp(-\mu^{\text{tot}} L) \cos^3\bar{\theta}(1 + \cos^2\bar{\theta})(s + \tfrac{1}{2}L)^{-2} \frac{1 - \exp(-\mu' L)}{\mu'}, \tag{11.10}$$

where

$$\mu' \equiv \mu^{\text{tot}}(\sec\bar{\theta} - 1). \tag{11.11}$$

This expression is a complicated function of r through (11.8). The total detected photon density due to the single pencil beam is

$$h(\mathbf{r}) = h_s(\mathbf{r}) + h_u(\mathbf{r}), \tag{11.12}$$

where $h_u(\mathbf{r})$, the unscattered component, is given by

$$h_u(\mathbf{r}) = \Phi_0 \exp(-\mu^{\text{tot}} L) = \Phi(L) \qquad (\mathbf{r} \text{ in beam area}). \tag{11.13}$$

Representative plots of $h_s(\mathbf{r})$ are given in Fig. 11.2.

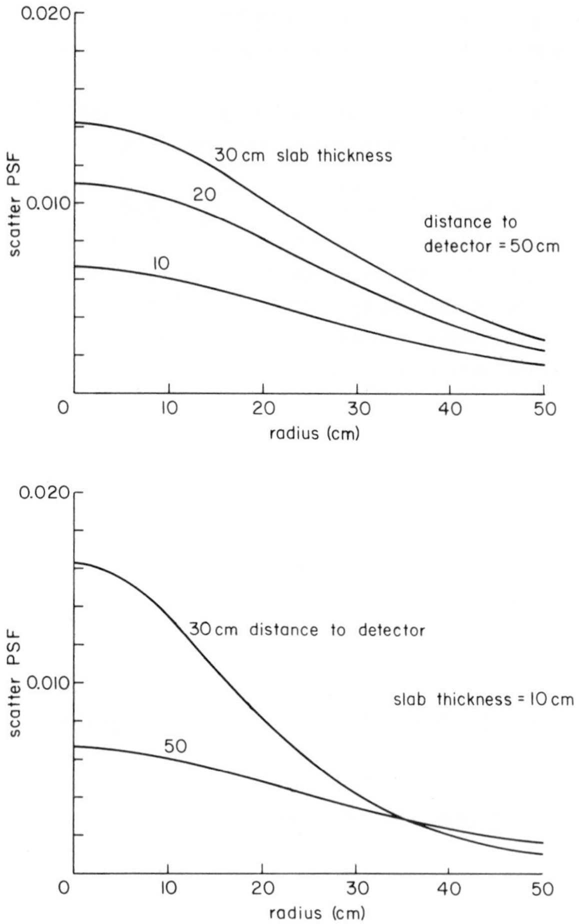

Fig. 11.2 Plots of the scatter PSF $h_s(\mathbf{r})$ from (11.10) for various slab thicknesses L and distances to the detector s. The ordinates are in units of $\frac{1}{2}r_0^2 n_e \mathscr{A} \Phi_0 \exp(-\mu^{\text{tot}} L)$.

There are two important points to be noted from this result. The first is that scatter gives rise to broad, structureless wings around a point image. [The pattern $h(\mathbf{r})$ just calculated can be regarded as the image of a low-contrast pointlike object of area $\mathscr{A}$ located somewhere along the pencil.] Although these wings appear to have very low amplitude, they soon become significant as the number of pencils in the beam is increased. For a very broad beam, the total scattered flux at any point on the detector is proportional to the area integral of $h_s(\mathbf{r})$, so even very small wings are important if they extend out a long way.

The second point, to be seen by comparing (11.10) and (11.13), is that the relative importance of $h_s(\mathbf{r})$ can be reduced by the simple expedient of increasing the air gap s. Since we have assumed that the primary beam is collimated (i.e., the source is a long distance to the left of the slab), increasing s has no effect on $h_u(\mathbf{r})$ but decreases $h_s(\mathbf{r})$ by the factor of $1/(s + \frac{1}{2}L)^2$.

11.2.3 Monte Carlo Analysis

Monte Carlo techniques are applicable to a wide variety of complicated transport problems. Basically, they amount to digitally tracing the fate of a large number of photons, using a random-number generator to determine when and where interactions occur and what their outcomes are.

As an example, consider a pointlike gamma-ray source embedded in a scattering medium. The computer launches a gamma-ray photon by randomly selecting its initial direction (e.g., by specifying the direction cosines). It then randomly determines how far the photon will go before an interaction takes place, whether the interaction is Compton or photoelectric, and for Compton interactions what the new direction cosines are. The usual Compton scattering formulas from Appendix C can be used to determine the energy of the scattered gamma ray. The process is continued in this way until the photon either dissipates all of its energy, escapes from the system altogether, or impinges on the detector. Then a new photon is launched and the process is repeated many times until an adequate statistical picture is assembled.

One difficulty with this procedure is that not all outcomes are equally likely at each step. For example, when an interaction occurs, the probability that it will be a Compton event is given by [see (C.6)]

$$\Pr(\text{Compton}) = Z\sigma^{\text{C}}/\sigma^{\text{tot}}, \tag{11.14}$$

while the probability that it will be photoelectric is

$$\Pr(\text{photo}) = \sigma^{\text{pe}}/\sigma^{\text{tot}}. \tag{11.15}$$

To account for these differing probabilities, the computer can be instructed to select a random number from a uniformly distributed set of random numbers in the interval (0, 1). If this random number turns out to be less than Pr(Compton), it is assumed that a Compton event occurs. Otherwise, if pair production is negligible, the event is taken to be photoelectric. This procedure will ensure that after a large number of events, the correct proportion of them will be Compton.

A more complicated procedure is required when there is a continuous range of choices possible. For example, right after an interaction, the computer must choose the path length $\mathbf{l}$ to be traversed before the next interaction. Any value from zero to infinity is possible. The probability density function for the random variable $\mathbf{l}$ is readily shown to be

$$\mathrm{pr}(l) = \bar{l}^{-1} \exp(-l/\bar{l}), \tag{11.16}$$

where $\bar{l}$ is the mean free path,

$$\bar{l} = (\mu^{\mathrm{tot}})^{-1}. \tag{11.17}$$

If we had a pool of random numbers distributed according to (11.16), we could simply select one of them without preference and use it for $\mathbf{l}$. However, digital random-number generators cannot readily be configured to have a specified density function, especially when the domain of the random variable is infinite. Usually, the generator will produce random numbers with uniform density in a finite interval, often $(0, 1)$. A simple trick suffices to convert this generated random number, call it $\mathbf{g}$, to the desired path length $\mathbf{l}$. The problem is to find a unique nonlinear transformation $l = l(g)$ mapping the random variable $\mathbf{g}$ of domain $(0, 1)$ to $\mathbf{l}$ having domain $(0, \infty)$. If the mapping is one-to-one, $\mathbf{l}$ can fall into the infinitesimal interval $(l, l + dl)$ only if $\mathbf{g}$ falls in $(g, g + dg)$. Hence

$$\mathrm{pr}(l)\, dl = \mathrm{pr}(g)\, dg \tag{11.18}$$

or

$$\mathrm{pr}(l) = \mathrm{pr}(g) \frac{dg}{dl}. \tag{11.19}$$

If $\mathbf{g}$ is uniformly distributed, $\mathrm{pr}(g) = 1$, so that

$$\frac{dg}{dl} = \mathrm{pr}(l) \tag{11.20}$$

or

$$g(l) = \int_0^l \mathrm{pr}(l')\, dl', \tag{11.21}$$

which, by (3.18), is simply the cumulative probability distribution function $\mathrm{Pr}(\mathbf{l} < l)$. Using (11.16), we find

$$g(l) = 1 - \exp(-l/\bar{l}), \tag{11.22}$$

from which a straightforward algebraic inversion yields

$$l(g) = -\bar{l} \ln(1 - g) \tag{11.23}$$

as the desired transformation.

The same procedure can be used with any specified probability density function. It can, for example, be used to properly weight the direction cosines of the scattered photon after a Compton event.

As a practical note, when using Monte Carlo analysis one should not take it for granted that a digital random-number generator indeed generates random numbers. A series of useful tests of the generator is described by Morin *et al.* (1979).

11.2.4 Formal Transport Theory; Derivation of the Boltzmann Equation

A very general (and usually correspondingly complicated) approach to scatter problems is formal transport theory based on the *Boltzmann equation* (Morse and Feshbach, 1953; Ishimaru, 1978). Originally developed in connection with the kinetic theory of gases, the Boltzmann equation is an integrodifferential equation for the total time derivative of a *phase-space distribution function* $f(\mathbf{p}, \mathbf{r}, t)$. Here $\mathbf{r}$ is a *three-dimensional* position vector and $\mathbf{p}$ is the momentum vector of a photon. The direction of $\mathbf{p}$ is the same as the direction of flight of the photon, while the magnitude of $\mathbf{p}$ is related to the photon energy $h\nu$ through

$$\mathrm{p} = h\nu/c = h/\lambda, \tag{11.24}$$

where c is the speed of light, h is Planck's constant, and ν and λ are, respectively, the frequency and wavelength of the photon.

The distribution function $f(\mathbf{p}, \mathbf{r}, t)$ is defined such that $f(\mathbf{p}, \mathbf{r}, t)\, d^3\mathrm{p}\, d^3\mathrm{r}$ is the average number of photons having coordinates x, y, z in the intervals $(x, x + dx)$, $(y, y + dy)$, $(z, z + dz)$, and momentum components p_x, p_y, p_z in the intervals $(\mathrm{p}_x, \mathrm{p}_x + d\mathrm{p}_x)$, $(\mathrm{p}_y, \mathrm{p}_y + d\mathrm{p}_y)$, $(\mathrm{p}_z, \mathrm{p}_z + d\mathrm{p}_z)$ at time t. In the language of kinetic theory, $d^3\mathrm{p}d^3\mathrm{r}$ is a cell in a six-dimensional *phase space*. The normalization of $f(\mathbf{p}, \mathbf{r}, t)$ is such that

$$\int_\infty d^3\mathrm{p} \int_\infty d^3\mathrm{r}\, f(\mathbf{p}, \mathbf{r}, t) = N(t), \tag{11.25}$$

where $N(t)$ is the total number of photons of all energies, directions, and locations at time t.

The volume density of photons, without regard to their energy, is given by

$$u(\mathbf{r}, t) = \int_\infty d^3\mathrm{p}\, f(\mathbf{p}, \mathbf{r}, t). \tag{11.26}$$

Note that $u(\mathbf{r}, t)\, d^3\mathrm{r}$ is the mean number of photons in the volume element $d^3\mathrm{r}$ at location $\mathbf{r}$.

The total net momentum per unit volume is given by

$$\mathbf{J}(\mathbf{r}, t) = \int_\infty \mathbf{p} f(\mathbf{p}, \mathbf{r}, t)\, d^3\mathrm{p}. \tag{11.27}$$

The Boltzmann equation has the general form

$$\frac{\partial f(\mathbf{p},\mathbf{r},t)}{\partial t} = \left.\frac{\partial f(\mathbf{p},\mathbf{r},t)}{\partial t}\right|_{\text{prop}} + \left.\frac{\partial f(\mathbf{p},\mathbf{r},t)}{\partial t}\right|_{\text{scat}} + \left.\frac{\partial f(\mathbf{p},\mathbf{r},t)}{\partial t}\right|_{\text{abs}} + \left.\frac{\partial f(\mathbf{p},\mathbf{r},t)}{\partial t}\right|_{\text{gen}}, \tag{11.28}$$

where the subscripts stand for propagation, scattering, absorption, and generation. The absorption term is the simplest one. We assume that the photon energy is below the pair-production threshold, so that the photoelectric effect is the only total-absorption process. By comparison with (C.4) from Appendix C, we have

$$\Delta f|_{\text{abs}} = -c\,\Delta t n_a \sigma^{\text{pe}} f(\mathbf{p},\mathbf{r},t) \tag{11.29a}$$

or

$$\left.\frac{\partial f}{\partial t}\right|_{\text{abs}} = -c n_a \sigma^{\text{pe}} f(\mathbf{p},\mathbf{r},t), \tag{11.29b}$$

where the incremental length dx in (C.4) has been replaced with $c\,\Delta t$, the distance each photon travels in time Δt, and n_a is the number of atoms per unit volume.

The scattering term in (11.28) contains one term just like (11.29), but with σ^{C} in place of σ^{pe}, to account for removal of photons from the phase space cell at $(\mathbf{p},\mathbf{r})$. However, this cell can also *gain* photons by scattering into it from other cells in phase space. The general form is

$$\left.\frac{\partial f}{\partial t}\right|_{\text{scat}} = -c n_e \sigma^{C} f(\mathbf{p},\mathbf{r},t) + c n_e \int_{\infty} s(\mathbf{p},\mathbf{p}') f(\mathbf{p}',\mathbf{r},t)\, d^3\text{p}', \tag{11.30}$$

where $s(\mathbf{p},\mathbf{p}')$ expresses the probability for scattering from the cell at $(\mathbf{p}',\mathbf{r})$ into the one at $(\mathbf{p},\mathbf{r})$. This probability can be related to the more familiar differential scattering cross section by

$$s(\mathbf{p},\mathbf{p}') = \left(\frac{1}{\text{p}'}\right)^2 \delta\left[\text{p} - \text{p}' - \left(\frac{\Delta\mathscr{E}}{c}\right)\right]\frac{d\sigma^{C}}{d\Omega'}, \tag{11.31}$$

where $\Delta\mathscr{E}$, the Compton energy loss, depends on the scattering angle (the angle between $\mathbf{p}$ and $\mathbf{p}'$) and on the initial energy $\text{p}'c$ as discussed in Section C.3. If the direction $\mathbf{p}$ is chosen as the polar axis for expressing $\mathbf{p}'$ in polar coordinates $(\text{p}', \theta'_{\text{p}}, \phi'_{\text{p}})$, then the solid angle $d\Omega'$ is given by $\sin\theta'_{\text{p}}\, d\theta'_{\text{p}}\, d\phi'_{\text{p}}$, and $d^3\text{p}' = \text{p}'^2\, d\text{p}'\, d\Omega'$. For the low-energy case where $\Delta\mathscr{E}$ is negligible, (11.30) reduces to

$$\left.\frac{\partial f}{\partial t}\right|_{\text{scat}} = -c n_e \sigma^{C} f(\mathbf{p},\mathbf{r},t) + c n_e \int_{4\pi} \left(\frac{d\sigma^{C}}{d\Omega'}\right) f(\mathbf{p}',\mathbf{r},t)\, d\Omega'. \tag{11.32}$$

Note that $d\sigma^{C}/d\Omega'$ is a function of the angle between $\mathbf{p}$ and $\mathbf{p}'$.

The propagation term in (11.28) accounts for movement of photons from one spatial region to another. A photon of momentum $\mathbf{p}$ has a velocity $c\hat{\mathbf{p}}$, where $\hat{\mathbf{p}} = \mathbf{p}/p$ is a unit vector in the direction of $\mathbf{p}$. If this photon is at point $\mathbf{r}$ at time t, it must be at point $\mathbf{r} + c\,\Delta t\hat{\mathbf{p}}$ at time $t + \Delta t$ if it is not scattered or absorbed. Therefore, as far as the propagation term is concerned,

$$f(\mathbf{p}, \mathbf{r} + c\,\Delta t\hat{\mathbf{p}}, t + \Delta t) = f(\mathbf{p}, \mathbf{r}, t). \tag{11.33}$$

Expanding the left-hand side of this equation in a Taylor series, we find

$$f(\mathbf{p}, \mathbf{r}, t) + (c\,\Delta t)\hat{\mathbf{p}} \cdot \nabla f(\mathbf{p}, \mathbf{r}, t) + \Delta t\,\partial f(\mathbf{p}, \mathbf{r}, t)/\partial t = f(\mathbf{p}, \mathbf{r}, t), \tag{11.34}$$

or

$$\left.\frac{\partial f(\mathbf{p}, \mathbf{r}, t)}{\partial t}\right|_{\text{prop}} = -c\hat{\mathbf{p}} \cdot \nabla f(\mathbf{p}, \mathbf{r}, t). \tag{11.35}$$

The remaining term in (11.28) accounts for generation of photons within the medium, for example by a radioactive isotope. If the only radiation sources are external to the medium, as we shall assume for now, the generation term is zero.

Combining (11.29), (11.30), and (11.35), and using $n_e = Zn_a$ and $\sigma^{\text{tot}} = \sigma^{\text{pe}} + Z\sigma^{\text{C}}$, we find

$$\frac{\partial f(\mathbf{p}, \mathbf{r}, t)}{\partial t} = -cn_a\sigma^{\text{tot}} f(\mathbf{p}, \mathbf{r}, t) - c\hat{\mathbf{p}} \cdot \nabla f(\mathbf{p}, \mathbf{r}, t) + \frac{cn_a}{Z}\int_\infty s(\mathbf{p}, \mathbf{p}')f(\mathbf{p}', \mathbf{r}, t)\,d^3p'. \tag{11.36}$$

11.2.5 Solutions of the Boltzmann Equation

Unless the radiation flux incident on the scattering medium is varying very rapidly (on a scale of nanoseconds), we do not need to solve the full time-dependent Boltzmann equation. Rather, we need only find the steady-state solution where $\partial f/\partial t = 0$. From (11.36), this means that

$$n_a\sigma^{\text{tot}} f(\mathbf{p}, \mathbf{r}) = -\hat{\mathbf{p}} \cdot \nabla f(\mathbf{p}, \mathbf{r}) + \frac{n_a}{Z}\int_\infty s(\mathbf{p}, \mathbf{p}')f(\mathbf{p}', \mathbf{r})\,d^3p', \tag{11.37}$$

where omission of the time argument in $f(\mathbf{p}, \mathbf{r})$ implies the steady-state solution.

It is often convenient (Ishimaru, 1978) to divide $f(\mathbf{p}, \mathbf{r})$ into two parts—the attenuated incident component $f_i(\mathbf{p}, \mathbf{r})$ and a diffuse or scattered component $f_d(\mathbf{p}, \mathbf{r})$:

$$f(\mathbf{p}, \mathbf{r}) = f_i(\mathbf{p}, \mathbf{r}) + f_d(\mathbf{p}, \mathbf{r}). \tag{11.38}$$

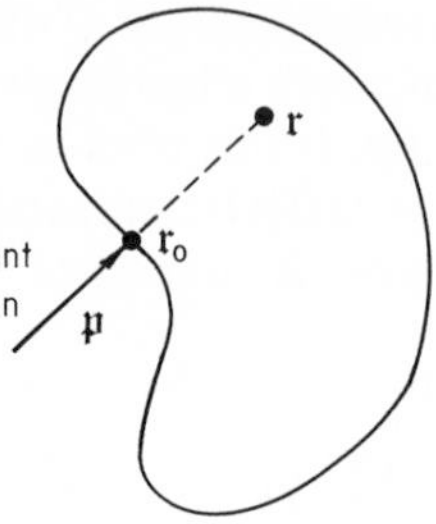

Fig. 11.3 Illustration of the meaning of the limits of integration in (11.40). A photon of momentum $\mathbf{p}$ that has travelled without scatter to point $\mathbf{r}$ must have entered the body at point $\mathbf{r}_0$.

The component $f_i(\mathbf{p}, \mathbf{r})$ is just the incident flux attenuated according to Beer's law. It is governed by the differential equation

$$\hat{\mathbf{p}} \cdot \nabla f_i(\mathbf{p}, \mathbf{r}) = -n_a \sigma^{tot} f_i(\mathbf{p}, \mathbf{r}), \tag{11.39}$$

which has the solution

$$f_i(\mathbf{p}, \mathbf{r}) = f_i(\mathbf{p}, \mathbf{r}_0) \exp\left(-\int_{\mathbf{r}_0}^{\mathbf{r}} n_a \sigma^{tot}\, dl \right). \tag{11.40}$$

Here $\mathbf{r}_0$ is the entrance point for a photon going in direction $\mathbf{p}$ and passing through point $\mathbf{r}$ (see Fig. 11.3). The integral is along the straight line from $\mathbf{r}_0$ to $\mathbf{r}$, and both n_a and σ^{tot} may vary in an arbitrary manner along this line.

Combining (11.37)–(11.39), we see that the diffuse component satisfies

$$\hat{\mathbf{p}} \cdot \nabla f_d(\mathbf{p}, \mathbf{r}) = -n_a \sigma^{tot} f_d(\mathbf{p}, \mathbf{r}) + \varepsilon_i(\mathbf{p}, \mathbf{r}) + \frac{n_a}{Z} \int_\infty s(\mathbf{p}, \mathbf{p}') f_d(\mathbf{p}', \mathbf{r})\, d^3p', \tag{11.41}$$

where $\varepsilon_i(\mathbf{p}, \mathbf{r})$ is an effective source generated by the incident flux:

$$\varepsilon_i(\mathbf{p}, \mathbf{r}) = \frac{n_a}{Z} \int_\infty s(\mathbf{p}, \mathbf{p}') f_i(\mathbf{p}', \mathbf{r})\, d^3p'. \tag{11.42}$$

The boundary condition on $f_d(\mathbf{p}, \mathbf{r})$ is that the diffuse component is generated entirely within the scattering medium. Therefore $f_d(\mathbf{p}, \mathbf{r})$ should be zero when $\mathbf{r}$ lies on the surface of the medium and $\mathbf{p}$ points inward.

Following Ishimaru, we can get something resembling a solution to (11.41) by noting that

$$\hat{\mathbf{p}} \cdot \nabla f_d(\mathbf{p}, \mathbf{r}) = \frac{df_d(\mathbf{p}, \mathbf{r})}{dl}, \tag{11.43}$$

where d/dl denotes a directional derivative along a line parallel to $\mathbf{p}$. With this notation, (11.41) has the form

$$\frac{df_d}{dl} + P f_d = Q(\mathbf{p}, \mathbf{r}), \tag{11.44}$$

where

$$P = -n_a \sigma^{\text{tot}}, \tag{11.45}$$

$$Q(\mathbf{p}, \mathbf{r}) = \frac{n_a}{Z} \int_\infty s(\mathbf{p}, \mathbf{p}') f_d(\mathbf{p}', \mathbf{r}) \, d^3p' + \varepsilon_i(\mathbf{p}, \mathbf{r}). \tag{11.46}$$

The general solution of (11.44) is

$$f_d(\mathbf{p}, \mathbf{r}) = K e^{-\alpha} + e^{-\alpha} \int_{\mathbf{r}_0}^{\mathbf{r}} Q(\mathbf{p}, \mathbf{r}') e^{\alpha'} \, dl', \tag{11.47}$$

where K is a constant,

$$\alpha = \alpha(\mathbf{r}) = \int_{\mathbf{r}_0}^{\mathbf{r}} n_a \sigma_{\text{tot}} \, dl, \tag{11.48}$$

and $\alpha' = \alpha(\mathbf{r}')$. To satisfy the boundary conditions, K must be zero. The final result is

$$f_d(\mathbf{p}, \mathbf{r}) = \int_{\mathbf{r}_0}^{\mathbf{r}} \exp(\alpha' - \alpha) \left(\frac{n_a}{Z} \int_\infty s(\mathbf{p}, \mathbf{p}') f_d(\mathbf{p}', \mathbf{r}') \, d^3p' + \varepsilon_i(\mathbf{p}, \mathbf{r}') \right) dl'. \tag{11.49}$$

Of course, this equation is not really a solution because it contains the unknown $f_d(\mathbf{p}, \mathbf{r})$ buried in a double integral on the right-hand side. It is, however, an integral equation for $f_d(\mathbf{p}, \mathbf{r})$ that can be used to derive various approximate solutions. As an example, let us again consider the single-scatter approximation introduced in Section 11.2.2. This approximation is incorporated into (11.49) by neglecting $f_d(\mathbf{p}', \mathbf{r}')$ on the right compared with the attenuated incident flux $f_i(\mathbf{p}', \mathbf{r}')$. In other words, the scattering term in the Boltzmann equation, in this limit, includes only previously unscattered photons. Equation (11.7) can then be recognized as a special case of (11.49).

An important attribute of (11.49) is that it provides a straightforward way of improving upon the single-scatter approximation by an iterative procedure. If we denote the integral on the right of (11.49) as a linear operator $\mathscr{L}$, we can write symbolically, using (11.42),

$$f_d = \mathscr{L}\{f\} = \mathscr{L}\{f_d + f_i\}. \tag{11.50}$$

The single-scatter limit is a first approximation of f_d, denoted $f_d^{(1)}$, and given by

$$f_d^{(1)} = \mathscr{L}\{f_i\}. \tag{11.51}$$

A second approximation can be obtained by using $f_d^{(1)}$ in the integral of (11.49), so that

$$f_d^{(2)} = \mathscr{L}\{f_d^{(1)} + f_i\}. \tag{11.52}$$

The process can in principle be continued in this way until acceptable accuracy is attained. At each step a complicated double integral must be evaluated. Furthermore the integrand depends on $\mathbf{p}$, so a huge number of integrations are required at each iteration.

11.2.6 The Diffusion Approximation

The diffusion approximation is the opposite extreme from the single-scatter approximation. In the latter we assume that each photon undergoes zero or one scattering event. The single-scatter approximation is thus most suitable when the thickness of the medium is small compared to $1/\mu^{\text{tot}}$. In the diffusion approximation, on the other hand, it is assumed that there are a very large number of scattering events. This is a good approximation if the thickness is large compared to $1/\mu^{\text{tot}}$.

If there are a large number of scattering events and there is a substantial energy loss on each event, then the resultant photon has very little energy left and will quite likely be photoelectrically absorbed. Therefore the diffusion approximation is of little use in the high-energy range where $\Delta\mathscr{E}$ is large (see Table 11.1). Its greatest applicability is in the energy range where $\Delta\mathscr{E}$ is negligible.

If $\Delta\mathscr{E}$ is negligible, the scattering term in the Boltzmann equation mixes together only photons having the same energy or magnitude of $\mathbf{p}$. We can therefore treat such groups of photons independently, which we emphasize by writing

$$f(\mathbf{p}, \mathbf{r}) = f_{\text{p}}(\hat{\mathbf{p}}, \mathbf{r}). \tag{11.53}$$

We also define a spatial density of photons of momentum p by

$$u_{\text{p}}(\mathbf{r}) = \int_{4\pi} f_{\text{p}}(\hat{\mathbf{p}}, \mathbf{r})\, d\Omega, \tag{11.54}$$

where $d^3\text{p} = \text{p}^2\, d\text{p}\, d\Omega$ so that the overall spatial density is [cf. (11.26)]

$$u(\mathbf{r}) = \int_0^\infty \text{p}^2 u_{\text{p}}(\mathbf{r})\, d\text{p}. \tag{11.55}$$

Similarly, the photons of (magnitude) momentum p have a net (vector) momentum density given by

$$\mathbf{J}_{\text{p}}(\mathbf{r}) \equiv \int_{4\pi} \mathbf{p} f_{\text{p}}(\hat{\mathbf{p}}, \mathbf{r})\, d\Omega, \tag{11.56}$$

so that the overall momentum density (11.27) is

$$\mathbf{J}(\mathbf{r}) = \int_0^\infty \text{p}^2 \mathbf{J}_{\text{p}}(\mathbf{r})\, d\text{p}. \tag{11.57}$$

The division into attenuated incident and diffuse components is still valid and applies to $u_{\text{p}}(\mathbf{r})$ and $\mathbf{J}_{\text{p}}(\mathbf{r})$ as well as $f_{\text{p}}(\hat{\mathbf{p}}, \mathbf{r})$:

$$f_{\text{p}}(\hat{\mathbf{p}}, \mathbf{r}) = f_{\text{p,i}}(\hat{\mathbf{p}}, \mathbf{r}) + f_{\text{p,d}}(\hat{\mathbf{p}}, \mathbf{r}); \tag{11.58}$$

$$u_{\text{p}}(\mathbf{r}) = u_{\text{p,i}}(\mathbf{r}) + u_{\text{p,d}}(\mathbf{r}) = \int_{4\pi} f_{\text{p,i}}(\mathbf{p}, \mathbf{r})\, d\Omega + \int_{4\pi} f_{\text{p,d}}(\hat{\mathbf{p}}, \mathbf{r})\, d\Omega; \tag{11.59}$$

$$\mathbf{J}_{\text{p}}(\mathbf{r}) = \mathbf{J}_{\text{p,i}}(\mathbf{r}) + \mathbf{J}_{\text{p,d}}(\mathbf{r}) = \int_{4\pi} \mathbf{p} f_{\text{p,i}}(\hat{\mathbf{p}}, \mathbf{r})\, d\Omega + \int_{4\pi} \mathbf{p} f_{\text{p,d}}(\hat{\mathbf{p}}, \mathbf{r})\, d\Omega. \tag{11.60}$$

The essence of the diffusion approximation is to assume that $f_{\mathfrak{p},\mathrm{d}}(\mathbf{p}, \mathbf{r})$ is almost independent of the direction of $\hat{\mathbf{p}}$. The small residual anistropy of $f_{\mathfrak{p},\mathrm{d}}(\hat{\mathbf{p}}, \mathbf{r})$ is in the direction of the net diffuse momentum density $\mathbf{J}_{\mathfrak{p},\mathrm{d}}(\mathbf{r})$. A general expression for $f_{\mathfrak{p},\mathrm{d}}(\hat{\mathbf{p}}, \mathbf{r})$ could be obtained as an expansion in Legendre polynomials about this preferred direction $\mathbf{J}_{\mathfrak{p},\mathrm{d}}$, but the diffusion approximation truncates this expansion with only the zeroth-order and first-order terms. Since the zeroth-order Legendre polynomial is a constant and the first-order one is just a cosine, we can write

$$f_{\mathfrak{p},\mathrm{d}}(\hat{\mathbf{p}}, \mathbf{r}) \approx A + B\mathbf{J}_{\mathfrak{p},\mathrm{d}}(\mathbf{r}) \cdot \hat{\mathbf{p}}. \tag{11.61}$$

The constant A is found by integrating both sides of (11.61) over all directions of $\hat{\mathbf{p}}$. The term proportional to B integrates to zero, and

$$\int_{4\pi} f_{\mathfrak{p},\mathrm{d}}(\hat{\mathbf{p}}, \mathbf{r})\, d\Omega = 4\pi A = u_{\mathfrak{p},\mathrm{d}}(\mathbf{r}). \tag{11.62}$$

To find B, we note that

$$\begin{aligned} J_{\mathfrak{p},\mathrm{d}}^2 &= \mathbf{J}_{\mathfrak{p},\mathrm{d}} \cdot \mathbf{J}_{\mathfrak{p},\mathrm{d}} = \mathbf{J}_{\mathfrak{p},\mathrm{d}} \cdot \int_{4\pi} \mathbf{p} f_{\mathfrak{p},\mathrm{d}}(\hat{\mathbf{p}}, \mathbf{r})\, d\Omega \\ &\approx \mathbf{J}_{\mathfrak{p},\mathrm{d}} \cdot \int_{4\pi} \mathbf{p}(A + B\mathbf{J}_{\mathfrak{p},\mathrm{d}} \cdot \hat{\mathbf{p}})\, d\Omega \\ &= B\mathfrak{p} \int_{4\pi} (\mathbf{J}_{\mathfrak{p},\mathrm{d}} \cdot \hat{\mathbf{p}})^2\, d\Omega = (4\pi/3)B\mathfrak{p}J_{\mathfrak{p},\mathrm{d}}^2. \end{aligned} \tag{11.63}$$

The last step follows readily if $\mathbf{J}_{\mathfrak{p},\mathrm{d}}$ is chosen as the polar axis. Hence

$$B = 3/(4\pi\mathfrak{p}), \tag{11.64}$$

so that (11.61) becomes

$$f_{\mathfrak{p},\mathrm{d}}(\hat{\mathbf{p}}, \mathbf{r}) \approx \frac{1}{4\pi} u_{\mathfrak{p},\mathrm{d}}(\mathbf{r}) + \frac{3}{4\pi\mathfrak{p}} \mathbf{J}_{\mathfrak{p},\mathrm{d}}(\mathbf{r}) \cdot \hat{\mathbf{p}}. \tag{11.65}$$

11.2.7 Derivation of the Diffusion Equation

If we include a generation term to allow for the possibility of radioactive isotopes within the body, the steady-state Boltzmann equation (11.37) becomes

$$\begin{aligned} n_a\sigma^{\mathrm{tot}} f_{\mathfrak{p}}(\hat{\mathbf{p}}, \mathbf{r}) = &-\hat{\mathbf{p}} \cdot \nabla f_{\mathfrak{p}}(\hat{\mathbf{p}}, \mathbf{r}) \\ &+ \frac{n_a}{Z} \int_{4\pi} \frac{d\sigma^{\mathrm{C}}}{d\Omega'} f_{\mathfrak{p}}(\hat{\mathbf{p}}', \mathbf{r})\, d\Omega' + \varepsilon_{\mathfrak{p}}(\mathbf{r}), \end{aligned} \tag{11.66}$$

where we have used the elastic form (11.32) in the scattering term, and

$$\left.\frac{\partial f_{\mathfrak{p}}(\hat{\mathfrak{p}}, \mathfrak{r}, t)}{\partial t}\right|_{\text{gen}} \equiv c\varepsilon_{\mathfrak{p}}(\mathfrak{r}). \tag{11.67}$$

It is assumed that the generation term is isotropic, so that $\varepsilon_{\mathfrak{p}}(\mathfrak{r})$ is independent of the direction of $\mathfrak{p}$, and that the generation rate is constant.

For the diffuse component $f_{\mathfrak{p},\mathrm{d}}(\hat{\mathfrak{p}}, \mathfrak{r})$, (11.66) becomes [cf. (11.41)]

$$n_{\mathrm{a}}\sigma^{\mathrm{tot}} f_{\mathfrak{p},\mathrm{d}}(\hat{\mathfrak{p}}, \mathfrak{r}) = -\hat{\mathfrak{p}} \cdot \nabla f_{\mathfrak{p},\mathrm{d}}(\hat{\mathfrak{p}}, \mathfrak{r}) + \varepsilon_{\mathrm{i}}(\mathfrak{p}, \mathfrak{r}) + \varepsilon_{\mathfrak{p}}(\mathfrak{r}) + \frac{n_a}{Z}\int_{4\pi} \frac{d\sigma^{\mathrm{C}}}{d\Omega'} f_{\mathfrak{p},\mathrm{d}}(\hat{\mathfrak{p}}', \mathfrak{r})\, d\Omega'. \tag{11.68}$$

Since the gradient operator ∇ acts only on the vector $\mathfrak{r}$, $\mathfrak{p}$ may be regarded as a constant vector as far as this operator is concerned, so that

$$\hat{\mathfrak{p}} \cdot \nabla f_{\mathfrak{p},\mathrm{d}}(\hat{\mathfrak{p}}, \mathfrak{r}) = \nabla \cdot [\hat{\mathfrak{p}} f_{\mathfrak{p},\mathrm{d}}(\hat{\mathfrak{p}}, \mathfrak{r})]. \tag{11.69}$$

Integrating (11.68) over all directions of $\hat{\mathfrak{p}}$ and using (11.31), (11.42), (11.54), (11.56), and (11.69), we find

$$n_{\mathrm{a}}\sigma^{\mathrm{tot}} u_{\mathfrak{p},\mathrm{d}}(\mathfrak{r}) = -(1/\mathfrak{p})\,\nabla \cdot \mathbf{J}_{\mathfrak{p},\mathrm{d}}(\mathfrak{r}) + (n_{\mathrm{a}}\sigma^{\mathrm{C}}/Z) u_{\mathfrak{p},\mathrm{i}}(\mathfrak{r}) + 4\pi\varepsilon_{\mathfrak{p}}(\mathfrak{r}) + (n_{\mathrm{a}}\sigma^{\mathrm{C}}/Z) u_{\mathfrak{p},\mathrm{d}}(\mathfrak{r}). \tag{11.70}$$

In this equation $\varepsilon_{\mathfrak{p}}(\mathfrak{r})$ and $u_{\mathfrak{p},\mathrm{i}}(\mathfrak{r})$ are known or easily calculated quantities, but $\mathbf{J}_{\mathfrak{p},\mathrm{d}}(\mathfrak{r})$ and $u_{\mathfrak{p},\mathrm{d}}(\mathfrak{r})$ are unknown. To get another equation involving these two unknowns, we substitute (11.65) into (11.68), yielding

$$\frac{1}{4\pi} n_{\mathrm{a}}\sigma^{\mathrm{tot}} u_{\mathfrak{p},\mathrm{d}} + \frac{3}{4\pi\mathfrak{p}} n_{\mathrm{a}}\sigma^{\mathrm{tot}} \mathbf{J}_{\mathfrak{p},\mathrm{d}} \cdot \hat{\mathfrak{p}} = -\frac{1}{4\pi}\hat{\mathfrak{p}} \cdot \nabla u_{\mathfrak{p},\mathrm{d}} - \frac{3}{4\pi\mathfrak{p}}\hat{\mathfrak{p}} \cdot \nabla(\mathbf{J}_{\mathfrak{p},\mathrm{d}} \cdot \hat{\mathfrak{p}}) + \varepsilon_{\mathrm{i}} + \varepsilon_{\mathfrak{p}} + \frac{n_{\mathrm{a}}}{4\pi Z} u_{\mathfrak{p},\mathrm{d}}\sigma^{\mathrm{C}} + \frac{n_{\mathrm{a}}}{Z}\frac{3}{4\pi\mathfrak{p}}\int_{4\pi}\frac{d\sigma^{\mathrm{C}}}{d\Omega'} \mathbf{J}_{\mathfrak{p},\mathrm{d}} \cdot \hat{\mathfrak{p}}'\, d\Omega'. \tag{11.71}$$

Making use of the fact that $d\sigma^{\mathrm{C}}/d\Omega'$ is a function of only the angle between $\hat{\mathfrak{p}}$ and $\hat{\mathfrak{p}}'$, we can transform the integral in (11.71) to

$$\int_{4\pi}\frac{d\sigma^{\mathrm{C}}}{d\Omega'} \mathbf{J}_{\mathfrak{p},\mathrm{d}} \cdot \hat{\mathfrak{p}}'\, d\Omega' = (\mathbf{J}_{\mathfrak{p},\mathrm{d}} \cdot \hat{\mathfrak{p}})\beta, \tag{11.72}$$

where

$$\beta = \int_{4\pi} \frac{d\sigma^{C}}{d\Omega'} (\hat{\mathbf{p}} \cdot \hat{\mathbf{p}}')\, d\Omega'. \tag{11.73}$$

The quantity β, a weighted average of the cosine of the scattering angle, measures the difference in probability of forward and backward scattering. When the approximation of (11.1) is used, β is zero.

Multiplying (11.71) by $\hat{\mathbf{p}}$ and integrating over Ω gives, for $\beta = 0$,

$$(n_a\sigma^{tot}/p)\mathbf{J}_{p,d} = -\tfrac{1}{3}\nabla u_{p,d} + \int_{4\pi} \hat{\mathbf{p}}\varepsilon_i(\mathbf{p}, \mathbf{r})\, d\Omega, \tag{11.74}$$

where we have used the identity (Ishimaru, 1978)

$$\int_{4\pi} \hat{\mathbf{p}}(\hat{\mathbf{p}} \cdot \mathbf{A})\, d\Omega = 4\pi\mathbf{A}/3, \tag{11.75}$$

with $\mathbf{A}$ being any constant vector (i.e., one independent of the direction $\hat{\mathbf{p}}$).

Equation (11.70) gives $u_{p,d}$ in terms of $\nabla \cdot \mathbf{J}_{p,d}$, while (11.74) gives $\mathbf{J}_{p,d}$ in terms of $\nabla u_{p,d}$. Taking the divergence of (11.74) and inserting it into (11.70) produces

$$\nabla^2 u_{p,d} - \kappa^2 u_{p,d} = 3\nabla \cdot \int_{4\pi} \mathbf{p}\varepsilon_i(\mathbf{p}, \mathbf{r})\, d\Omega - \left(\frac{3n_a^2\sigma^{tot}\sigma^{C}}{Z}\right) u_{p,i}(\mathbf{r}) - 12\pi n_a\sigma^{tot}\varepsilon_p(\mathbf{r}), \tag{11.76}$$

where

$$\kappa^2 = 3n_a^2\sigma^{tot}(\sigma^{tot} - \sigma^{C}/Z) = 3n_a^2\sigma^{tot}\sigma^{pe}. \tag{11.77}$$

Except for a factor of $\sqrt{3}$, κ is the geometric mean of the total linear attenuation coefficient $n_a\sigma^{tot}$ and the linear attenuation coefficient for photoelectric absorption $n_a\sigma^{pe}$.

Equation (11.76) is the *diffusion equation*, an inhomogeneous linear differential equation for the diffuse component of the photon density, $u_{p,d}(\mathbf{r})$. The first two terms on the right-hand side are effective source terms produced by an external x-ray source. They may be calculated from equations (11.40), (11.42), and (11.54) if the incident flux and the properties of the scattering medium are given. The last term on the right-hand side in (11.76) accounts for radiation sources inside the scattering medium. After (11.76) is solved, the diffuse momentum flux $\mathbf{J}_{p,d}(\mathbf{r})$ can be calculated from (11.74) and the full distribution function follows from (11.58) and (11.65).

Boundary conditions and methods of solution of the diffusion equation are given by Ishimaru (1978), but the conditions for its validity (elastic scattering, large objects) are difficult to satisfy in practical radiographic problems.

11.3 THE IMPORTANCE OF SCATTERED RADIATION

11.3.1 Deterministic Image Properties

Scattered radiation enters into the analytical description of a radiographic system in much the same way as septal penetration radiation (see Section 4.6.2). The overall PSF $p_{\text{tot}}(\mathbf{r})$ consists of a primary or unscattered component $p_{\text{pri}}(\mathbf{r})$ and a scatter component $p_{\text{scat}}(\mathbf{r})$. The primary PSF was calculated for various systems in Chapter 4. It represents the point image formed by photons that have not undergone any interactions, either in the patient's body or in the shielding and collimating structure of the imaging system. The scatter PSF, on the other hand consists of photons that have undergone one or more Compton scattering events. [$p_{\text{scat}}(\mathbf{r})$ is often shift variant, but we shall not acknowledge that fact in the notation.] Since the scattered and unscattered photons form two mutually exclusive classes, it follows that $p_{\text{tot}}(\mathbf{r})$ can be written as a simple sum, just as in the case of septal penetration:

$$p_{\text{tot}}(\mathbf{r}) = p_{\text{pri}}(\mathbf{r}) + p_{\text{scat}}(\mathbf{r}). \tag{11.78}$$

The general character of the scatter PSF was indicated in Section 11.2. As exemplified by Fig. 11.2, $p_{\text{scat}}(\mathbf{r})$ is a broad, slowly varying function. It is often a good approximation to represent it as a Gaussian of the form

$$p_{\text{scat}}(\mathbf{r}) = A_s T \exp(-\pi \beta_s^2 r^2), \tag{11.79}$$

where T is the exposure time and A_s and β_s are parameters depending on the photon energy, and the properties of the scattering medium and the imaging system. (A_s has dimensions of 1/area, while β_s is a spatial frequency, dimensions 1/length.) One can, for example, obtain the Gaussian representation by using the expansion

$$\sec\theta \approx 1 + \tfrac{1}{2}\theta^2 \tag{11.80}$$

in (11.6)

Since the Fourier transform of a Gaussian is also a Gaussian, the transfer function for the scattered radiation is given by

$$P_{\text{scat}}(\boldsymbol{\rho}) = \mathscr{F}_2\{p_{\text{scat}}(\mathbf{r})\} = P_{\text{scat}}(0)\exp(-\pi\rho^2/\beta_s^2), \tag{11.81}$$

where, by the central ordinate theorem (B.15),

$$P_{\text{scat}}(0) = \int_\infty p_{\text{scat}}(\mathbf{r})\, d^2r = A_s T/\beta_s^2. \tag{11.82}$$

We may define a scatter-to-primary ratio (SPR) by

$$\mathrm{SPR} = \frac{\int_\infty p_{\mathrm{scat}}(\mathbf{r})\, d^2r}{\int_\infty p_{\mathrm{pri}}(\mathbf{r})\, d^2r} = \frac{P_{\mathrm{scat}}(0)}{P_{\mathrm{pri}}(0)}. \tag{11.83}$$

Even if the object is more complicated than a single point, the SPR is still given by (11.83) if the PSFs are shift invariant. To demonstrate this point, note that

$$\frac{\int_\infty [p_{\mathrm{scat}}(\mathbf{r}) ** f(\mathbf{r})]\, d^2r}{\int_\infty [p_{\mathrm{pri}}(\mathbf{r}) ** f(\mathbf{r})]\, d^2r} = \frac{P_{\mathrm{scat}}(0)F(0)}{P_{\mathrm{pri}}(0)F(0)} = \mathrm{SPR}. \tag{11.84}$$

On the other hand, if either p_{pri} or p_{scat} is shift variant, then SPR is a function of the object distribution $f(\mathbf{r})$.

As one way of investigating $p_{\mathrm{tot}}(\mathbf{r})$, let us assume that $p_{\mathrm{pri}}(\mathbf{r})$ can also be described by a Gaussian:

$$p_{\mathrm{pri}}(\mathbf{r}) = A_{\mathrm{p}} T \exp(-\pi\beta_{\mathrm{p}}^2 r^2). \tag{11.85}$$

This would be a good approximation for a transmission radiography system with a Gaussian focal spot, or for a nuclear medicine system where p_{pri} is dominated by the detector response, which is often Gaussian. In other cases, the main virtue of (11.85) is analytic simplicity. With this all-Gaussian model, $\mathrm{SPR} = A_{\mathrm{s}}\beta_{\mathrm{p}}^2/A_{\mathrm{p}}\beta_{\mathrm{s}}^2$, and the overall MTF is given by

$$\begin{aligned}\mathrm{MTF}_{\mathrm{tot}} &= \frac{P_{\mathrm{tot}}(\boldsymbol{\rho})}{P_{\mathrm{tot}}(0)} = \frac{P_{\mathrm{pri}}(\boldsymbol{\rho}) + P_{\mathrm{scat}}(\boldsymbol{\rho})}{P_{\mathrm{pri}}(0) + P_{\mathrm{scat}}(0)} \\ &= (1 + \mathrm{SPR})^{-1}[\exp(-\pi\rho^2/\beta_{\mathrm{p}}^2) + \mathrm{SPR}\cdot\exp(-\pi\rho^2/\beta_{\mathrm{s}}^2)]. \end{aligned} \tag{11.86}$$

This function is plotted in Fig. 11.4. Since the scatter MTF is always much narrower than the primary MTF ($\beta_{\mathrm{s}} \ll \beta_{\mathrm{p}}$), the effect of scatter is to reduce the contrast at intermediate spatial frequencies in the range between β_{s} and β_{p}. For frequencies small compared to β_{p} but large compared to β_{s}, the contrast reduction is

$$\frac{P_{\mathrm{tot}}(\boldsymbol{\rho})}{P_{\mathrm{pri}}(\boldsymbol{\rho})} \approx \frac{1}{1 + \mathrm{SPR}}, \qquad \beta_{\mathrm{s}} \ll \rho \ll \beta_{\mathrm{p}}. \tag{11.87}$$

As an example of the applicability of this result, consider a typical transmission radiography system where β_{p} may be 5 mm^{-1}. The scatter PSF will usually have a width of many centimeters, so that $\beta_{\mathrm{s}} \approx 0.01\ \mathrm{mm}^{-1}$ is not unreasonable. Then (11.87) shows that sinusoidal objects with spatial periods in the range from a millimeter or so to a few centimeters will have their

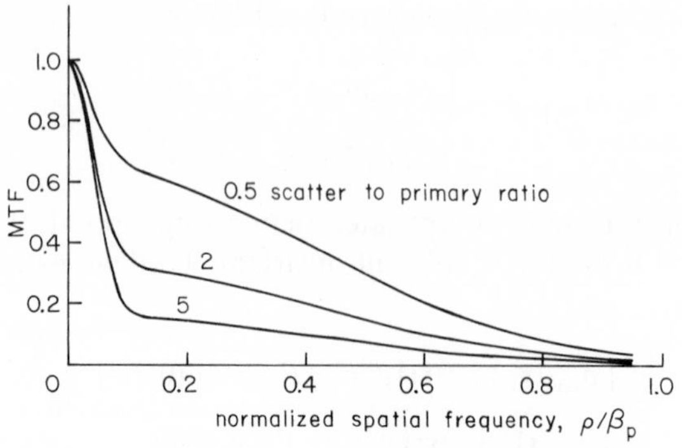

Fig. 11.4 MTF for a model in which both the scatter PSF and the primary PSF are Gaussian functions.

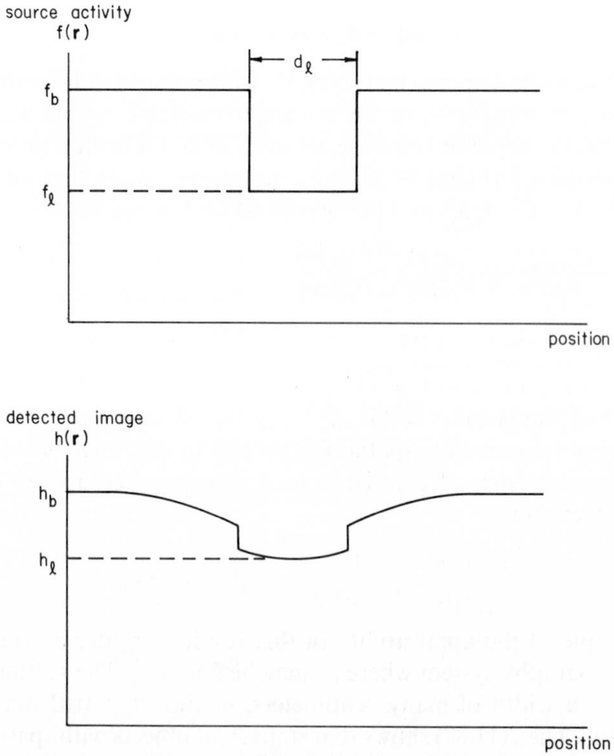

Fig. 11.5 Top: Broad, uniform source with a cold lesion of diameter d_l. Bottom: Image of the source when the only image degradation is a Gaussian scatter PSF.

modulation or contrast reduced by a factor of $(1 + \text{SPR})^{-1}$. If no precautions are taken, SPR can easily range up to 10.

Of course, scatter problems can also be analyzed entirely in the space domain. To illustrate, let us consider the nuclear-medicine problem illustrated in Fig. 11.5, which is intended to represent a liver scan with a cold, low-contrast lesion in a uniform background. The source function is

$$f(\mathbf{r}) = f_b + (f_l - f_b)\,\text{circ}(2r/d_l), \tag{11.88}$$

where subscripts b and l refer to "background" and "lesion." The detected image $h(\mathbf{r})$ is $f(\mathbf{r})$ filtered with $p_{tot}(\mathbf{r})$. Assuming unit magnification, we may write

$$h(\mathbf{r}) = f(\mathbf{r}) ** p_{tot}(\mathbf{r}) = f(\mathbf{r}) ** p_{pri}(\mathbf{r}) + f(\mathbf{r}) ** p_{scat}(\mathbf{r}). \tag{11.89}$$

We continue to use the Gaussian model for both p_{pri} and p_{scat}, and assume that the primary resolution is adequate to sharply image the lesion. The primary PSF can then be approximated by a delta function,

$$p_{pri}(\mathbf{r}) \approx (A_p T/\beta_p^2)\,\delta(\mathbf{r}). \tag{11.90}$$

By contrast, we assume that the scatter PSF is so broad that the lesion is completely unresolved by the scattered radiation, or $\beta_s d_l \ll 1$. This means that when p_{scat} is convolved with $f(\mathbf{r})$, the circ function in (11.88) can be treated as a delta function, so that

$$p_{scat}(\mathbf{r}) ** \text{circ}(2r/d_l) \approx \tfrac{1}{4}\pi d_l^2 p_{scat}(\mathbf{r}). \tag{11.91}$$

However, the background is assumed to be absolutely uniform, extending to infinity, so the approximation of (11.91) does not apply to the background term.

With these approximations, (11.89) becomes

$$\begin{aligned} h(\mathbf{r}) \approx\ & (A_p T/\beta_p^2)[f_b - \Delta f\,\text{circ}(2r/d_l)] \\ & + (A_s T/\beta_s)^2 f_b - \Delta f(\pi d_l^2/4) A_s T \exp(-\pi \beta_s^2 r^2), \end{aligned} \tag{11.92}$$

where $\Delta f = f_b - f_l$. Referring to Fig. 11.5, we see that

$$h_b = h(\mathbf{r} \to \infty) = \left(\frac{A_p T}{\beta_p^2} + \frac{A_s T}{\beta_s^2}\right) f_b, \tag{11.93}$$

$$h_l = h(\mathbf{r} = 0) = h_b - \Delta f\left(\frac{A_p T}{\beta_p^2} + \frac{\pi d_l^2}{4} A_s T\right). \tag{11.94}$$

Hence, with (11.82) and (11.83),

$$\frac{\Delta h}{h_b} = \frac{h_b - h_l}{h_b} = \frac{1 + (\frac{1}{4}\pi d_l^2)\beta_s^2\,\text{SPR}}{1 + \text{SPR}} \cdot \frac{\Delta f}{f_b}. \tag{11.95}$$

Once again, the contrast is reduced by a factor of $(1 + \text{SPR})^{-1}$. The extra term in the numerator, $(\pi d_l^2/4)\beta_s^2$ SPR, is probably negligible since we have assumed that $\beta_s d_l \ll 1$. However, the interpretation of this extra term is interesting. It represents the small fraction of the object spectrum that falls within the passband of the low-pass filter $p_{\text{scat}}(\mathbf{r})$. It does not appear in (11.87) because that equation applies to an object spectrum that is nonzero only at the specific frequency $\boldsymbol{\rho}$, rather than a spectrum like $\mathscr{F}_2\{\text{circ}(2r/d_l)\}$ that extends from zero to some finite "cutoff" frequency (of order $1/d_l$ in this case).

The procedures of this section can in principle be extended to more complicated objects and more general PSFs, but the analysis quickly becomes very involved. A particular difficulty arises when three-dimensional objects are considered, so that p_{scat} is not only shift variant within a single object plane, but also depends parametrically on the depth z of the plane. However, the main conclusion reached in this section remains generally valid: the contrast is always reduced by scatter.

11.3.2 Noise Due to Scatter

It is straightforward to include the effects of scatter in the noise analysis presented in Chapter 10. The noise in a processed image $\mathbf{u}^\dagger(\mathbf{r})$ depends on the PSF of the processing filter, $p_f(\mathbf{r})$, and on the mean spatial density of detected photons $h(\mathbf{r})$. It makes no difference whether a photon that contributes to $h(\mathbf{r})$ traveled to the detector plane in a straight line from the source or suffered one or more interactions en route. [We are assuming here that all photons are recorded in a binary fashion so that they either contribute to $h(\mathbf{r})$ or they do not. There would be an additional noise if photons of different energy contributed differently to the image (see Section 5.5.1).] Quite generally, the noise variance in $\mathbf{u}^\dagger(\mathbf{r})$ is given by (10.10). If we divide $h(\mathbf{r})$ into primary and scattered components, this equation reads

$$\sigma_{u^\dagger}^2(\mathbf{r}) = [p_f(\mathbf{r})]^2 ** [h_{\text{pri}}(\mathbf{r}) + h_{\text{scat}}(\mathbf{r})]. \tag{11.96}$$

Similarly, the mean value of $\mathbf{u}^\dagger(\mathbf{r})$ is given by (10.11) as

$$\langle \mathbf{u}^\dagger(\mathbf{r}) \rangle = p_f(\mathbf{r}) ** [h_{\text{pri}}(\mathbf{r}) + h_{\text{scat}}(\mathbf{r})]. \tag{11.97}$$

If we define SNR in the same way as in Chapter 10, we have

$$\text{SNR}(\mathbf{r}) = \frac{\langle \mathbf{u}^\dagger(\mathbf{r}) \rangle}{\sigma_{u^\dagger}(\mathbf{r})} = \frac{p_f ** (h_{\text{pri}} + h_{\text{scat}})}{[p_f^2 ** (h_{\text{pri}} + h_{\text{scat}})]^{1/2}}. \tag{11.98}$$

If both h_{pri} and h_{scat} are slowly varying by comparison with p_f and p_f^2, this equation reduces to

$$\text{SNR}(\mathbf{r}) \approx (A_{\text{eff}})^{1/2}[h_{\text{pri}}(\mathbf{r}) + h_{\text{scat}}(\mathbf{r})]^{1/2}, \tag{11.99}$$

where A_{eff} is the effective noise-averaging area given by [cf. (10.151)]

$$A_{\text{eff}} = \left(\int_{\infty} p_f(\mathbf{r})\, d^2 r \right)^2 \Big/ \int_{\infty} [p_f(\mathbf{r})]^2\, d^2 r. \tag{11.100}$$

The SNR is thus the square root of the total counts in the area A_{eff}.

Many authors adopt a different definition for SNR in scatter problems. They argue that the scatter photons contribute no useful "signal" information, so the signal should be defined as just $p_f(\mathbf{r}) ** h_{\text{pri}}(\mathbf{r})$. With this definition we have

$$\begin{aligned} \text{SNR}'(\mathbf{r}) &\equiv \frac{p_f(\mathbf{r}) ** h_{\text{pri}}(\mathbf{r})}{\sigma_{u^\dagger}(\mathbf{r})} \approx (A_{\text{eff}})^{1/2} \frac{h_{\text{pri}}(\mathbf{r})}{[h_{\text{pri}}(\mathbf{r}) + h_{\text{scat}}(\mathbf{r})]^{1/2}} \\ &= [A_{\text{eff}} h_{\text{pri}}(\mathbf{r})]^{1/2} \left(1 + \frac{h_{\text{scat}}(\mathbf{r})}{h_{\text{pri}}(\mathbf{r})} \right)^{-1/2}, \end{aligned} \tag{11.101}$$

where the last two expressions again require that h_{pri} and h_{scat} vary slowly over the area A_{eff}.

The quantity $h_{\text{scat}}(\mathbf{r})/h_{\text{pri}}(\mathbf{r})$ is a *local* scatter-to-primary ratio, not to be confused with the integral SPR given by (11.83) or (11.84). Only in the rather extreme case where the object $f(\mathbf{r})$ is slowly varying compared to the broad scatter PSF $p_{\text{scat}}(\mathbf{r})$ can we approximate $h_{\text{scat}}(\mathbf{r})/h_{\text{pri}}(\mathbf{r})$ by SPR.

Whichever definition is used, the SNR depends greatly on the nature of the object distribution. For example, consider a scintillation camera of unit magnification viewing a source distribution $f(\mathbf{r})$ in a scattering medium. If $f(\mathbf{r})$ is a point source $\delta(\mathbf{r})$, we have

$$h_{\text{pri}}(\mathbf{r}) = \delta(\mathbf{r}) ** p_{\text{pri}}(r) = p_{\text{pri}}(\mathbf{r}), \tag{11.102}$$

$$h_{\text{scat}}(\mathbf{r}) = \delta(\mathbf{r}) ** p_{\text{scat}}(\mathbf{r}) = p_{\text{scat}}(\mathbf{r}). \tag{11.103}$$

On the Gaussian model of Section 11.3.1, the local scatter-to-primary ratio at the center of the point image is just

$$\frac{h_{\text{scat}}(0)}{h_{\text{pri}}(0)} = \frac{p_{\text{scat}}(0)}{p_{\text{pri}}(0)} = \frac{A_{\text{s}}}{A_{\text{p}}} = \frac{\beta_{\text{s}}^2}{\beta_{\text{p}}^2} \cdot \text{SPR}. \tag{11.104}$$

Since $\beta_{\text{p}}^2 \gg \beta_{\text{s}}^2$, the local scatter-to-primary ratio at $\mathbf{r} = 0$ may be much less than one even when the integral ratio SPR is larger than one. This means that the scattered photons are spread out over the detector plane and do not seriously affect a point image.

The situation is very different for larger objects. We now let $f(\mathbf{r})$ be a uniform disk,

$$f(\mathbf{r}) = f_0 \, \text{circ}(2r/d_0). \tag{11.105}$$

If we assume that $\beta_s \ll 1/d_0 \ll \beta_p$, we find

$$h_{pri}(\mathbf{r}) \approx (f_0 A_p T/\beta_p^2)\,\mathrm{circ}(2r/d_0), \tag{11.106}$$

$$h_{scat}(\mathbf{r}) \approx (\pi d_0^2/4)(f_0 A_s T)\exp(-\pi\beta_s^2 r^2), \tag{11.107}$$

and

$$\frac{h_{scat}(0)}{h_{pri}(0)} = \frac{\pi}{4}\frac{A_s}{A_p}\beta_p^2 d_0^2 = \tfrac{1}{4}\pi\beta_s^2 d_0^2\ \mathrm{SPR}. \tag{11.108}$$

Thus the local scatter ratio at the center of the disk image increases rapidly as the disk diameter d_0 is increased, and the SNR degrades accordingly.

The same conclusion applies to transmission imaging, except that there d_0 should be interpreted as the diameter of the irradiated portion of the object.

11.4 CONTROL OF SCATTERED RADIATION

11.4.1 Transmission Imaging

Scattered radiation may be minimized in transmission radiography by:

1. limiting the area of the incident beam;
2. using an air gap between the scattering medium and the detector;
3. using a collimating grid between the scattering medium and the detector;
4. optimizing the spectrum of the incident x rays.

The efficacy of the first two methods can be seen from the single-scatter model introduced in Section 11.2.2. There we showed that a small pencil beam of x rays produces a broad exposure pattern on the detector. As long as this exposure pattern is broader than the incident beam, the total scatter exposure at any point is directly proportional to the beam area. Of course the beam area must be large enough to encompass everything of medical interest in the region being imaged, but making it larger than necessary increases the scatter fraction as well as the integrated patient dose.

The single-scatter discussion also showed the advantage of an air gap between the patient and the detector. Each volume element in the patient's body acts as a source of scattered radiation, and the detected scatter intensity falls off as the inverse square of the distance from the volume element to the detector. In Fig. 11.6 this distance is approximately the perpendicular distance s_2. Unscattered radiation, on the other hand, falls off approxi-

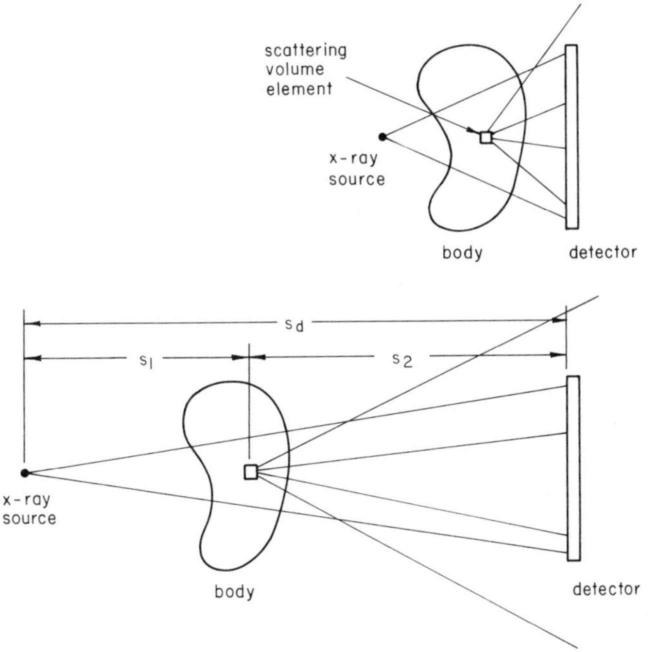

Fig. 11.6 Illustration of how an air gap can reduce the scatter-to-primary ratio in transmission radiography.

mately as $1/s_d^2$, where s_d is the perpendicular distance from the source to the detector plane. The local scatter-to-primary ratio thus varies as $(s_d/s_2)^2$.

Similar conclusions hold for the integral SPR. A circular detector of diameter d_{det} subtends a solid angle Ω_s from an axial scattering element, where

$$\Omega_s = 2\pi(1 - \cos\theta_s), \tag{11.109}$$

$$\theta_s = \tan^{-1}(d_{det}/2s_2). \tag{11.110}$$

Similarly, the solid angle subtended from the primary x-ray source is

$$\Omega_p = 2\pi(1 - \cos\theta_p), \tag{11.111}$$

$$\theta_p = \tan^{-1}(d_{det}/2s_d). \tag{11.112}$$

For a given scattering medium, the SPR is proportional to Ω_s/Ω_p. If the angles θ_p and θ_s are small, we have

$$\frac{\Omega_s}{\Omega_p} \approx \frac{\theta_s^2}{\theta_p^2} \approx \left(\frac{s_d}{s_2}\right)^2. \tag{11.113}$$

Thus the total detected scatter flux and the integral SPR are both reduced as s_2 is increased. However, there is little benefit in making s_2 very much larger than s_1; as soon as s_1 is negligible, $s_2 \approx s_d$ and the detector subtends approximately the same solid angle from the x-ray source as from the scattering element. Further increases in s_2 leave the SPR unchanged.

Of course, as discussed in Section 4.3.3, other considerations enter into the choice of s_1 and s_2 as well. If s_2/s_1 is increased, the focal spot of the x-ray tube must be smaller to maintain the same spatial resolution, but the resolution of the detector need not be as good [see (4.58) and (4.59)].

The third way to control scatter, the use of a grid, is illustrated in Fig. 11.7. In its simplest form, the grid is a series of parallel slats made of tungsten or other high-atomic-number material, and perhaps spaced apart with fiberboard or some other material with low-x-ray absorption. For an x-ray source a long distance away from the detector, the incident beam is essentially collimated. If $w \gg t$, very few of the unscattered photons strike the slats, and the primary image is largely unaffected by the grid. The only degradation of the primary image is a set of very fine lines, the shadows of the slats. This problem can be eliminated by making the grid frequency $1/w$ very large or by moving the grid uniformly parallel to the detector during exposure.

Scattered radiation, on the other hand, is no longer collimated, and most of it is blocked by the grid.

The calculation of the acceptance angle of the grid for scattered radiation is analogous to calculation of the geometric efficiency of a parallel-hole collimator for nuclear medicine. We showed in Section 4.5.4 that this efficiency is almost independent of the distance of the source from the face

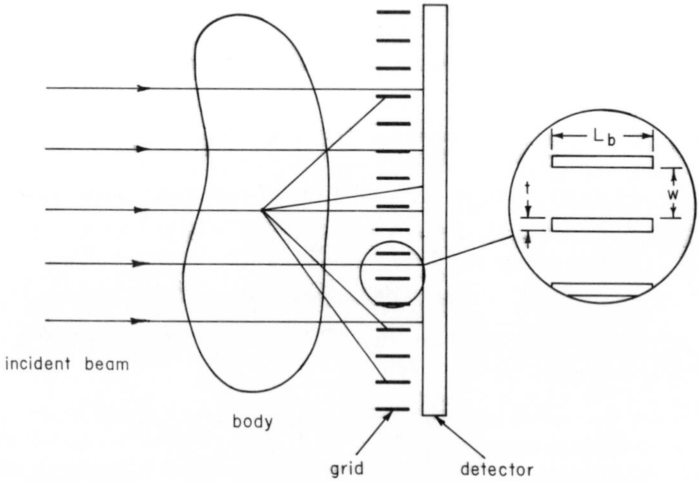

Fig. 11.7 A scatter-rejecting grid suitable for collimated radiation.

of the collimator. As the source moves away, the efficiency of each bore decreases but the number of bores that can accept radiation increases in a compensating manner [see (4.167)]. The same arguments apply to the grid, so we may as well calculate its acceptance solid angle by assuming the scatter source is in direct contact with the grid. Considering an isotropic distribution of scattered flux for simplicity, we find

$$\Omega_s = \int_0^{\pi} d\phi \int_{\pi/2 + W/2L_b}^{\pi/2 - W/2Lb} \sin\theta \, d\theta = \frac{\pi w}{L_b}. \tag{11.114}$$

If the slat thickness t is not negligible, this equation should also be multiplied by a packing fraction $w/(w + t)$. The quantity L_b/w is called the *grid ratio* (GR). Typical values of GR are 8 to 12.

Since a large detector in close proximity to a source subtends 2π steradians, we see that*

$$\frac{\mathrm{SPR}_{\mathrm{grid}}}{\mathrm{SPR}_{\mathrm{no\ grid}}} = \frac{\pi w/L_b}{2\pi} = \frac{1}{2\mathrm{GR}}. \tag{11.115}$$

If the reduction factor of (11.115) is inadequate, two crossed grids can be used. This combination is equivalent to a two-dimensional collimator, for which $\Omega_s = w^2/L_b^2$, giving

$$\frac{\mathrm{SPR}_{\mathrm{grid}}}{\mathrm{SPR}_{\mathrm{no\ grid}}} = \frac{w^2/L_b^2}{2\pi} = \frac{1}{2\pi(\mathrm{GR})^2} \tag{11.116}$$

The only reason not to make GR very large is the practical difficulty of making sure that the bores are properly aimed at the primary x-ray source. With a large GR, a slight tilt would greatly reduce the primary transmittance. A similar practical problem arises when the x-ray source is not a long distance from the grid. In that case it is common to use a *focused grid* as shown in Fig. 11.8.

Closely related to the grid is the scanning slit assembly shown in Fig. 11.9. The fore slit serves to define a narrow fan of x rays, while the aft slit rejects most of the scattered radiation. The two slits move at different velocities in such a way that they remain in line with the source. The time-averaged exposure on the detector is largely free of scatter.

The only drawback to this scheme is the relatively long time required to make a full exposure. Barnes and Brezovich (1979) have developed the method further by using several slits in each mask, creating what they call

* In practice, this equation somewhat overstates the reduction factor. Because of the forward peak in the scattering cross section and the finite size of the detector, the reduction will be less than 2GR. Furthermore, (11.115) applies only to the integral SPR; the grid is somewhat less effective, depending on the beam area, in reducing the local scatter-to-primary ratio.

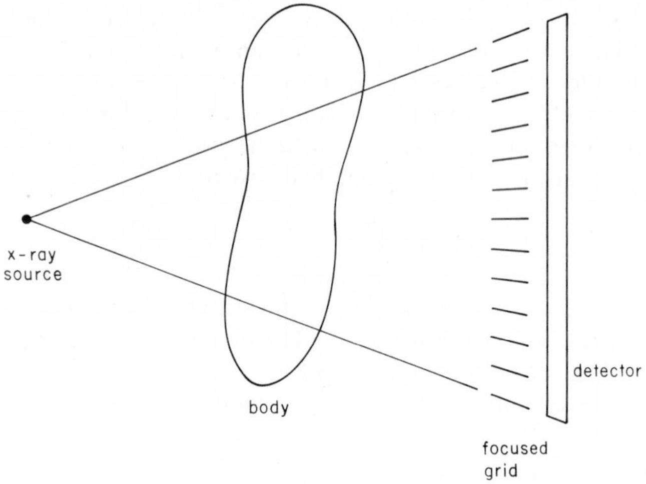

Fig. 11.8 Focused grid for scatter rejection when the x-ray source is at a finite distance from the detector.

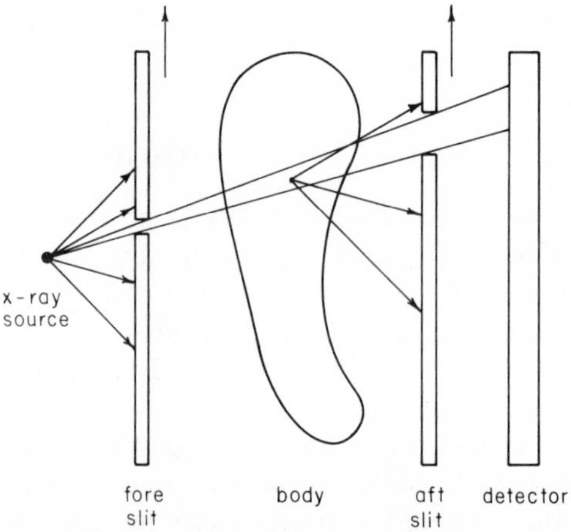

Fig. 11.9 Scanning slit assembly for scatter rejection.

a scanning multiple-slit assembly, or SMSA, and thereby reducing the exposure time. Some of their results are tabulated in Table 11.2.

Except for the scanning motion, the geometry of Fig. 11.9 is very similar to that of a fan-beam CT machine, which should also be largely immune to scatter. The old pencil-beam first-generation CT scanners, in fact, represent very nearly the best possible radiographic geometry for scatter rejection since the detector subtends such a small solid angle. But even with a fan beam, most of the scatter is out of the plane of the fan and hence misses

TABLE 11.2[a]

Scatter-to-Primary Ratios for Various Scatter-Reduction Techniques and X-Ray Tube Voltages[b]

Scatter-reduction technique	X-ray tube voltage 60 kVP	80 kVP	100 kVP	120 kVP
None	5.5	6.6	7.2	7.1
8:1 grid	0.72	1.0	1.2	1.4
12:1 grid	0.48	0.62	0.76	0.87
SMSA	0.16	0.20	0.22	0.22

[a] Taken from Barnes and Brezovich (1979).
[b] Using an 18-cm thick, 30 × 30 cm Lucite phantom.

the detector array. A collimator in front of the detectors improves matters further by eliminating certain multiply scattered photons.

The final method of scatter control in transmission radiography is optimization of the x-ray spectrum. High-energy photons interact with soft tissue predominantly by Compton scattering. Furthermore the differential scattering cross section is forward peaked (i.e., in the direction of the detector), so it might be expected that scattering problems would be particularly bad at high energies. However, higher energy photons have smaller total interaction cross sections and hence suffer fewer interactions in the body for a given number of transmitted photons. This effect reduces the scattered flux but also reduces the contrast in the primary image. Low-energy photons give a high-contrast primary image but are strongly absorbed in the body. The primary absorption process is photoelectric at very low energies ($\lesssim$40 keV). Scattered radiation could therefore be greatly diminished just by keeping the photon energy below about 40 keV, but this would not be acceptable in terms of patient dose for radiographs of thick body parts.

The choice of an optimum photon energy or spectrum is thus a complicated trade-off involving noise, dose, detector characteristics, scatter, image contrast, and the specific diagnostic information needed. More discussion of the problem is given by Motz and Danos (1978) and Muntz (1979).

11.4.2 Emission Imaging

The geometrical remedies for scatter in transmission imaging—airgaps, grids, scanning slits, etc.—are not applicable in emission imaging. The fundamental difference is that we know the location of the primary source in transmission imaging, but not in emission imaging. Photons coming from a particular volume element in the body in a nuclear image could equally well be photons originating from radioactive nuclei in that element or scattered photons from distant sources. There is no way to geometrically discriminate against scatter without the risk of also blocking desired primary photons.

On the other hand, nuclear imaging systems can use the powerful tool of energy discrimination. This method usually cannot be applied in transmission imaging because: (1) the photon arrival rate is much too high to allow processing individual photons; (2) the energy loss on each scattering event is very small at the low energies used in diagnostic radiology; (3) x-ray tubes emit a broad spectrum of energies, so it is impossible to reliably distinguish primary and scattered photons on the basis of their energy.

None of these difficulties applies in nuclear medicine. The isotopes used often emit most of their gamma rays with a single well-defined energy, and there is an appreciable energy loss on scatter. For example, the average loss for a 150-keV gamma ray is 27 keV, leaving the scattered photon an energy of 123 keV. There is no difficulty in discriminating between 123 and 150 keV with any well-designed scintillation detector, and semiconductor detectors can discriminate even much smaller differences. Furthermore the count rate in most nuclear medicine procedures is less than 10^5 counts/sec, allowing ample time for the electronics to process individual photons and accept or reject them on the basis of energy.

We may estimate the effect of energy discrimination on the integral SPR by using the single-scatter model. If the initial gamma-ray energy is $\mathscr{E}_0$ and the energy discriminator is set to reject photons below $\mathscr{E}_0 - \Delta\mathscr{E}$, then there is some maximum scattering angle $\theta_m(\Delta\mathscr{E})$ that could have occurred for any accepted photon. From (C.15)

$$\frac{1}{\mathscr{E}_0 - \Delta\mathscr{E}} - \frac{1}{\mathscr{E}_0} = \frac{1}{m_0 c^2}\{1 - \cos[\theta_m(\Delta\mathscr{E})]\}, \qquad (11.117)$$

or, if $\Delta\mathscr{E}/\mathscr{E}_0$ is small,

$$\frac{\Delta\mathscr{E}}{\mathscr{E}_0^2} \approx \frac{1}{m_0 c^2}\{1 - \cos[\theta_m(\Delta\mathscr{E})]\}. \qquad (11.118)$$

Since the primary photons are emitted isotropically, the distribution of once-scattered photons (in a thick scattering medium) is also isotropic even though the differential scattering cross section $d\sigma^C/d\Omega$ depends on scattering angle. Some small fraction of the scattered photons, determined by the geometry of the imaging system, are detected. This fraction is independent of the scattering angle θ and is the same as for unscattered photons. In other

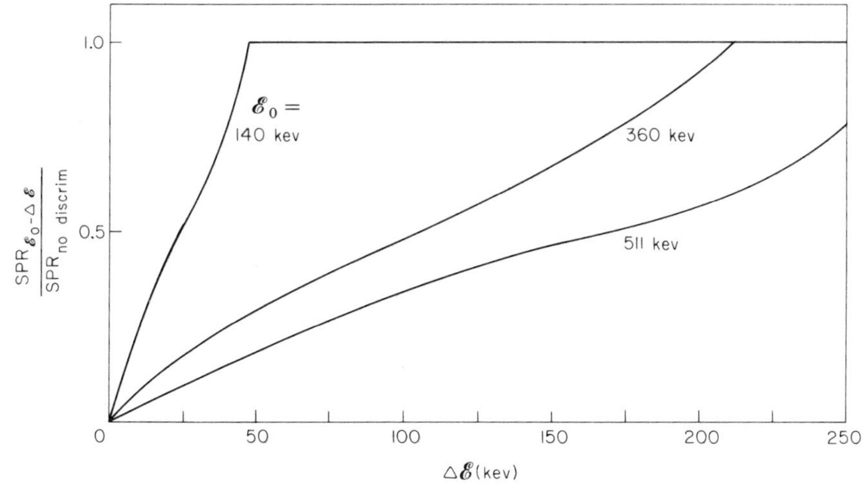

Fig. 11.10 Effect of energy discrimination on scatter-to-primary ratio in the single-scatter approximation [see (11.119)].

words, photons that have been scattered through, say, 30° are just as likely to be collected as unscattered photons since their initial directions were isotropically random. Therefore, the SPR with the energy threshold set at $\mathscr{E}_0 - \Delta\mathscr{E}$ is related to the SPR without energy discrimination by

$$\frac{SPR_{\mathscr{E}_0-\Delta\mathscr{E}}}{SPR_{\text{no discrim}}} = \frac{2\pi \int_0^{\theta_m(\Delta\mathscr{E})} (d\sigma^C/d\Omega)\sin\theta\, d\theta}{2\pi \int_0^{\pi} (d\sigma^C/d\Omega)\sin\theta\, d\theta}. \qquad (11.119)$$

If we use the low-energy limit (11.1) for $d\sigma^C/d\Omega$, this ratio of SPRs becomes

$$\frac{SPR_{\mathscr{E}_0-\Delta\mathscr{E}}}{SPR_{\text{no discrim}}} = \tfrac{1}{2} - \tfrac{3}{8}\cos[\theta_m(\Delta\mathscr{E})] - \tfrac{1}{8}\cos^3[\theta_m(\Delta\mathscr{E})]. \qquad (11.120)$$

More generally, (11.119) can be evaluated from the data given in Fig. C.7 and C.12. The ratio $SPR_{\mathscr{E}_0-\Delta\mathscr{E}}/SPR_{\text{no discrim}}$ is plotted in Fig. 11.10 for several values of $\mathscr{E}_0$.

Many experimental studies of the effect of energy discrimination on imaging performance have been performed. A typical example is shown in Fig. 11.11. The general effect of better energy discrimination is to reduce the wings on the PSF and to restore the MTF at intermediate spatial frequencies. For this reason, there is considerable interest in building a nuclear camera based on semiconductor detectors, such as germanium, which have good energy resolution.

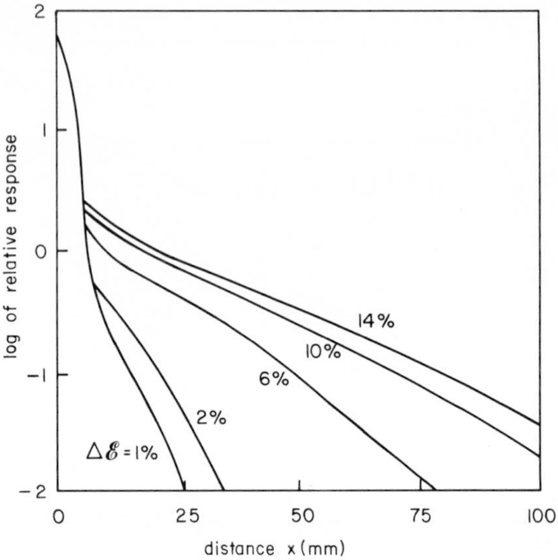

Fig. 11.11 Line spread function for a 140-keV source in a scattering medium for a detector with 3-mm spatial resolution and different degrees of energy discrimination. (Courtesy of J. W. Steidley.)

11.5 USES OF SCATTERED RADIATION

To this point we have regarded scattered radiation as something to be eliminated, but it is also possible to make good use of it. One way, called Compton radiography (Lale, 1959; Clark and van Dyk, 1969), is illustrated in Fig. 11.12. A ring source of ^{99m}Tc is used to irradiate a thin slice of the brain with 140-keV gamma rays. Except for multiple-scatter events, only 90° scattered rays can pass through the collimator. The energy window of the Anger camera is set at 109 keV, which is the energy of the gamma rays after 90° scattering.

Compton radiography provides a map of the Compton scattering cross-section, which is proportional to electron density, in the irradiated plane. This is basically the same information as in a CT scan at high energy, but Compton radiography may permit reduced patient dose. [See, however, the very pessimistic appraisal by Battista and Bronskill (1981).]

A variation on this theme, suggested by Leunbach (1977), is shown in Fig. 11.13. Here the incident radiation is collimated to a thin pencil beam which is viewed by two collimated detectors. For one position of the source and detectors, the system measures the electron density at the intersection

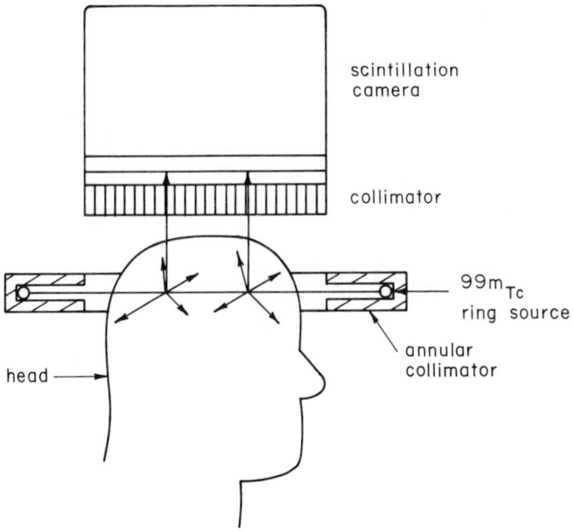

Fig. 11.12 Geometry for Compton radiography with a ring source.

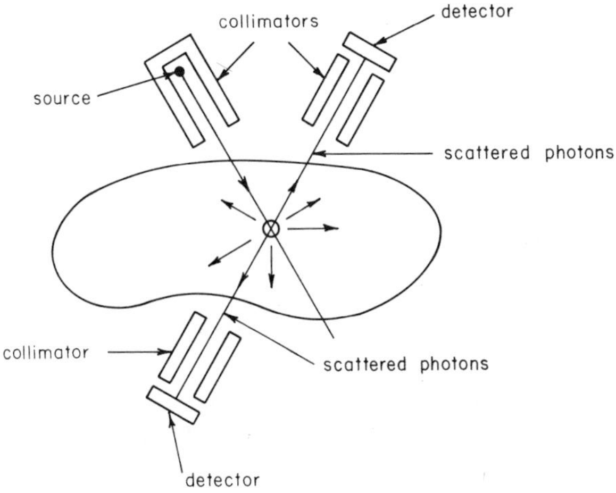

Fig. 11.13 Compton radiography system proposed by Leunbach (1977).

region defined by the incident beam and the field of view of the detectors. By scanning the whole source-detector assembly, a 2D or 3D image can be built up. This instrument can image any organ of the body in any section. A density discrimination of 1% is claimed.

It is also possible to form an image using fluorescent x rays rather than Compton scattered gamma rays (Hoffer *et al.*, 1969). In the system shown

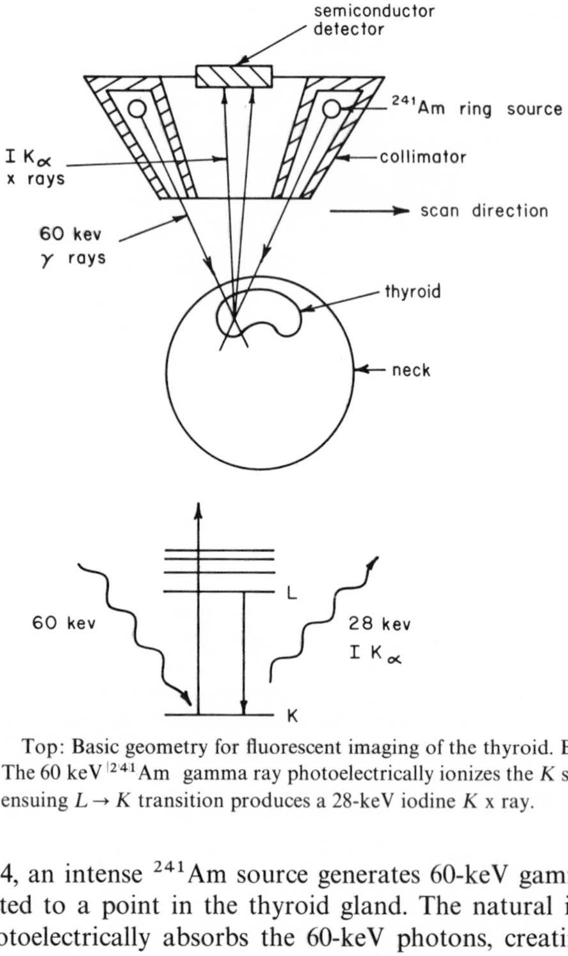

Fig. 11.14 Top: Basic geometry for fluorescent imaging of the thyroid. Bottom: Energy-level diagram. The 60 keV ^{241}Am gamma ray photoelectrically ionizes the K shell of an iodine atom, and the ensuing $L \rightarrow K$ transition produces a 28-keV iodine K x ray.

in Fig. 11.14, an intense ^{241}Am source generates 60-keV gamma rays that are collimated to a point in the thyroid gland. The natural iodine in the thyroid photoelectrically absorbs the 60-keV photons, creating vacancies in the K shell that are quickly filled with the emission of characteristic iodine K_α radiation at 28 keV. These fluorescent x rays are detected by a semiconductor detector. An image is built up by scanning the source-detector assembly.

This system provides unique information—the distribution of natural, stable iodine in the thyroid gland. It is thus complementary to nuclear medicine techniques using radioactive isotopes of iodine that measure the differential uptake of iodine by the thyroid.

In principle, fluorescent imaging could also be used for other high-atomic-number elements, but no other is present in the body in sufficient concentration. It is also possible to use stable isotopes as tracers in the same way as radioactive isotopes are used in nuclear medicine.

References

Abramowitz, M., and Stegun, I. A. (1970). "Handbook of Mathematical Functions with Formulas, Graphs and Mathematical Tables," National Bureau of Standards, Applied Mathematics Series, No. 55. U.S. Gov. Print. Off., Washington, D.C.

Abbott, E. A. (1952). "Flatland," 6th ed. Dover, New York.

Akcasu, A. Z., May, R. S., Knoll, G. F., Rogers, W. L., Koral, K. F., and Jones, L. W. (1974). Coded aperture gamma ray imaging with stochastic apertures. *Opt. Eng.* **13**, 117.

Alvarez, R. E., and Macovski, A. (1976). Energy-selective reconstructions in x-ray computerized tomography. *Phys. Med. Biol.* **21**, 733–744.

Anger, H. O. (1958). Scintillation camera. *Rev. Sci. Instrum.* **29**, 27.

Anger, H. O. (1964). Scintillation camera with multichannel collimators. *J. Nucl. Med.* **5**, 515–531.

Anger, H. O. (1967). *In* "Instrumentation in Nuclear Medicine" (G. J. Hine, ed.), Vol. 1, pp. 485–552. Academic Press, New York.

Anger, H. O. (1968). Sensitivity and resolution of the scintillation camera. *In* "Fundamental Problems in Scanning" (A. Gottschalk and R. N. Beck, eds.), pp. 117–144. Thomas, Springfield, Illinois.

Anger, H. O. (1974). Tomography and other depth-discrimination techniques. *In* "Instrumentation in Nuclear Medicine" (G. J. Hine and J. A. Sorenson, eds.), Vol. 2, pp. 61–100. Academic Press, New York.

Anger, H. O., and Davis, D. H. (1964). Gamma-ray detection efficiency and image resolution in sodium iodide. *Rev. Sci. Instrum.* **35**, 693.

Anger, H. O., Mortimer, R. K., and Tobias, C. A. (1956). Visualization of gamma-ray emitting isotopes in the human body. *Proc. Int. Conf. Peaceful Uses At. Energy, 1st, Geneva, 1955* **14**, 204.

Arnold, B. A., and Bjärngard, B. E. (1979). The effect of phosphor K x-rays on the MTF of rare-earth screens. *Med. Phys.* **6**, 500–503.

Arnold, B. A., Eisenberg, H, and Bjärngard, B. E. (1976). The LSF and MTF of rare-earth oxysulfide intensifying screens. *Radiology* **121**, 473–477.

Arnold, B. A., Eisenberg, H., and Bjärngard, B. E. (1978). Measurements of reciprocity law failure in green-sensitive x-ray films. *Radiology* **126**, 493–498.

Attix, F. H., ed. (1972). "Topics in Radiation Dosimetry," Supplement 1. Academic Press, New York.

Attix, F. H., and Roesch, W. C., eds. (1966). "Radiation Dosimetry," 2nd ed., Vol. 2. Academic Press, New York.

Attix, F. H., and Roesch, W. C., eds. (1968). "Radiation Dosimetry," 2nd ed., Vol. 1. Academic Press, New York.

Attix, F. H., and Tochilin, E., eds. (1969). "Radiation Dosimetry," 2nd ed., Vol. 3. Academic Press, New York.

Bailey, N. A., Crepeau, R. L., and Lasser, E. C. (1974). Fluoroscopic tomography. *Invest. Radiol.* **9**, 96–103.

Barber, D. C. (1973). Collimator transfer function for single bore and multichannel focusing collimators. *Int. J. Appl. Radiat. Isot.* **25**, 193.

Barnes, G. T., and Brezovich, I. A. (1979). The design and performance of a scanning multiple slit assembly. *Med. Phys.* **6**, 197.

Barrett, H. H. (1972). Fresnel zone plate imaging in nuclear medicine. *J. Nucl. Med.* **13**, 382.

Barrett, H. H., and DeMeester, G. D. (1974). Quantum noise in fresnel zone plate imaging. *Appl. Opt.* **13**, 1100.

Barrett, H. H., and Horrigan, F. A. (1973). Fresnel zone plate imaging of gamma rays; Theory. *Appl. Opt.* **12**, 2686.

Barrett, H. H., DeMeester, G. D., Wilson, D. T., and Farmelant, M. H. (1973). Recent advances in fresnel zone-plate imaging. *In* "Medical Radioisotopes Scintigraphy," Vol. 1. IAEA, Vienna.

Barrett, H. H., Stoner, W. W., Wilson, D. T., and DeMeester, G. D. (1974). Coded apertures derived from the fresnel zone plate. *Opt. Eng.* **13**, 539.

Barrett, H. H., Gordon, S. K., and Hershel, R. S. (1976). Statistical limitations in transaxial tomography. *Comput. Biol. Med.* **6**, 307.

Battista, J. J. and Bronskill, M. J. (1981). Compton scatter imaging of transverse sections: An overall appraisal and evaluation for radiotherapy planning, *Phys. Med. Biol.* **26**, 81–99.

Beck, R. N. (1964a). A theory of radioisotope scanning systems. *In* "Medical Radioisotope Scanning," Vol. 1, pp. 35–56. IAEA, Vienna.

Beck, R. N. (1964b). Collimators for radioisotope scanning systems. *In* "Medical Radioisotope Scanning," Vol. 1, pp. 211–231. IAEA, Vienna.

Beck, R. N. (1968a). The scanning system as a whole: General considerations. *In* "Fundamental Problems in Scanning," (A. Gottschalk, R. N. Beck, eds.) Chap. 3. Thomas, Springfield, Illinois.

Beck, R. N. (1968b). Collimation of gamma rays. *In* "Fundamental Problems in Scanning," (A. Gottschalk, R. N. Beck, eds.) Chap. 6, pp. 71–92. Thomas, Springfield, Illinois.

Beck, R. N. (1969). Effects of scattered radiation on scintillation detector response. *In* "Medical Radioisotope Scintigraphy," Vol. 1, pp. 595–616. IAEA, Vienna.

Biberman, L. M., ed. (1973). "Perception of Displayed Information." Plenum, New York.

Blackwell, H. R. (1946). Contrast thresholds of the human eye. *J. Opt. Soc. Am.* **36**, 624.

Bracewell, R. (1965). "The Fourier Transform and Its Applications." McGraw-Hill, New York.

Bracewell, R. N., and Riddle, A. C. (1967). Inversion of fan-beam scans in radio astronomy. *Astrophys. J.* **150**, 427–434.

Brown, C. M. (1972). Multiplex imaging and random arrays. Ph.D. Thesis, Univ. of Chicago, Chicago, Illinois.

Brown, C. M. (1974). Multiplex imaging with multiple-pinhole cameras. *J. Appl. Phys.* **45**, 4.

Brownell, G. L., and Burnham, C. A. (1974). Recent developments in positron scintigraphy. *In* "Instrumentation in Nuclear Medicine" (G. J. Hine and J. A. Sorenson, eds.), Vol. 2, pp. 135–159. Academic Press, New York.

Brownell, G. L., Correia, J. A., and Zamenhof, R. G. (1978). Positron instrumentation. *Recent Adv. Nucl. Med.* **5**, 1–69.

Budinger, T. F., and Gullberg, G. T. (1977). Transverse section reconstruction of gamma-ray emitting radionuclides in patients. *In* "Reconstruction Tomography in Diagnostic Radiology and Nuclear Medicine" (M. M. Ter-Pogossian, M. E. Phelps, G. L. Brownell, J. R. Cox, D. O. Davis, and R. G. Evens, eds.), pp. 315–342. Univ. Park Press, Baltimore, Maryland.

Burgess, A. E. (1978). An empirical equation for screen MTFs. *Med. Phys.* **5**, 199–204.

Causer, D. A. (1974). The design of parallel hole gamma camera collimators. *Int. J. Appl. Radiat. Isot.* **26**, 355.

Ceglio, N. M., Attwood, D. T., and George, E. V. (1977a). Zone plate coded imaging on a microscopic scale. *J. Appl. Phys.* **48**, 1563.

Ceglio, N. M., Attwood, D. T., and George, E. V. (1977b). Zone plate coded imaging of laser produced plasmas. *J. Appl. Phys.* **48**, 1566.

Chang, L. T. (1976). Radionuclide imaging with coded apertures and three-dimensional image reconstruction from focal plane tomography. Ph.D. Thesis, Univ. of California, Berkeley.

Chang, L. T., Kaplan, S. N., Macdonald, B., Perez-Mendez, V., and Shiraishi, L. (1974). A method of tomographic imaging using a multiple pinhole coded aperture. *J. Nucl. Med.* **15**, 1063.

Chiu, M. Y. (1980). Three-dimensional radiographic imaging. Ph.D. Thesis, Univ. of Arizona, Tucson.

Chiu, M. Y., Barrett, H. H., Simpson, R. G., Chou, C., Arendt, J. W., and Gindi, G. R. (1979). Three-dimensional radiographic imaging with a restricted view angle. *J. Opt. Soc. Am.* **69**, 1323.

Chiu, M. Y., Barrett, H. H., and Simpson, R. G. (1980). Three-dimensional reconstruction from planar projections, *J. Opt. Soc. Am.* **70**, 755–761.

Cho, Z. H., Cohen, M. B., Singh, M., Eriksson, L., Chan, J., MacDonald, N., and Spolter, L. (1977). Performance and evaluation of the circular ring transverse axial positron camera (CRTAPC). *IEEE Trans. Nucl. Sci.* **24**, 532–543.

Chou, C., and Barrett, H. H. (1978). Gamma ray imaging in fourier space. *Opt. Lett.* **3**, 5.

Clark, R. L., and van Dyk, G. (1969). Compton scattered gamma rays in diagnostic radiology. *In* "Medical Radioisotope Scintigraphy," Vol. 1, pp. 247–260. IAEA, Vienna.

Coltman, J. W. (1954). Specification of imaging properties by response to sine wave input. *J. Opt. Soc. Am.* **44**, 468.

Cormack, A. M. (1963). Representation of a function by its line integrals with some radiological applications. *J. Appl. Phys.* **34**, 2722–2727.

Dainty, J. C., and Shaw, R. (1974). "Image Science: Principles, Analysis, and Evaluation of Photographic-Type Imaging Processes." Academic Press, New York.

Davenport, W. B., Jr. (1970). "Probability and Random Processes." McGraw-Hill, New York.

Davenport, W. B., Jr., and Root, E. L. (1958). "An Introduction to the Theory of Random Signals and Noise." McGraw-Hill, New York.

Derenzo, S. E., Zaklad, H., and Budinger, T. F. (1977). Analytical study of a high-resolution positron ring detector system for transaxial reconstruction tomography. *In* "Reconstruction Tomography in Diagnostic Radiology and Nuclear Medicine" (M. M. Ter-Pogossian, M. E. Phelps, G. L. Brownell, J. R. Cox, Jr., D. O. Davis, and R. G. Evans, eds.), pp. 343–358. Univ. Park Press, Baltimore, Maryland.

Derenzo, S. E., Budinger, T. F., Huesman, R. H., Cahoon, J. L., and Vuletich, T. (1980). Imaging properties of a positron tomograph with 280 BGO crystals, *Nucl. Sci. Symp., Orlando, Florida, November 5 –7.* LBL#11858. [Also *IEEE Trans. Nucl. Sci.* **28**(1), 1981 81–89.]

DeVries, H. (1943). The quantum character of light and its bearing upon threshold of vision, the differential sensitivity and visual acuity of the eye. *Physica* (*Utrecht*) **10**, 553.

Dick, C. E. and Motz, J. W. (1981). Image information transfer properties of x-ray fluorescent screens, *Med. Phys.* **8**(3), 337–346.

Dicke, R. H. (1968). Scatter-hole cameras for x-rays and gamma rays. *Astrophys. J.* **153**, L101.

Dirac, P. A. M. (1958). "The Principles of Quantum Mechanics." Oxford Univ. Press, London and New York.

Dixon, R. L., and Ekstrand, K. E. (1976). Heuristic model for understanding x-ray film characteristics. *Med. Phys.* **3**, 340–345.

Doi, K. (1965). Optical transfer functions of the focal spot of x-ray tubes. *Am. J. Roentgenol., Radium Ther. Nucl. Med.* **94**, 712.

Doi, K. (1969). Wiener spectrum analysis of quantum statistical fluctuations and other noise sources in radiography. *In* "Television in Diagnostic Radiology" (R. D. Mosley, Jr. and J. H. Rust, eds.). Aesculapius Publ., Birmingham, Alabama.

Doi, K., and Rossmann, K. (1975). Effect of focal spot distribution on blood vessel imaging in magnification radiography. *Radiology* **114**, 435.

Egan, J. P. (1975). "Signal Detection Theory and ROC Analysis." Academic Press, New York.

Egan, J. P., and Clarke, F. R. (1966). Psychophysics and signal detection. *In* "Experimental Methods and Instrumentation in Psychology" (J. B. Sidowsky, ed.), pp. 211–246. McGraw-Hill, New York.

Evans, R. D. (1968). X-ray and γ-ray interactions. *In* "Radiation Dosimetry" (F. H. Attix and W. C. Roesch, eds.), Vol. 1, Chap. 3. Academic Press, New York.

Fano, U. (1946). On the theory of ionization yield of radiations in different substances. *Phys. Rev.* **70**, 44.

Fano, U. (1948). Ionization yield of radiations, II. The fluctuations in the number of ions. *Phys. Rev.* **72**, 26.

Farmelant, M. H., DeMeester, G. D., Wilson, D. T., and Barrett, H. H. (1975). Initial clinical experiences with a fresnel zone plate imager. *J. Nucl. Med.* **16**, 183.

Fenimore, E. E., and Cannon, T. M. (1978). Coded aperture imaging with uniformly redundant arrays. *Appl. Opt.* **17**, 337–347.

Fried, D. L. (1965). Noise in photoemission current. *Appl. Opt.* **4**, 79.

Frieden, B. R. (1975). Image enhancement and restoration. *In* "Picture Processing and Digital Filtering" (T. W. Huang, ed.), pp. 179–248. Springer-Verlag, Berlin and New York.

Frieser, H. (1960). Spread function and contrast transfer function of photographic layers. *Photogr. Sci. Eng.* **4**, 324–329.

Gaskill, J. D. (1978). "Linear Systems, Fourier Transforms, and Optics." Wiley, New York.

Gerchberg, R. W. (1974). Super-resolution through error energy reduction. *Opt. Acta* **21**, 709.

Gilbert, P. (1972). Iterative methods for the three-dimensional reconstruction of an object from projections. *J. Theor. Biol.* **36**, 105–117.

Goitein, M. (1972). Three-dimensional density reconstruction from a series of two-dimensional projections. *Nucl. Instrum. Methods* **101**, 509–518.

Goodenough, D. J. (1972). Radiographic applications of signal detection theory. Ph.D. Thesis, Univ. of Chicago, Chicago, Illinois.

Goodenough, D. J. (1975). Objective measures related to ROC curves. *Proc. Soc. Photo-Opt. Instrum. Eng., Appl. Opt. Instrum. Med. III* **47**, 134.

Goodenough, D. J., Rossmann, K., and Lusted, L. B. (1972). Radiographic applications of signal detection theory. *Radiology* **105**, 199.

Goodenough, D. J., Rossmann, K., and Lusted, L. B. (1973). Factors affecting the detectability of a simulated radiographic signal. *Invest. Radiol.* **8**, 339.

Goodenough, D. J., Rossmann, K., and Lusted, L. B. (1974). Radiographic applications of receiver operating characteristic (ROC) curves. *Radiology* **110**, 89.

Goodman, J. W. (1968). "Introduction to Fourier Optics." McGraw-Hill, New York.

Gordon, R. (1974). A tutorial on ART (Algebraic Reconstruction Techniques). *IEEE Trans. Nucl. Sci.* **21**, 78–93.

Gordon, R., Bender, R., and Herman, G. T. (1970). Algebraic reconstruction techniques (ART) for three-dimensional electron microscopy and x-ray photography. *J. Theor. Biol.* **29**, 471–481.

Grant, D. G. (1972). Tomosynthesis: A three dimensional radiographic imaging technique. *IEEE Biomed. Trans.* **19**, 20–28.

Green, D. M., and Swets, J. A. (1974). "Signal Detection Theory and Psychophysics." Krieger, Huntington, New York.

Greivenkamp, J. E., Swindell, W., Gmitro, A. F., and Barrett, H. H. (1981). Incoherent optical processor for x-ray transaxial tomography, *Appl. Opt.* **20**, 264–273.

Hanbury Brown, R., and Twiss, R. Q. (1956). Correlation between photons and two coherent beams of light. *Nature* (*London*) **178**, 4541.

Harding, G., Bertram, U., and Weiss, H. (1978). Towards optimum blurring in spiral tomography. *Med. Phys.* **5**, 280–284.

Harris, C. C., Bell, P. R., Satterfield, M. M., Ross, D. A., and Jordan, J. C. (1964). The design and performance of a large high-resolution focusing collimator. *In* "Medical Radioisotope Scanning," Vol. 1, pp. 193–208. IAEA, Vienna.

Heitler, W. (1966). "The Quantum Theory of Radiation," 2nd ed. Oxford Univ. Press, London and New York.

Helstrom, C. W. (1967). Image restoration by the method of least squares. *J. Opt. Soc. Am.* **57**, 3.

Herman, G. T. (1979). Correction for beam hardening in computed tomography. *Phys. Med. Biol.* **24**, 81–106.

Herman, G. T. (1980). "Image Reconstruction from Projections." Academic Press, New York.

Herman, G. T., Lent, A., and Rowland, S. W. (1973). ART: Mathematics and applications. A report on the mathematical foundations and on the applicability to real data of the Algebraic Reconstruction Techniques. *J. Theor. Biol.* **42**, 1–32.

Herz, R. H. (1969). "The Photographic Action of Ionizing Radiations." Wiley (Interscience), New York.

Hiramoto, T., Tanaka, E., and Nohara, N. (1971). A scintillation camera based on delay-line time conversion. *J. Nucl. Med.* **12**, 160–165.

Hoffer, P. B., Charleston, D. B., Beck, R. N., and Gottschalk, A. (1969). Fluorescent scanning. *In* "Medical Radioisotope Scintigraphy," Vol. 1, p. 261. IAEA, Vienna.

Holman, B. L., Idoine, J. D., Sos, T. A., Tancrell, R., and DeMeester, G. (1977). Tomographic scintigraphy of regional myocardial perfusion. *J. Nucl. Med.* **18**, 764–769.

Honda, T., and Tsujiuchi, J. (1975). Restoration of linear-motion blurred pictures by image scanning method. *Opt. Acta* **22**, 6–9.

Huesman, R. H., Gullberg, G. T., Greenberg, W. L., and Budinger, T. F. (1977). "RECLBL Library Users Manual: Donner Algorithms for Reconstruction Tomography." Lawrence Berkeley Laboratory, University of California.

International Commission on Radiation Units and Measurements (1971). "Radiation Quantities and Units," No. 19.

International Commission on Radiation Units and Measurements (1980). "Radiation Quantities and Units," No. 33 (supercedes No. 19).

Ishimaru, A. (1978). "Wave Propagation and Scattering in Random Media," Vol. 1. Academic Press, New York.

Jackson, J. D. (1975). "Classical Electrodynamics," 2nd ed. Wiley, New York.

Jahns, M. F. (1981). The influence of penetrating radiation on collimator performance. *Phys. Med. Biol.* **26**, 113–124.

Jerri, A. J. (1977). The Shannon sampling theorem—Its various extensions and applications: A review. *Proc. IEEE* **65**, 1565.

Johns, H. E., and Cunningham, J. R. (1969). "The Physics of Radiology," 3rd ed. Thomas, Springfield, Illinois.

Kelly, J. G., Stalker, K. T., McArthur, D. A., Chu, K. W., and Powell, J. E. (1979). Theory and application of the coded aperture fuel motion detection systems, *Proc. Int. Meeting Fast Reactor Safety Technology, Seattle, Washington, August 19–23* **5**, 2302.

Keyes, J. W., Orlandea, N., Heetderks, W. J., Leonard, P. F., and Rogers, W. L. (1977). The humongotron-A scintillation-camera transaxial tomograph. *J. Nucl. Med.* **18**, 381–387.

Keyes, J. W., Leonard, P. F., Svetkoff, D. J., Brody, S. L., Rogers, W. L., and Lucchesi, B. R. (1978). Myocardial imaging using emission computed tomography. *Radiology* **127**, 809–812.

Keyes, W. I. (1975). The fan-beam gamma camera. *Phys. Med. Biol.* **20**, 489.

Kijewski, P. K., and Bjärngard, B. E. (1978). Correction for beam hardening in computed tomography. *Med. Phys.* **5**, 209–216.

Kircos, L. T., Leonard, P. F., and Keyes, J. W. (1978). An optimized collimator for single-photon computed tomography with a scintillation camera. *J. Nucl. Med.* **19**, 322–323.

Klauder, J. R., Price, A. C., Darlington, D., and Albersheim, W. J. (1960). The theory and design of chirp radars. *Bell Syst. Tech. J.* **39**, 745.

Klein, C. A. (1968). Semiconductor particle detectors: A reassessment of the Fano factor situation. *IEEE Trans. Nucl. Sci.* **15**, 214–225.

Kock, M., and Tiemens, U. (1973). Tomosynthesis: A holographic method for variable depth display. *Opt. Commun.* **7**, 260–265.

Koral, K. F., and Rogers, W. L. (1979). Application of ART to time-coded emission tomography. *Phys. Med. Biol.* **24**, 879.

Koral, K. F., Rogers, W. L., and Knoll, F. G. (1975). Digital tomographic imaging with a time-modulated pseudorandom coded aperture and an Anger camera. *J. Nucl. Med.* **16**, 402.

Kuhl, D. E., Edwards, R. Q., Ricci, A. R., Yacob, R. J., Mich, T. J., and Alavi, A. (1976). The Mark IV system for radionuclide computed tomography of the brain. *Radiology* **121**, 405–413.

Kujoory, M. A., Miller, E. L., Barrett, H. H., Gindi, G. R., and Tamura, P. N. (1980). Coded-aperture imaging of gamma ray sources with an off-axis rotating slit. *Appl. Opt.* **19**, 4186–4195.

Kulberg, G. H., and van Dijk, N. (1972). Improved resolution of the Anger scintillation camera through the use of threshold preamplifiers. *J. Nucl. Med.* **13**, 169–171.

Lale, P. G. (1959). The examination of internal tissues using gamma-ray scatter with a possible extension for megavoltage therapy. *Phys. Med. Biol.* **4**, 159.

Leith, E. N., and Upatnieks, J. (1962). Reconstructed wavefronts and communication theory. *J. Opt. Soc. Am.* **52**, 10.

Leunbach, I. (1977). Three-dimensional imaging and tomography using Compton scatter. *In* "Medical Radionuclide Imaging," Vol. 1, p. 263. IAEA, Vienna.

Levitan, E. (1979). On true 3-D object reconstruction from line integrals. *Proc. IEEE* **67**, 1679–1680.

Littleton, J. L., Durizch, M. L., and Geary, J. C. (1976). "Tomography: Physical Principles and Clinical Applications." Williams & Wilkins, Baltimore, Maryland.

Loevinger, R. (1981). "A formalism for calculation of absorbed dose to a medium from photon and electron beams," *Med. Phys.* **8**, 1–12.

Lorrain, P., and Corson, D. R. (1970). "Electromagnetic Fields and Waves," 2nd ed. Freeman, San Francisco, California.
Lusted, L. B. (1968). "Introduction to Medical Decision Making." Thomas, Springfield, Illinois.
Macdonald, B., Chang, L. T., Perez-Mendez, V., and Shiraishi, L. (1974). Gamma-ray imaging using a Fresnel zone plate aperture, multiwire proportional chamber, and computer reconstruction. *IEEE Trans. Nucl. Sci.* **21**, 672.
MacIntyre, W. J., Fedoruk, S. O., Harris, C. C., Kuhl, D. E., and Mallard, J. A. (1969). Sensitivity and resolution in radioisotope scanning. *In* "Medical Radioisotope Scintigraphy," Vol. 1, p. 391. IAEA, Vienna.
McKeighen, R. E. (1980). A review of gamma camera technology for medical imaging. *In* "Imaging for Medicine" (Sol Nudelman and Dennis D. Patton, eds.), pp. 119–163, Plenum, New York.
Marchand, E. W. (1964). Derivation of the point spread function from the line spread function. *J. Opt. Soc. Am.* **54**, 915.
Mather, R. L. (1957). Gamma-ray collimator penetration and scattering effects. *J. Appl. Phys.* **28**, 1200.
May, R. S., Akcasu, Z., and Knoll, G. F. (1974). Gamma-ray imaging with stochastic apertures. *Appl. Opt.* **13**, 2589.
Mees, C. E. K., and James, T. H. (1966). "The Theory of the Photographic Process," 3rd ed., Macmillan, New York.
Mertz, L. (1974). Applicability of the rotation collimator to nuclear medicine. *Opt. Commun.* **12**, 216.
Mertz, L., and Young, N. O. (1961). Fresnel transformation of images. *Proc. Int. Conf. Opt. Instrum.*, p. 305.
Messiah, A. (1961). "Quantum Mechanics." North-Holland Publ., Amsterdam.
Metz, C. E. (1969). A mathematical investigation of radioisotope scan image processing. Ph.D. Thesis, Univ. of Pennsylvannia, Philadelphia.
Metz, C. E. (1978). Basic principles of ROC analysis. *Semin. Nucl. Med.* **8**, 283.
Metz, C. E., and Beck, R. N. (1974). Quantitative effects of stationary linear image processing on noise and resolution of structure in radionuclide images. *J. Nucl. Med.* **15**, 164.
Miller, E. (1978). Radially symmetrical coded apertures. M.S. Thesis, Univ. of Arizona, Tucson.
Miracle, S., Yzuel, M. J., and Millán, S. (1979). A study of the point spread function in scintillation camera collimators. *Phys. Med. Biol.* **24**, 372.
Moody, N. F., Paul, W., and Joy, M. L. G. (1970). A survey of medical gamma-ray cameras. *Proc. IEEE* **58**, 217.
Morin, R. L., Raeside, D. E., Goin, J. E., and Widman, J. C. (1979). Monte Carlo advice. *Med. Phys.* **6**, 305.
Morse, P. M., and Feshbach, H. (1953). "Methods of Theoretical Physics," Part I. McGraw-Hill, New York.
Motz, J. W., and Danos, M. (1978). Image information content and patient exposure. *Med. Phys.* **5**, 8–22.
Mozley, J. M. (1968). The modulation transfer function for scanners. *In* "Fundamental Problems in Scanning" (A. Gottschalk and R. Beck, eds.), p. 301. Thomas, Springfield, Illinois.
Muehllehner, G. (1971). A tomographic scintillation camera. *Phys. Med. Biol.* **16**, 87–96.
Muntz, E. P. (1979). Analysis of the significance of scattered radiation in reduced dose mammography, including magnification effects, scatter suppression, and focal spot and detector blurring. *Med. Phys.* **6**, 110–117.
Nalcioglu, O., and Cho, Z. H. (1978). Reconstruction of 3D objects from cone beam projections. *Proc. IEEE* **66**, 1584.

Newell, R. R., Saunders, W., and Miller, E. (1952). Multichannel collimators for gamma-ray scanning with scintillation counters. *Nucleonics* **10**, 36–40.

Ohyama, N., Honda, T., and Tsujiuchi, J. (1981). Tomogram reconstruction using advanced coded-aperture imaging, *Opt. Commun.* **36**, 434–438.

Orlov, S. S. (1975a). Theory of three-dimensional reconstruction, I. Conditions for a complete set of equations. *Kristallografiya* **20**, 511–515 [Engl. transl., *Sov. Phys.—Crystallogr.* **20**, 312].

Orlov, S. S. (1975b). Theory of three-dimensional reconstruction, II. The recovery operator. *Kristallografiya* **20**, 701–709 [Engl. transl., *Sov. Phys.—Crystallogr.* **20**, 429].

Papoulis, A. (1962). "The Fourier Integral and Its Applications." McGraw-Hill, New York.

Papoulis, A. (1965). "Probability, Random Variables, and Stochastic Processes." McGraw-Hill, New York.

Papoulis, A. (1975). A new algorithm in spectral analysis and band-limited extrapolation. *IEEE Trans. Circuits Syst.* **22**, 735.

Patton, D. D. (1978). Decision making in nuclear medicine. *Semin. Nucl. Med.* **8**, 272–282.

Ra, J. B., and Cho, Z. H. (1981). Generalized true three-dimensional reconstruction algorithms. *Proc. IEEE* **69**, 668–670.

Ramachandran, G. N., and Lakshminarayanan, A. V. (1971). Three-dimensional reconstruction from radiographs and electron micrographs: Application of convolutions instead of Fourier transforms. *Proc. Natl. Acad. Sci. U.S.A.* **68**, 2236–2240.

Rao, G. U. V., and Fatouros, P. (1978). The relationship between resolution and speed of x-ray intensifying screens. *Med. Phys.* **5**, 205–208.

Rao, G. U. V., and Wagner, H. N. (1967). Effect of an analog rate-meter on the modulation transfer function in radioisotope scanning. *Radiology* **88**, 504.

Rao, G. U. V., Fatouros, P. P., and James, A. E. (1978). Physical characteristics of modern radiographic screen-film systems. *Invest. Radiol.* **13**, 460–489.

Renaud, L., Joy, M. L. G., and Gilday, D. L. (1979). Fourier multiaperture emission tomography. *J. Nucl. Med.* **20**, 986.

Riederer, S. J., Pelc, N. J., and Chesler, D. A. (1978). The noise power spectrum in computed tomography. *Phys. Med. Biol.* **23**, 446.

Rogers, W. L., Han, K. S., Jones, L. W., and Beierwaltes, W. H. (1972). Application of a Fresnel zone plate to gamma-ray imaging. *J. Nucl. Med.* **13**, 612.

Rogers, W. L., Koral, K. F., Mayans, R., Leonard, P. F., Thrall, J. H., Brady, T. J., and Keyes, J. W. (1980). Coded-aperture imaging of the heart. *J. Nucl. Med.* **21**, 371–378.

Rose, A. (1948a). The sensitivity performance of the human eye on an absolute scale. *J. Opt. Soc. Am.* **38**, 196.

Rose, A. (1948b). Television pickup tubes and the problem of vision. *Adv. Electron.* **1**, 131.

Rosell, F. A., and Willson, R. H. (1973). Recent psychophysical experiments and the display signal-to-noise ratio concept. *In* "Perception of Displayed Information" (L. Biberman, ed.) pp. 167–232. Plenum, New York.

Rossmann, K. (1963). Spatial fluctuations of x-ray quanta and the recording of radiographic mottle. *Am. J. Roentgenol., Radium Ther. Nucl. Med.* **90**, 863.

Rossmann, K. (1968). The spatial frequency spectrum: A means for studying the quality of radiographic imaging systems. *Radiology* **90**, 1.

Rossmann, K. (1969). Image quality. *Radiol. Clin. North Am.* **7**, 419.

Rotenberg, A. D., and Johns, H. W. (1965). Collimator efficiency and design. *Phys. Med. Biol.* **10**, 51–65.

Schnitzler, A. D. (1973). Analysis of noise-required contrast and modulation in image-detecting and display systems. *In* "Perception of Displayed Information" (L. Biberman, ed.), pp. 119–166. Plenum, New York.

Selwyn, E. W. H. (1935). A theory of graininess. *Photogr. J.* **75**, 571.

Shepp, L. A. (1980). Computerized tomography and nuclear magnetic resonance. *J. Comput. Assist. Tomog.* **4**, 94–107.

Shepp, L. A., and Logan, B. F. (1974). The Fourier reconstruction of a head section. *IEEE Trans. Nucl. Sci.* **21**, 21–43.

Shulman, A. R. (1970). "Optical Data Processing." Wiley, New York.

Sibilia, C., and Bertolotti, M. (1981). The photon anticorrelation effect in the stimulated annihilation process of electron–positron pairs. *Opt. Acta* **28**, 503–514.

Simpson, R. G. (1978). Annular coded-aperture system for nuclear medicine. Ph.D. Thesis, Univ. of Arizona, Tucson.

Simpson, R. G., and Barrett, H. H. (1980). Coded-aperture imaging. *In* "Imaging in Diagnostic Medicine" (S. Nudelman, ed.), pp. 217–311. Plenum, New York.

Simpson, R. G., Barrett, H. H., and Fisher, H. D. (1977). Decoding techniques for use with annular coded apertures. *In* "Applications of Holography and Optical Data Processing" (E. Marom, A. A. Friesem, and E. Weiner-Avnear, eds.), pp. 119–128. Pergamon, Oxford.

Snyder, H. L. (1973). Image quality and observer performance. *In* "Perception of Displayed Information" (L. Biberman, ed.), pp. 87–118. Plenum, New York.

Stalker, K. T. and Kelly, J. G. (1980). Coded aperture imaging system for nuclear fuel motion detection, *1980 Int. Opt. Comput. Conf. SPIE* **231**.

Stoner, W. W., Sage, J. P., Braun, M., Wilson, D. T., and Barrett, H. H. (1976). Transmission imaging with a coded source. *Proc. ERDA X-Gamma Ray Symp., Ann Arbor, Mich.* pp. 133–136.

Swank, R. K. (1973a). Absorption and noise in x-ray phosphors. *J. Appl. Phys.* **44**, 4190.

Swank, R. K. (1973b). Calculation of modulation transfer functions of x-ray fluorescent screens. *Appl. Opt.* **12**, 1865–1870.

Swets, J. A., and Pickett, R. A. (1979). Evaluation of diagnostic devices in clinical medicine: A general protocol. Rep. No. 3819, Bolt Beranek and Newman, Inc., Cambridge, Massachusetts.

Swindell, W. (1970). A noncoherent optical analog image processor. *Appl. Opt.* **9**, 2459.

Swindell, W., Greivenkamp, J. E., Gmitro, A. F., and Barrett, H. H. (1981). A low-cost computed tomographic scanner. *Radiology* **139**, 499–501.

Tam, K. C., Perez-Mendez, V., and Macdonald, B. (1979). Three-dimensional object reconstruction in emission and transmission tomography with limited angular input. *IEEE Trans. Nucl. Sci.* **26**, 2797.

Tanaka, E. (1979). Generalized correction functions for convolutional techniques in 3D image reconstruction. *Phys. Med. Biol.* **24**, 157.

Tanaka, E., and Iinuma, T. A. (1975). Image processing for coded aperture imaging and an attempt at rotating slit imaging. *Proc. Int. Conf. Inf. Process. Scintigr. 4th, Orsay*, pp. 43–55

Tanaka, E., Hiramoto, T., and Nohara, N. (1970). Scintillation cameras based on new position arithmetics. *J. Nucl. Med.* **9**, 542–549.

Ter-Pogossian, M. M. (1967). "The Physical Aspects of Diagnostic Radiology." Harper (Hoeber), New York.

Tipton, M. D., Dowdy, J., Stokely, E. M. (1976). Background suppression of multiple pinhole-coded aperture scintigrams. *Proc. Int. Conf. Med. Phys. AAPM, 4th, Ottawa, July 1976.*

Tipton, M. D. (1978). The odcat: One dimensional coded aperture tomography *Rec. Fut. Devel. Med. Imaging SPIE* **152**.

Tsui, B. M. W., Beck, R. N., Metz, C. E., and Doi, K. (1980). Transfer function analysis of the total image-forming process in nuclear medicine, *J. Appl. Photogr. Eng.* **6**, 131–140.

Turin, G. L. (1960). An introduction to matched filters. *IRE Trans. Inf. Theory* **6**, 311.

U.S. Department HEW (1970). "Radiological Health Handbook," Rev. ed. U.S. Gov. Print. Off., Washington, D.C.

van Roosbroeck, W. (1965). Theory of the yield and Fano factor of electron-hole pairs generated in semiconductors by high-energy particles. *Phys. Rev.* **139**, A1702.

Venema, H. W. (1979). X-ray absorption, speed, and luminescent efficiency of rare earth and other intensifying screens. *Radiology* **130**, 765–771.

Vest, C. M., and Steel, D. G. (1978). Reconstruction of spherically symmetric objects from silt-imaged emission: Application to spatially resolved spectroscopy. *Opt. Lett.* **3**, 54.

Vogel, R. A., Kirch, D., LeFree, M., and Steele, P. (1978). A new method of multiplanar emission tomography using a seven pinhole collimator and an Anger scintillation camera. *J. Nucl. Med.* **19**, 648.

Vyborny, C. J., Metz, C. E., Koi, K., and Haus, A. G. (1978). Calculated characteristic x-ray reabsorption in radiographic screens. *J. Appl. Photogr. Eng.* **4**, 172–177.

Wagner, R. F. (1977). Noise equivalent parameters in general medical radiography: The present picture and future pictures. *Photogr. Sci. Eng.* **21**, 252–262.

Wagner, R., and Sandrik, J. M. (1979). An introduction to digital noise analysis. *In* "The Physics of Medical Imaging" (A. G. Haus, ed.), pp. 524–546. Am. Assoc. Phys. Med., New York.

Wagner, R. F., Weaver, K. E., Denny, E. W., and Bostrom, R. G. (1974). Toward a unified view of radiological imaging systems, Part 1: Noiseless images. *Med. Phys.* **1**, 11–24.

Walton, P. W. (1973). An aperture imaging system with instant decoding and tomographic capabilities. *J. Nucl. Med.* **14**, 861.

Whitehead, F. R. (1977). Quantitative analysis of minimum detectable lesion-to-background uptake ratios for nuclear medicine imaging systems. *In* "Medical Radionuclide Imaging," Vol. 1, p. 409. IAEA, Vienna.

Wiener, N. (1933). "The Fourier Integral and Certain of Its Applications." Cambridge Univ. Press, London and New York.

Wiener, N. (1949). "Extrapolation, Interpolation, and Smoothing of Stationary Time Series." Wiley, New York.

Wilks, R. J., Mallard, J. R., and Taylor, C. G. (1969). The Collywobbler—A moving collimator image-processing device for stationary detectors in radioisotope scanning. *Br. J. Radiol.* **42**, 705–709.

Wilson, D. T., DeMeester, G. D., Barrett, H. H., and Barsack, E. (1973). A new configuration for coded-aperture imaging. *Opt. Commun.* **8**, 384.

Wouters, A., Simon, K. M., and Hirschberg, J. G. (1973). Direct method of decoding multiple images. *Appl. Opt.* **12**, 1871.

Young, N. O. (1963). Photography without lenses or mirrors. *Sky Telescope* **25**, 8.

Author Index

Numbers in italics indicate the pages on which complete references can be found.

C

D

E

F

G

H

Subject Index

G

H

I

K

L

Q

R

S